Alternative Medicine Guide

The Supplement Shopper

by GREGORY POULS, D.C.,

and MAILE POULS, Ph.D.,

with BURTON GOLDBERG

FUTURE MEDICINE PUBLISHING

TIBURON, CALIFORNIA

Future Medicine Publishing, Inc.
1640 Tiburon Blvd., Suite 2
Tiburon, CA 94920
www.alternativemedicine.com

Senior Editor: John Anderson
Associate Editor: China Williams
Art Director: Anne Walzer
Production Manager: Gail Gongoll

Manufactured in the United States of America.

10 9 8 7 6 5 4 3 2 1

Library of Congress Cataloging-in-Publication Data
Pouls, Gregory.
    The supplement shopper / by Gregory Pouls and Maile Pouls
    with Burton Goldberg.
        p.   cm.
    Includes bibliographical references and index.
    At head of title: Alternative medicine guide.
    ISBN 1-887299-17-3 (pbk.)
    1. Dietary supplements--Therapeutic use Encyclopedias. 2. Herbs--
Therapeutic use Encyclopedias.   I. Pouls, Maile.   II. Goldberg,
Burton, 1926-   .   III. Title.   IV. Title: Alternative medicine guide.
RM258.5.P68   1999
615.5--dc21   99-12466
                                                                       CIP

Contents

PART ONE–
An Introduction to Supplements

PART TWO–
An A-Z of Health Conditions:
Nutrients and Herbal Remedies

PART THREE—
Supplements as Preventive Medicine

About the Authors

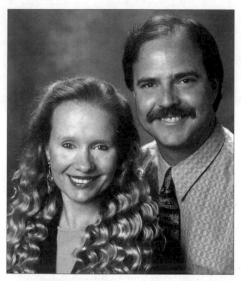

Maile Pouls, Ph.D., a clinical nutritionist who specializes in enzyme and nutritional therapy, is co-founder of the Health Enhancement Center in Santa Cruz, California. A nationally recognized health educator, Dr. Pouls publishes, with her husband, Gregory, the newsletter *Your Nutritionist*. She also maintains the website www.yournutrition.com, which provides information about general nutrition, and Healthy Alternatives Plus, a line of nutritional products that she developed. In her clinical practice, she utilizes 68 enzyme and nutrient formulas, and over 3,000 different therapeutic vitamin, mineral, and herbal products, including her own line of products. Dr. Pouls focuses on treating the underlying nutritional/biochemical causes of disease, rather than treating only symptoms.

To contact **Drs. Gregory and Maile Pouls:** Health Enhancement Center, 2222 East Cliff Drive, Suite 4B, Santa Cruz, CA 95062; tel: 831-477-1100; fax: 831-425-2222; website: http://www.yournutrition.com; e-mail: drpouls@cruzio.com. For the newsletter *Your Nutritionist:* tel: 800-962-4414 or 831-477-1040; fax: 831-477-1040.

Gregory Pouls, D.C., a chiropractor and nutritional product formulator, is co-founder and director of the Health Enhancement Center, the newsletter *Your Nutritionist*, and the website www.yournutrition.com. His primary research focus is on advancements in clinical nutrition and the effects of human-made chemicals on health and the natural environment. Dr. Pouls has researched and reviewed the product lines of environmentally concerned manufacturers (such as manufacturers of air/water filtration systems, natural cleaning products, and chemical-free personal care products). Comprehensive information about these products and the environmental problems that they help alleviate will be available to the public in the fall of 1999 at the website www.naturaldetox.com.

Acknowledgments

We would like to acknowledge the doctors, authors, and research scientists who educated us, personally or through their published works, thereby forming the foundation for this book:

Richard Anderson, N.D., N.M.D.

Nancy Appleton, Ph.D.

James Balch, M.D.

Phyllis Balch, C.N.C.

Jeffrey Bland, Ph.D.

James Breneman, M.D.

Gabriel Cousens, M.D.

William Lee Cowden, M.D.

William Crook, M.D.

Andrea Dworkin, N.D.

Samuel S. Epstein, M.D.

Alan Gaby, M.D.

Ralph Golan, M.D.

Burton Goldberg

Elson Haas, M.D.

Christopher Hobbs, L.Ac.

Edward Howell, M.D.

William Kellas, Ph.D.

Dharma Singh Khalsa, M.D.

Philip Landrigan, M.D.

Lita Lee, Ph.D.

Howard Loomis, D.C.

Daniel Mowrey, Ph.D.

Michael Murray, N.D.

Herbert Needleman, M.D.

Gary Null, Ph.D.

Linda Rector Page, N.D., Ph.D.

John Robbins

Humbart Santillo, N.D.

Maurice Shils, M.D., Sc.D.

Steven Sinatra, M.D.

Michael Tierra, L.Ac., O.M.D.

Melvyn Werbach, M.D.

Jonathan Wright, M.D.

Ruth Winters, M.S.

User's Guide

One of the features of this book is that it is interactive, thanks to the following icons:

This means you can turn to the listed pages elsewhere in this book for more information.

Many times the text mentions a medical term that requires explanation. We don't want to interrupt the text, so instead we put the explanation in the margins under this icon.

This tells you where to contact a physician, group, or publication mentioned in the text. This is an editorial service to our readers. All items are based on recommendations from the clinical practice of physicians in this book. The publisher has no financial interest in any clinic, physician, or product discussed in this book.

This sign tells you there may be some risks, uncertainties, side effects, or special contraindications regarding a procedure or substance.

Here we refer you to our book, *Alternative Medicine Definitive Guide to Cancer,* for more information on a particular topic.

Here we refer you to our book, *Alternative Medicine Definitive Guide to Headaches,* for more information on a particular topic.

Here we refer you to our book, *Alternative Medicine Guide to Heart Disease,* for more information on a particular topic.

Here we refer you to our book, *Alternative Medicine Guide to Chronic Fatigue, Fibromyalgia, and Environmental Illness* for more information on a particular topic.

Here we refer you to our book, *Alternative Medicine Guide to Women's Health 1,* for more information on a particular topic. This book covers infertility, endometriosis, vaginitis, menstrual problems, ovarian cysts, PMS, fibroids, and urinary tract infections.

Here we refer you to our book, *Alternative Medicine Guide to Women's Health 2,* for more information on a particular topic. This book covers breast cancer, fibrocystic breasts, environmental illness, chronic fatigue, fibromyalgia, depression, and osteoporosis.

Here we refer you to our book, *The Enzyme Cure,* for more information on enzymes and how they can be used to relieve health problems.

Important Information–This book is presented as an educational tool to assist in the understanding, assessment, and selection of treatments and preventative measures regarding health problems. It should not be used as a substitute for qualified medical advice, particularly by pregnant women, with respect to diagnosis or treatment. Consult your physician or other licensed health-care professional before undertaking any treatment. The reaction to different nutritional supplements and herbs varies among individuals. Many of the nutrients described in this book in relation to specific health conditions are not understood, nor are they endorsed, by any government or regulatory agency. The authors and publisher disclaim any responsibility for the reaction of any individual to, or the efficacy of, any treatment described in this book. Branded products and services are evaluated solely on the authors' experience. Reference to them does not imply any endorsement over other branded products and services.

Taking Control of
Your Own Health

MANY PRACTITIONERS of conventional medicine continue to dispute the health benefits of nutritional supplements, claiming that nature's cures are "unscientific" and potentially "dangerous." They usually fail to mention that adverse reactions from prescription drugs kill over 100,000 Americans each year, according to Stephen Fried's book *Bitter Pills: Inside the Hazardous World of Legal Drugs* (Bantam Books, 1998). Fried's book reports that drug side effects are the leading cause of death in the United States. To me, that calls into question a suspect allegiance between the American Medical Association and an $85-billion pharmaceutical industry.

Thankfully, Americans are realizing that they don't need to be sick or even die from drug reactions in the name of health. According to a survey conducted by Landmark Healthcare, based in Sacramento, California, 42% of the American population is using alternative medicine. People are discovering that there are alternatives to conventional medicine that treat underlying causes of disease rather than mask symptoms. They are rejecting the side effects and pain caused by medicine that is supposed to alleviate suffering. And most importantly, they are taking charge of their health by demanding coverage of alternative therapies by health insurance providers and increased availability of over-the-counter nutritional supplements.

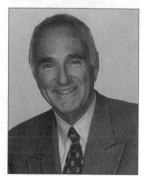

Walk down your grocery store aisle and you will see shelves lined with vitamins, minerals, herbs, and other remedies that would have been almost impossible to get prior to the 1994 Dietary Supplement Health and Education Act (DSHEA). That act lifted regulatory barriers and allowed supplements to bypass the federal food and drug testing procedures. While the change is good for people who need access to natural remedies, it creates a problem for a consumer trying to choose the best product. Many people who would benefit from supplements are not using them because they are afraid to make an unwise choice and don't know where to begin to learn about nutrition.

My advice to you is to begin right here with *The Supplement Shopper*. I've chosen two experts to write this book: Maile Pouls, Ph.D., a clinical nutritionist who specializes in enzyme and nutritional therapy, and her husband, Gregory Pouls, D.C., a chiropractor and nutritional product formulator.

Drs. Pouls have consulted with medical doctors, biochemists, research analysts, and the production managers for more than 300 reputable companies. They have collected data regarding the most effective, well-documented, and widely accepted products and compared the claims of the company with published studies by the foremost medical doctors and clinical professionals. In their own practice, they have used over 3,000 products to treat patients. Through careful observation and recording of their patients' individual body chemistry, physical symptoms, and overall well-being, they have been able to select the best nutritional supplements and manufacturers.

In this book, you will also learn the underlying causes of over 50 health conditions and the nutrients that support the affected organs and body systems. But keep in mind that vitamins and similar products are meant to supplement and augment nutrients already being consumed through a balanced diet of organic vegetables, fruits, whole grains, and meat and dairy products.

I urge you, above all, to take control of your own health. The tools are simple: eat right, use nutritional supplements wisely, don't use prescription drugs (except when absolutely necessary), detoxify, and exercise. Stop thinking of health as the absence of illness—start thinking of health as the presence of vitality. God Bless.

—Burton Goldberg

Visit our website at
www.alternativemedicine.com

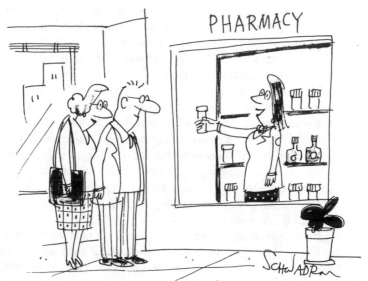

"THIS IS A REAL MIRACLE DRUG. IT COSTS THE SAME THIS YEAR AS IT DID LAST YEAR."

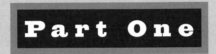

Part One

An Introduction to Supplements

CHAPTER

1

Using Supplements Wisely

"W hy am I always sick?" ask many of our new patients in our nutritional and chiropractic practices. They recount to us their disjointed attempts at health-conscious living and resulting disappointment as the latest "fad" fails. Our patients are frustrated because they want to subscribe to the tenets of good health but don't know where to begin.

A well-balanced diet is the first and probably most difficult step towards well-being. Statistically, studies have concluded that almost two-thirds of an average American's diet is made up of fats and refined sugars that provide "empty" calories with little nutritional value and even harmful cumulative effects on the body. Refined sugars decrease immune function and increase the risk of heart disease. Consumption of high levels of saturated fat, found in fried foods and margarine, contributes to high blood cholesterol levels and the inhibition of essential fatty acids required for many body functions.

The remaining one-third of the average diet is responsible for providing the bulk of essential nutrients needed for health and well-being. That is not an easy task when numerous modern techniques for food processing actually strip away nutrients. The process of refining flour substantially decreases levels of dietary fiber and important vitamins needed for energy. Foods also contain preservatives, chemicals, and flavor enhancers, some of which may contribute to neuro-degenerative diseases. Even healthy dietary alternatives such as fresh fruits and vegetables are usually grown in nutrient-poor soils that are unable to provide important enzymes and minerals. Today, a whole bushel of apples may be needed to keep the doctor away.

In America, we have an overabundance of food but an under-abundance of nutrition. We rarely encounter severe nutritional deficiencies such as rickets and scurvy or hear of an American child suffering from malnutrition. But we have probably all experienced insomnia, mood swings, and the inability to concentrate—all signs of a deficiency in B vitamins. The symptoms of nutritional deficiencies encompass many of today's common ailments: general body ache, chronic infections, digestive problems (heartburn, gas, bloating), fatigue, headaches, premenstrual syndrome (PMS), allergies, attention deficit disorder, anxiety, and depression.

Nutritional supplementation (including vitamins, minerals, herbs, homeopathic remedies, and superfoods) is one of the many therapies we use to correct the ailments listed above. Supplements can be used in accordance with proper dietary habits to obtain the daily levels of nutrients specific to an individual, to treat diseases or health conditions, or to cope with environmental or lifestyle stresses such as smoking, air pollution, emotional and psychological factors, or recovery from surgery.

It is also important to know your individual nutritional needs. The rate at which nutrients need to be replaced through diet is dependent upon the individual's genetics, gender, exercise level, general health, and stress factors (emotional, psychological, and intake of alcohol and drugs). There is no magic bullet or "super" nutrient that works the same for everyone all of the time.

We recommend consulting an alternative medicine practitioner to determine nutritional deficiencies and biochemical imbalances. These can be tested through blood, urine, saliva, and stool analysis. If you are unable to locate a doctor that will provide this service, contact the Great Smokies Diagnostic Laboratory (see Appendix, pp. 484-485) for a consumer-direct health screening test.

Digestive competence should also be examined to determine the body's ability to extract nutrients from food and supplements. We find that 90% of our patients have digestive problems that contribute to their nutritional deficiencies. Without correcting imbalances in the digestive tract, a well-balanced diet and nutritional supplementation can not adequately nourish the body.

Finally, lifestyle factors need to be evaluated by a qualified practitioner. Chronic stress can quickly deplete the nutritional stores of an individual by affecting energy regulation, hormone production, and immune system functioning. Stress reduction, sufficient amounts of rest and exercise, and resolution of psychological problems are powerful tools for regaining health.

To obtain **referrals to physicians trained in nutritional medicine, contact:** American Holistic Health Association, P.O. Box 17400, Anaheim, CA 92817-7400; tel: 714-779-6152; website: www.ahha.org. American College of Advancement in Medicine, P.O. Box 3427, Laguna Hills, CA 92654; tel: 949-583-7666.

A Healthy Diet

Eating a well-balanced diet of organic, whole, unprocessed foods is an important component of preventing illness, slowing aging, and correcting nutritional deficiencies. The correct ratios of carbohydrates, fats, and proteins that people should consume is a constant source of disagreement for nutritionists and doctors. Adding to the debate, we recommend a diet that consists of 50% carbohydrates, 30% fats, and 20% proteins.

Fiber and starches, which are complex carbohydrates, have more nutritional value than simple, sugar carbohydrates. Foods rich in complex carbohydrates include vegetables, whole grains, and milk and dairy products. These foods are more beneficial if raised or processed under organic (non-chemical) conditions.

Contrary to popular belief, some fats are good for you, but not all fats are created equal. Of the three kinds of fats (saturated, polyunsaturated, and monounsaturated), polyunsaturated are the healthiest because they are a dietary source of essential fatty acids (EFAs, see "An A-Z Nutrient Guide," pp. 24-62). The two principal types of EFAs are omega-3 and omega-6 oils. Foods rich in omega-3 include oils derived from fish, such as salmon and cod, as well as flaxseed, canola, and walnut oils. Plant and vegetable oils such as safflower, corn, peanut, and sesame are high in omega-6. Evening primrose, black currant, and borage oils contain the most therapeutic form of omega-6 oil.

Healthy sources of protein are foods that contain all the essential amino acids (the building blocks of proteins). These "complete" proteins are milk, eggs, cheese, meat, fish, and poultry. Green leafy vegetables, grains, and beans (legumes) are a source of some important amino acids, but not all, and are therefore referred to as "incomplete" proteins. These proteins can be combined with complementary foods such as brown rice, corn, nuts, seeds, or whole-grain wheats to form complete proteins. We recommend obtaining proteins primarily from vegetable sources. Of the animal proteins, poultry and fish are healthier sources than red meat and dairy, which should be eaten infrequently and in small portions. For all dietary sources of protein, choose organic products.

Supplements: An Overview

A product that is ingested orally and contains vitamins, minerals, herbs, amino acids, or other nutrients from food qualifies as a dietary supplement, according to the 1994 Congressional Dietary

Recommended Daily Allowances

The generally accepted reference standard for nutritional adequacy in the United States is the U.S. Recommended Daily Allowance (U.S. RDA). Developed by a group of government-sponsored scientists, its function is to provide levels of essential nutrients that prevent classic deficiency diseases (rickets, scurvy, or beriberi) and set marginal daily guidelines for average population groups. Since the scientists disagreed on exact RDAs, they built within the guidelines instructions to keep reviewing and updating the RDAs every four years as new information is discovered.

The RDAs have since been adjusted to include higher levels of essential nutrients, but a growing number of scientists have begun to dispute the validity of nutritional guidelines. They maintain that the standards may not be appropriate to prevent mild deficiency reactions such as nervousness, insomnia, mental exhaustion, improper immune function, or proneness to injury. New evidence about the wide variance of nutritional needs for each individual further highlights the inaccuracies of the standards. The nutritional needs of growing children, for instance, do not match those of menopausal women, athletes, or the elderly; then, too, it is important to consider the unique individual needs within a specific age group. Another frequent criticism of the RDAs is that they do not take into account nutrient-deficient food, modern food handling, and environmental factors.[1]

Some scientists support additional revisions of the RDAs to include larger doses of nutrients for the purposes of preventing illness and reducing the effects of environmental pollutants. To accomodate for each individual's nutritional needs, these scientists suggest that nutritional screening tests be used to determine specific and unique deficiencies that might deviate from the revised guidelines.

Supplement Health and Education Act. Supplements are not considered drugs under this act and do not need to be reviewed by the Food and Drug Administration (FDA) before entering the market.

The FDA, however, regulates the information a manufacturer can provide about a product. Manufacturers can not claim that a product will treat or diagnose a disease; for example, claiming that a product treats osteoporosis is illegal. But they can claim that calcium lowers the risk of osteoporosis when scientific studies (reviewed by the FDA) support the link between the nutrient and the health condition. They can also make structure-function claims, which describe the role or

Supplements can be used in accordance with proper dietary habits to obtain the daily levels of nutrients specific to an individual, to treat diseases or health conditions, or to cope with environmental or lifestyle stresses (such as smoking, air pollution, emotional and psychological factors, or recovery from surgery).

function of a nutrient in the body. For instance, a product is allowed to state "calcium builds strong bones." Every structure-function claim must be followed by a disclaimer: "This statement has not been evaluated by the Food and Drug Administration. This product is not intended to diagnose, treat, cure, or prevent any disease."

What to Look For—Here is a brief checklist of things you should know when shopping for supplements:

• **Know your nutrients:** vitamins, minerals, bioflavonoids—the list is never-ending. See "An A-Z Nutrient Guide" (Chapter 2) for an overview of the role of these and other nutrients in the body and specific recommendations for supplementation.

• **Know the nutritional deficiencies involved in illness:** for this, refer to the specific health condition listed in Part II: An A-Z of Health Conditions. Or, for general health maintenance questions, refer to Part III: Supplements as Preventive Medicine.

• **Look for a reputable manufacturer:** this book lists over 100 companies that produce consistently reliable products, which are available across the country.

• **Look for an informative label:** a product's label should tell you all of its ingredients (including bulking agents and fillers), expiration date (ingredients can lose their potency over time), and the manufacturer's name and address. See "How to Read a Dietary Supplement Label" (pp. 22-23) for a diagram of label anatomy.

What Form to Take and When—No matter how beneficial the nutrient, it is useless if the body can't break it down into absorbable molecules. This depends on two factors: the form of the supplement (tablets, capsules, powders, etc.) and the time that the supplement is ingested.

When taking supplements, be sure to drink enough water to help assimilation and prevent side effects.

Common Forms: Tablets that are "heat-pressed," or hard and shiny, are extremely difficult for the body to break down. Often they pass through the system in a solid state.

For most supplements, the easiest to assimilate are loose powders (which can be mixed with juice or sprinkled on food) or softgel capsules (which are chewed before swallowing). Equally efficacious are herbal tinctures and most homeopathic remedies, which come in sublingual tablets held under the tongue until dissolved.

For children who turn their noses up to anything that doesn't look sweet, try chewable, flavored wafers. When choosing chewable products, make sure that only natural flavorings are used.

Timing: If you are taking high doses, do not take the supplements all at once, but divide them into smaller amounts ingested throughout the day. Usually there is a maximum amount of the nutrient, vitamin or otherwise, that can be absorbed at one time. See "An A-Z Nutrient Guide" (Chapter 2) for more information about when to take your supplements.

How to Read a Dietary Supplement Label

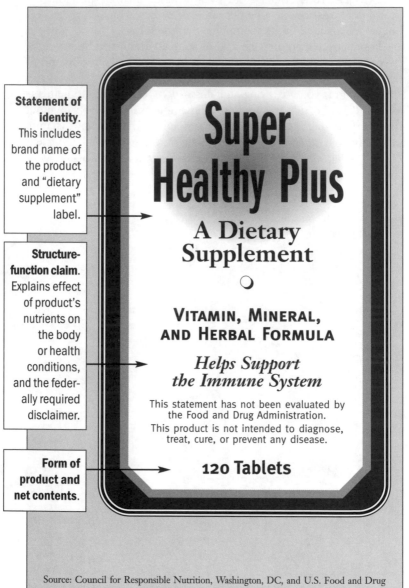

Statement of identity. This includes brand name of the product and "dietary supplement" label.

Structure-function claim. Explains effect of product's nutrients on the body or health conditions, and the federally required disclaimer.

Form of product and net contents.

Super Healthy Plus

A Dietary Supplement

VITAMIN, MINERAL, AND HERBAL FORMULA

Helps Support the Immune System

This statement has not been evaluated by the Food and Drug Administration. This product is not intended to diagnose, treat, cure, or prevent any disease.

120 Tablets

Source: Council for Responsible Nutrition, Washington, DC, and U.S. Food and Drug Administration's Center for Food Safety and Applied Nutrition, Washington, DC.

Directions for use: take one capsule daily.

SUPPLEMENT FACTS

Serving Size: one capsule

	Amount Per Serving	% Daily Value
Vitamin A (as beta carotene)	5000 IU	100%
Vitamin C (from ascorbic acid)	60 mg	100%
Vitamin E (as d-alpha tocopheryl)	30 IU	100%
Zinc (as zinc citrate)	23 mg	
Echinacea (powdered root)	200 mg	*
Goldenseal (powdered root)	80 mg	*

* Daily value not established

Other ingredients: *gelatin, water, binders, and coatings*

Manufacturer's
or distributor's name,
address, and zip code

Directions.
Recommended by manufacturer. It is not advised to exceed this amount without recommendations from a health-care professional.

Supplement facts panel.
Lists serving size, amount contained in each tablet or capsule (if the serving size is one tablet) and active ingredients. Also includes "Daily Value," the percentage of the recommended daily intake for each nutrient. An asterisk indicates that a Daily Value is not established for that nutrient.

Other ingredients.
A complete list of all ingredients used to formulate the supplement. Ingredients are listed in descending order of predominance and by common name or proprietary blend.

Name and address of **manufacturer.**

CHAPTER 2

An A-Z Nutrient Guide

Essential nutrients are absolutely necessary for human life but can not be manufactured by the body. Derived from food sources, essential nutrients include eight amino acids, at least 13 vitamins, and at least 15 minerals, plus certain fatty acids, water, and carbohydrates. There are also many non-essential nutrients, or cofactors, that are manufactured by the body under healthy conditions. Non-essential nutrients work with the essential nutrients to break down and convert food into cellular energy, regulate metabolic reactions such as the body's physical and mental functions, and provide the building blocks of the body's structural parts, including bones, muscles, connective tissues, and organs.

Amino Acids

Amino acids are the building blocks of proteins; in fact, proteins are actually chains of amino acids linked together, each one having a specific function. Proteins are in turn the building blocks of the body. Twenty-two amino acids are vital to the body's growth, development, and maintenance. Some are manufactured in the body while others, called essential amino acids, must be obtained from the diet or nutritional supplements. Semi-essential amino acids can be made by the body in amounts that are adequate to maintain basic protein requirements, however, additional dietary sources are required during times of growth or stress.

Recommendations—Amino acid deficiency may be an underlying factor, often undetected, for many common disorders. Vegetarians and vegans (vegetarians who eat no dairy products) often have difficulty meeting dietary protein requirements, and should take an amino acid complex supplement. Amino acid supplementation is also valuable to athletes, bodybuilders, people in mentally or physically stressful professions, and dieters who are trying to prevent sugar or carbohydrate cravings.

We recommend buying supplements that are labeled "USP pharmaceutical grade," L-crystalline, free-form amino acids. The term "USP" means that the product meets the standards of purity and

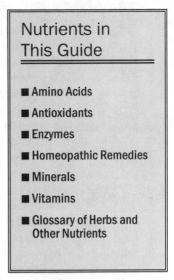

Nutrients in This Guide

- Amino Acids
- Antioxidants
- Enzymes
- Homeopathic Remedies
- Minerals
- Vitamins
- Glossary of Herbs and Other Nutrients

potency set by the United States Pharmacopeia. The term *free-form* refers to the highest level of purity of the amino acid. The *L* refers to one of the two forms in which most amino acids come, designated D- and L- (as in D-lysine or L-lysine). The L-form amino acids are proper for human biochemistry, as proteins in the human body are made from this form. The exception is phenylalanine, which consists of a combination of the D- and L- forms (thus its full name DL-phenylalanine).

We do not recommend that people take individual amino acids for extended or indefinite periods as this can create an imbalance of other amino acids in the body and possibly cause other health conditions. If individual amino acids are going to be used to support specific health conditions, we recommend following this course of treatment with a complex of free-form amino acids to ensure balanced amino acid nutrition. Please consult a qualified health-care professional before beginning such therapies. Individual amino acids often come with warnings or precautions for women who are pregnant or for people with certain health conditions.

The amino acids discussed here and throughout this book are the L-form, unless otherwise noted.

For maximum assimilation, amino acid supplements should be taken on an empty stomach at least one hour before a meal. To improve their utilization, take a multivitamin and multimineral complex containing vitamins B (especially B2 and B6 or B complex), C, and E.[2]

The Essential Amino Acids

■ **Isoleucine** aids in energy production, hemoglobin (carries oxygen in blood) formation, and in the regulation of energy from blood sugars. Since it assists in the metabolism and formation of muscles, isoleucine is a useful supplement for bodybuilders (weight-lifters), when taken with balanced proportions of leucine and valine.

■ **Leucine** helps heal injured or weakened muscles, fractured or weakened bones, and skin conditions or injuries. Leucine can also be used as a nutritional support for post-surgery recovery. It reduces excessive blood sugar levels (important for diabetics) and is a good source of fuel during prolonged workouts or exercise. Leucine (with balanced proportions of isoleucine and valine) assists in the metabolism and formation of muscles.

■ **Lysine** assists in the formation of antibodies (immune cells which inhibit viruses), enzymes, and hormones, which are all necessary for the repair of damaged or unhealthy connective tissues. Lysine helps develop bones by assisting in the metabolism of calcium from the intestinal tract and is also important for the formation of collagen, a vital protein component of bones, cartilage, connective tissues, and skin. It is useful for treating canker and cold sores and other herpes virus outbreaks. Lysine is also useful for building muscles and for recovering from surgery or muscular or sports injuries.

■ **Methionine** is the source of organic sulfur (which must be constantly replaced) and is a potent antioxidant (SEE QUICK DEFINITION). It helps prevent excessive accumulation of fats in the liver and vascular system, detoxify heavy metals and toxins, and protect against the damaging effects of radiation on the body. Methionine also aids in relieving fatigue, reducing histamine release (which may help prevent allergies), and preventing premature hair loss.

■ **Phenylalanine** is a precursor, or building block, of the neurotransmitters (chemical nerve messengers) dopamine and norepinephrine, which regulate mood, promote alertness, and enhance memory and cognitive function. It is used for certain types of depression, headaches (especially migraine), menstrual cramps, weight gain or obesity (phenylalanine acts as a natural appetite suppressant), and Parkinson's disease (a loss of muscle control due to abnormally low levels of dopamine).

See **Antioxidants**, pp. 30-31.

■ **Threonine** is an immune-stimulating amino acid,

promoting thymus gland growth and activity (antibody production). Often deficient in vegetarians, threonine is important for the production of elastin (elastic connective tissue), collagen, and cell membranes (especially connective tissues). It also helps control the accumulation of fat in the liver.

■ **Tryptophan,** a precursor to the neurotransmitter serotonin (which regulates mood and sleep patterns), is a sleep aid and mood elevator/antidepressant. Unfortunately, the FDA banned over-the-counter tryptophan in 1989. However, an alternative, 5-hydroxy-tryptophan or 5-HTP (a highly purified extract of *Griffonia simplicifolia*, a West African plant containing tryptophan) is available and produces results similar to tryptophan.

⟩CAUTION⟨

Consult a qualified health-care practitioner before taking tryptophan or 5-HTP. Pregnant women should not take either supplement.

■ **Valine** can be used by the body to produce energy and is important for the formation, metabolism, and repair of muscle tissue. It has a natural stimulating effect and can benefit bodybuilders if used in balanced proportions with leucine and isoleucine. It is also used in the treatment of drug addictions when amino acid deficiencies are also present.

Semi-Essential Amino Acids

■ **Arginine** is most needed during times of growth (childhood or pregnancy) and great stress. It stimulates the release of human growth hormone (HGH) and is important for muscle metabolism, increasing muscle mass while decreasing body fat. Athletes should take arginine and ornithine for their muscle-building and post-injury recovery effects. It also combats physical and mental fatigue, enhances immune function by increasing thymus gland production of T cells (cells of the immune system), is necessary to produce collagen (a structural protein of the connective tissue), and aids in the general detoxification of ammonia (a common by-product of human metabolism). But arginine-containing foods or supplements can aggravate certain diseases such as herpes simplex virus.

■ **Histidine** is essential for the growth and repair of tissues, especially during childhood and pregnancy; it also helps maintain the fatty (myelin) sheath insulating nerves. Important in the development and production of red and white blood cells, histidine is useful for treating anemia. Histidine has also been used to treat allergies, cardiovascular disease, rheumatoid arthritis, and digestive-tract ulcers. It helps prevent cataracts, increase libido (by raising histamine levels, which are related to sexual function), remove toxic metals from the body, and protect the body from radiation damage.

Non-Essential Amino Acids

Even though the following amino acids are termed "non-essential"—meaning they can be manufactured by the body—it is entirely possible that, due to nutritional deficiencies or metabolic problems, the body cannot produce any or enough of them. If this occurs, as with essential amino acid deficiencies, specific functions will not be performed and the body will begin to work less efficiently.

■ **Alanine** promotes immunity by increasing production of immunoglobulins and antibodies (SEE QUICK DEFINITION). It assists the body in metabolizing glucose, which serves as fuel for the brain, nervous system, and muscles, as well as energy. Hypoglycemia may be associated with low alanine levels. Alanine assists in the metabolism of organic acids in the body and is important for the makeup of vitamin B5 (pantothenic acid).

■ **Aspartic acid** is involved in the formation and function of DNA and RNA, protects the liver, promotes proper cell function, and supports immunity by improving antibody production. It also helps increase stamina and reduce fatigue. Aspartic acid has been used clinically to treat certain nerve and brain conditions, including depression.

■ **Citrulline,** found mainly in the liver, is metabolized by the body to form arginine. It promotes the detoxification of ammonia, stimulates the immune system, and assists with recovery from fatigue, illness, or injury.

■ **Cysteine** is part of the keratin protein found in hair, nails, and skin. It protects against radiation damage and helps shield the brain and liver from toxic heavy metals (lead, mercury, cadmium) and the damaging effects of alcohol, cigarettes, and drugs. It supports the immune system by helping to prevent infection and promotes healing of respiratory conditions. Cysteine is used to treat rheumatoid arthritis and arteriosclerosis (hardening of the arteries) and is also used to promote hair growth.

■ **Cystine** is important for the formation of healthy hair and skin. It supports the immune system by stimulating the production of white blood cells and aids in the healing process after burns or surgery. Cystine has been used to treat certain respiratory conditions including bronchitis, but is not generally used clinically because it can accumulate in the system and cause kidney problems.

■ **Glutamic acid** is a neurotransmitter important for brain metabolism. It assists in transporting potassium across the blood-brain barrier and in detoxifying ammonia from the brain. Important for the metabolism of other amino acids, fats and sugars, glutamic acid is useful for balancing hypoglycemia (low blood sugar) and overcoming fatigue. Glutamic acid has been used to treat numerous brain and nervous conditions.

■ **Glutamine** assists in improving mental alertness and memory. It can readily pass through the blood-brain barrier and be converted into glutamic acid (see above). It also increases GABA (gamma-aminobutyric acid), a central nervous system neurotransmitter important for brain function and mental ability. It has been used to treat alcoholism and alcohol poisoning, mental illness, and degenerative brain conditions. Glutamine helps stop alcohol and sugar cravings and aids in the absorption of minerals into the tissues. Glutamine assists in the formation of muscles and prevention of muscle wasting in chronically ill people.

■ **Glycine** has a calming effect on the brain and is important for central nervous system function. It supports immune function, promotes the healing of wounds, and assists in the conversion of stored sugars into energy. Glycine is used as a sweetener and as an ingredient in many antacid products. Glycine is also a building block for other non-essential amino acids.

■ **Ornithine** stimulates the release of growth hormone. When taken with arginine and carnitine, it has the effect of increasing muscle mass while decreasing body fat (helpful for weight loss and/or bodybuilding). Ornithine is needed for a healthy liver, as it detoxifies ammonia from the liver and is involved in liver regeneration. It supports immune function and tissue repair and healing.

Ornithine should not be taken by children, pregnant or nursing women, or schizophrenics, unless under the supervision of a licensed health-care professional.

■ **Proline** assists in the production of collagen and works with vitamin C to heal and repair cartilage, the heart muscles, joints, and tendons. Proline acts as a source of stored energy for the liver and muscles.

■ **Serine** is a component of brain proteins and the fatty (myelin) sheaths that protect nerves. It is a source of stored energy for the liver and muscles and helps metabolize fats, oils, and fatty acids. It also is important for the growth of muscles and a healthy immune system (by improving antibody protection). It is used in skin creams as a natural moisturizer.

■ **Taurine** is the primary amino acid building block for other amino acids and is crucial for the proper assimilation and utilization of calcium, magnesium, potassium, and sodium. It is important in the formation of bile and is a component of white blood cells, skeletal and heart muscles, and the tissues of the central nervous system. Taurine supports normal brain function, and has been used to help control hyperactivity, epilepsy, and nervous system imbalance caused by alcohol or drug abuse. It has been used to treat atherosclerosis (fatty buildup in the arteries), heart disorders, high blood pressure, hypoglycemia (low blood sugar), and seizures.

■ **Tyrosine** is a building block of the neurotransmitters norepinephrine and dopamine, which help regulate mood, feelings, appetite, anxiety, and depression. It helps regulate the adrenal, pituitary, and thyroid glands, assists in the production of melanin (substance responsible for hair and skin color), and increases muscle growth while reducing body fat (ideal for weight loss and/or bodybuilding). It also assists in the formation of red and white blood cells.

Antioxidants

An antioxidant (meaning "against oxidation") is a natural biochemical substance that protects living cells against damage from harmful free radicals (SEE QUICK DEFINITION). Antioxidants work to neutralize free radicals, which, if left uncontrolled, can lead to cellular aging, degeneration, arthritis, heart disease, cancer, and other illnesses.

Recommendations—Environmental pollution and stressful lifestyles make daily supplementation with antioxidants a necessity. Extra supplementation may be required if you smoke cigarettes, exercise regularly, eat a diet high in fat or oil, are exposed to second-hand smoke, chemical pollutants or irritants, frequent X rays or radiation, or to high doses of UV (ultraviolet) rays from the sun. When antioxidants are taken in combination, they are more effective than when they are used individually.

Before supplementing with beta carotene, consult a health-care professional if you have alcoholic liver disease, smoke cigarettes, or are exposed to asbestos. For selenium, do not exceed doses of 300 mg to 400 mg per day; possible side effects include anemia, poor appetite, and liver cirrhosis.[3]

Types of Antioxidants

- **Amino acids:** cysteine, glutathione, methionine
- **Bioflavonoids:** anthocyanin bioflavonoids (in fruit, especially grapes, cranberries, and bilberries), citrus bioflavonoids (in grapefruit, lemons, and oranges), oligometric proanthocyanidins (OPC) in pycnogenol (pine bark or grape seed extract)

See the Glossary of Herbs and Other Nutrients, pp. 40-62, for more information about **antioxidant nutrients**.

- **Carotenes:** alpha and beta carotene (in red, yellow, and dark green fruits and vegetables), lycopene (in red fruits and vegetables, such as red grapefruit and tomatoes)
- **Dietary sources:** cayenne pepper, garlic, turmeric
- **Herbs:** astragalus, bilberry, ginkgo, green tea, milk thistle, sage
- **Minerals:** copper, manganese, selenium, zinc
- **Vitamins:** A, B1, C, and E, coenzyme Q10, NADH (nicotinamide adenine dinucleotide)
- **Enzymes:** catalase, glutathione peroxidase, superoxide dismutase (SOD)
- **Hormone:** melatonin

Enzymes

Enzymes are specialized living proteins fundamental to all living processes in the body, necessary for every chemical reaction and the normal activity of our organs, tissues, fluids, and cells. In the body, there are over 3,000 different kinds of enzymes, each with distinctly different tasks.[4] Metabolic enzymes help produce energy for cellular functions and also assist in clearing the body of toxins and cellular debris. Enzymes involved in digestion include food enzymes (which are responsible for predigestion in the mouth and stomach) and pancreatic enzymes (which carry on digestion in the intestines).

The main food enzymes include protease, which digests proteins; amylase, digests carbohydrates; lipase, digests fats; cellulase, digests fiber; and disaccharidase, digests sugars.

Pancreatic digestive enzymes (including amylase, lipase, and protease) are produced and stored in the pancreas. When food is being

Enzymes are specialized living proteins fundamental to all living processes in the body, necessary for every chemical reaction and the normal activity of our organs, tissues, fluids, and cells.

processed by the digestive organs, the pancreas will contribute appropriate amounts of the digestive enzyme needed to break down a fat, protein, carbohydrate, or sugar. Each of the food nutrients must be broken down into molecular size to be able to pass through the intestinal wall and enter the bloodstream. From the blood, they can be delivered to various tissues in the body as nutrients. These enzymes also work well as anti-inflammatory agents or scavengers for viruses and other foreign particles in the blood.

Eating a diet high in raw foods takes the load off the pancreas to supply all the necessary digestive enzymes. Enzymes are killed by high cooking temperatures, so it is important to eat raw, live enzyme-rich foods. Unfortunately, many Americans eat a diet primarily composed of cooked, refined, nutrient- and enzyme-deficient (dead) food. Years of eating such a diet results in an overdrawn pancreatic "account" of digestive enzymes.

First, this causes digestive complications, such as bad breath, bloating, belching, poor digestion and assimilation of nutrients, as well as stomach and colon pain, flatulence, and nutritional deficiencies. Second, lacking the enzymes it needs for digestion, the body draws enzymes from white blood cells in the immune system. If this becomes a regular occurrence, immunity is compromised and illness and digestive imbalances occur.

The effects of poor digestion include nutritional deficiencies and most digestive and pancreatic disorders eventually contribute to food or airborne allergies, autoimmune disorders, bacterial or viral infections, or inflammatory or degenerative conditions.

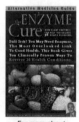

For more about **enzymes**, see *The Enzyme Cure* (Future Medicine Publishing, 1998; ISBN 1-887299-22-X); to order, call 800-333-HEAL.

Recommendations—To aid in digestion, take supplements of digestive enzymes (food or pancreatic enzymes), one-half hour prior to a meal. Supplements of food enzymes are usually derived from plant sources such as aspergillus, a type of fungus. Supplements of pancreatic enzymes are usually derived from animal sources but we have found that they work only in a small portion of the digestive tract due to a limited pH (acidity) range. We recommend plant-derived enzymes that work in a broader pH range and throughout the entire gastrointestinal tract. When supplementing with metabolic enzymes, choose a product that has an enteric coating, so that it can pass safely through the stomach acid to the small intestine for absorption in the latter phases of digestion. If metabolic enzymes are dissolved in the stomach, they become less effective.

Homeopathic Remedies

The word homeopathy comes from the Greek word *homios*, which means "like" or "similar," and *pathos*, which means "suffering." Homeopathic remedies are generally dilutions of natural substances from plants, minerals, and animals. It is based on the following three principles:

- **Like cures like:** this means that the same substance that in large doses produces the patient's totality of symptoms will in smaller doses cure the patient.
- **The more a remedy is diluted, the greater its potency:** counter to the belief that higher dosages have greater effects, homeopathic remedies are diluted with pure water or alcohol and then vigorously shaken (succussing) to produce higher potencies. On the labels of homeopathic remedies will appear the potency of each ingredient, such as sulphur 12X. This means that sulphur has undergone 12 successive dilutions and succussions.
- **An illness is specific to the individual:** there is a specific homeopathic remedy for the specific symptoms of an illness. If a patient has a headache that originates in the front of the head and moves into the eyes, the remedy will differ from a headache originating in the back of the head. Remedies are specifically matched to symptom patterns or "profiles" to help stimulate the body's innate healing response.

There are thousands of homepathic remedies available over-the-counter. Single remedy preparations contain only one homeopathic remedy, while combination remedies contain multiple remedies to cover a broad range of symptoms. The body will assimilate what it needs in combination remedies and discard what is not necessary, without side effects. In this book, single or combination remedies derived from plants are specified as phyto-homeopathic.

Recommendations—Homeopathic remedies work on a deeper level in the body when nutrients or drugs have failed. We recommend homeopathy for acute conditions (such as severe viral infections or muscle injuries), for health conditions that have not responded to other therapies, or for people who cannot swallow large capsules. For best results, homeopathic remedies should be used according to the directions at the prescribed dosage and time. Smoking, consumption of alcohol, coffee, some teas, and toothpaste or other oral products that contain mint or aromatic oils may reduce the effectiveness of the remedy.

Minerals

Research has now found between 75 and 80 different minerals in the tissues of animals and humans. At least 60 of these minerals have been scientifically documented as essential cofactors for enzyme reactions, as aids in the uptake and utilization of vitamins necessary for the formation of DNA and RNA, and as structural components of the skeleton. As with essential amino acids, these minerals are termed "essential" because the body cannot make them and they must be obtained from diet or nutritional supplements.

In order to have a healthy body, the concentration of minerals must be specifically maintained. Due to the poor nutritional quality of the standard American diet (high in fat, sugar, refined carbohydrates, and processed foods) and the poor mineral content of American soil, it can no longer be taken for granted that sufficient minerals can be obtained from food sources.

Recommendations—Multimineral complexes need to contain the amounts and ratios of minerals appropriate to the health condition and lifestyle of the individual. Take mineral supplements at a different time than your highest fiber meal of the day, as fiber can decrease mineral absorption. Absorption of zinc is especially impaired by the phytates in beans, cereals, and pasta.

We recommend mineral supplements for people of all ages, with a few notes of caution:

• People with kidney problems should be especially careful when supplementing with minerals. Do not supplement with calcium if you have renal failure.

• Single minerals should be taken with care because certain minerals require others for assimilation and function. Another danger of supplementing with single minerals is the possibility of skewing mineral balance. Iron and copper are potent oxidants and should be taken with care after consulting a health-care professional. Zinc supplements should not be taken in excess of 100 mg a day, as it may cause immunosuppression, which leads to greater susceptibility to infections.[5]

Types of Minerals

The following are brief descriptions of the minerals most often cited in this book and their most common functions and uses in the body:

■ **Calcium,** the most abundant mineral in the body is essential for healthy bones and teeth, and for preventing osteoporosis, high blood pressure, insomnia, PMS, and panic attacks. The most absorbable forms of calcium are calcium ascorbate, calcium citrate, calcium malate, calcium glycinate, and calcium derived from crystalline hydroxyapatite. Calcium citrate is the specific form of calcium that we recommend for people with a history of kidney stones. In clinical studies, calcium citrate has helped prevent the recurrence of kidney-stone formation in almost 90% of the study subjects.[6] The least absorbable forms are calcium carbonate and calcium derived from oystershells. Some calcium supplement products derived from calcium carbonate and oystershells can be contaminated with lead. Be sure to buy products that are derived from purified sources.

Mineral supplements are available in three forms: colloidal, chelated colloidal, or ionic. Colloidal minerals are derived from rocks, the same source as mineral-rich foods. Usually available in powdered form, colloidals are not readily absorbed into the bloodstream. By attaching a protein molecule to the colloidal mineral (chelated colloidal), the absorption of the supplement is slightly improved. Many doctors recommend chelated colloidal supplements, but products that have a high sodium or aluminum content should be avoided. For our own patients, we prefer using liquid ionic minerals, because they are easily absorbed and ready to be used by the body without undergoing a conversion process.

■ **Copper** is required for RNA/DNA function, cellular respiration, and strength of the elastic fibers in blood vessels, skin, and vertebral discs.

■ **Germanium** enhances oxygen availability and the immune system, increasing the activity of NK (natural killer) cells, T cells, and macrophages.

■ **Iodine** is essential for proper function of the thyroid gland and prevents hypothyroidism (underproduction of thyroid hormones).

■ **Iron** is a cofactor and activator for enzymes. It is also an essential component of hemoglobin, the pigment in red blood cells which is responsible for the transport of oxygen in the body.

■ **Magnesium** is essential for cellular communication, enzyme reactions, and structural function. It also prevents headaches, changes in heart rhythm and electrical activity, nerve/muscle problems, tremors, and arteriosclerosis (hardening of the arteries).

■ **Manganese** is essential for forming numerous enzymes, hormones, and proteins.

■ **Molybdenum,** found in the kidneys and liver, activates the essential enzymes involved in metabolism and detoxification.

■ **Phosphorus,** the second most prevalent mineral in the body, is involved in virtually every metabolic function and is essential for bones and teeth.

■ **Potassium** is essential for cell health and numerous electro-chemical and enzyme systems.

■ **Selenium,** an important antioxidant, inhibits oxidation/rancidity of body fats and prevents age/liver spots as well as various heart, liver, immune, and muscle conditions.

■ **Silica** supports collagen formation and keeps arteries, hair, nails, and skin healthy.

■ **Sulfur** (found in bones, cartilage, hair, nails, skin, tendons, and sulfur-bearing amino acids) helps maintain antibodies, enzymes, hemoglobin, and hormones.

■ **Zinc** (found in the bones, DNA and RNA, eyes, kidneys, nails, skin, pancreas, prostate gland, and semen) activates metal-containing enzymes, helps synthesize nucleic acid and protein, and supports immune function. *Precautions: Do not exceed 100 mg per day of zinc; possible side effects include immunosuppression, or an increased susceptibility to infections.*

Vitamins

Supplementing with vitamins is advisable for the same reasons we need to take mineral supplements—poor diet and agricultural soil quality (see Minerals, above). There are two main categories of vitamins: fat-soluble and water-soluble.

The fat-soluble vitamins are A, D, E, and K. These oil-based nutrients are more readily stored in body tissues (primarily the liver and fatty tissues) than other types of nutrients.

Water-soluble nutrients include vitamins C and B complex. Water-soluble vitamins need to be replaced regularly as they are not stored well in the tissues of the body, but are usually excreted in one to four days.

Recommendations—Take fat-soluble vitamins with the one daily meal that contains the most fat. Look for supplements that are mycelized or emulsified, meaning that the size of the oil droplet has been reduced in order to increase absorption. As health problems caused by toxicity can occur with the overuse of fat-soluble vitamins, we advise caution in supplementing with higher than recommended dosages (see specific vitamins for precautions).

Types of Vitamins
The following are the actions and properties of the vitamins most frequently recommended in this book:

■ **Vitamin A** is a fat-soluble vitamin that prevents night-blindness and supports optical tissues and systems; it also supports the immune system and protects the body from colds, flu, and infections. Vitamin A is important for the health and healing of the hair, skin, and tissues of the mouth, and for the formation of bones, teeth, and sperm. *Precautions: Do not exceed 50,000 IU per day; possible side effects include weight loss, skin difficulties, bone pain, and bleeding.*[7]

■ **Vitamin B complex** contains various ratios of individual B vitamins to nutritionally support the brain, eyes, hair, intestines, liver, mouth, muscles, and skin; assist in energy production; and help reduce fatigue. B complex vitamins are often recommended to repair damaged nerves and to treat anxiety syndromes, diminished mental functions, and depression. Stress levels, diet, and lifestyle can cause the body to use B vitamins relatively quickly. Deficiency of B vitamins impairs immunity and reduces resistance to infection.[8]

■ **Vitamin B1** (thiamin) plays a key metabolic role in energy production; supports the nervous system and brain function; and improves circulation, blood formation, and digestion. It is also an antioxidant.

■ **Vitamin B2** (riboflavin) is important for energy production, supports cellular growth and respiration, assists in the formation of red blood cells and antibodies (immune cells), and promotes healthy hair, nails, and skin. Vitamin B2 benefits vision and is important for pregnancy.

■ **Vitamin B3** (niacin, niacinamide, nicotinic acid) increases circulation and aids in the metabolism of carbohydrates, fats, and proteins. It is also needed for the formation of sex hormones, supports the intestines and nervous system, benefits skin conditions such as acne, and helps lower high cholesterol levels. Headaches, poor memory, mental illness, and vertigo can be relieved by vitamin B3.

■ **Vitamin B5** (pantothenic acid), known as an "anti-stress" vitamin, is vital for adrenal gland function. It is also used for conditions involving stress and fatigue, allergies, arthritis, asthma, headaches, insomnia, psoriasis, post-operative shock, anemia, depression, and anxiety.

■ **Vitamin B6** (pyridoxine) is important for the nervous system, brain function, formation of RNA and DNA, and antibody production. Because B6 balances hormones and water levels (B6 is a mild diuretic) it is useful for premenstrual syndrome (PMS), painful periods, fatigue, and morning sickness in women. Vitamin B6 also helps relieve allergies, arthritis, asthma, autism, neuritis, epilepsy and convulsions, Parkinson's, schizophrenia, learning disabilities, and carpal tunnel syndrome. *Precautions: Taking more than 300 mg per day may cause liver and neurologic toxicity.*[9]

■ **Vitamin B12** (cyanocobalamin, cobalamin) is the only vitamin that contains cobalt (mineral cofactor and activator of enzymes). It is important for the nervous system, proper digestion and assimilation of foods, and the formation of red blood cells (assisting in the utilization of iron). Useful for fatigue, B12 helps increase energy levels.

■ **Vitamin B15** (pangamic acid) is an antioxidant and energy stimulant; often used to treat mental retardation, Down syndrome, atherosclerosis (fatty deposits along the arteries), emphysema, and liver cirrhosis.

■ **Biotin** (a member of the B vitamin family) supports the bones, glands, and nerves, and enhances the utilization of insulin (helpful for diabetics). Biotin is used by the body to metabolize carbohydrates, fats, and proteins, produce fatty acids, strengthen hair and nails and prevent baldness and the graying of hair (if a biotin deficiency exists). It is also used to treat skin conditions such as dermatitis, dandruff, eczema, psoriasis (especially in children), and seborrhea.

■ **Choline** (a member of the B vitamin family) is a brain nutrient used in the transmission of nerve signals. It also works with inositol to emulsify fats and prevent fat buildup in the liver. Choline is useful for Alzheimer's disease, cirrhosis of the liver, dizziness, headaches, heart palpitations, hepatitis, memory problems, Parkinson's disease, ringing in the ears, and stroke.

■ **Folic acid** (folacin, folate; members of the B vitamin family) is important for red blood cell formation, breakdown and utilization of proteins, and proper cell division, which is especially important in the early stages of pregnancy (folic acid prevents spina bifida and neural tube defects). It is also useful for acne, anemia, atherosclerosis, canker sores, cervical cancer, cervical dysplasia, dermatitis, diarrhea, fatigue, gingivitis, gout, immune weakness, infection, old age, osteoporosis, periodontal disease, pregnancy, restless leg syndrome, and skin ulcers.

■ **Inositol** (a member of the B vitamin family) is important for bone marrow, eyes, and intestines. It assists in metabolizing fats in the blood and liver and lowers cholesterol. Together with biotin and choline, inisotol helps control arteriosclerosis (hardening of the arteries), hypertension, and male pattern baldness. It is useful for people suffering from multiple sclerosis (often deficient in inositol) and diabetics with pain, numbness, and nerve degeneration.[10]

■ **Para-aminobenzoic acid** (PABA, a member of the B vitamin family) is important for the skin, hair pigment (color), and blood cell formation. PABA aids in the metabolism and assimilation of amino acids (proteins) and is essential for the growth of "friendly" intestinal bacteria and supports their production of vitamin B12. It protects the skin from sunburn and cancer caused by excessive ultraviolet light (sunshine) and is useful for burns and vitiligo (depigmentation of the skin).

■ **Vitamin C** is an antioxidant involved in more than 300 biological processes in the body. It is important for immune function, formation of collagen (found in bones, capillary walls, cartilage, joint linings, ligaments, vertebral discs, and teeth), iron absorption, useful for healing wounds and burns, lowering cholesterol, preventing constipation, easing arthritis and rheumatism, and preventing blood clots, bruising, and atherosclerosis. People who will immediately benefit from supplementation of vitamin C include alcohol drinkers, athletes, elderly, pregnant or lactating women or people with recurrent infections or chronic disease or who use antibiotics or prescription medications.

Ascorbic acid, the synthetic (or man-made) form of vitamin C, is tolerated by most people, but can be irritating to people with sensitive digestive systems. If you are sensitive to ascorbic acid, consider using buffered vitamin C (combined with potassium or sodium to reduce acidity) or esterified vitamin C (which is more expensive but more readily absorbed than other forms of C). Natural sources of vitamin C include acerola berries, rose hips, or citrus fruits. To increase absorption of vitamin C, take equal amounts of citrus or other bioflavonoids. *Precautions: Pregnant women should not take more than five grams (5,000 mg) of vitamin C per day because it can cause "rebound scurvy" in the newborn child. People with chronic renal failure or on hemodialysis should consult a health-care practitioner before supplementing with vitamin C.*[11]

■ **Vitamin D** (calciferol), known as the "sunshine" vitamin, it is created in the skin by exposure to the sun's ultraviolet rays. Vitamin D assists in the metabolism and assimilation of calcium and phosphorus (which are both important for bone formation) from the digestive tract. Vitamin D's regulation of calcium is also important for the health of the developing heart and nervous system, for proper thyroid gland function, and for normal blood clotting. It is helpful for the prevention and treatment of diminished immunity, calcium deficiencies, osteoporosis, and conditions involving the eyes, including conjunctivitis and glaucoma. People who immediately benefit from vitamin D supplementation include breast-feeding women (especially during winter months because of less sunlight), the elderly (especially if housebound), vegetarians and vegans, and women who have had a series of pregnancies. *Precautions: Do not take doses higher than 3,000 IU per day; possible side effects include kidney impairment, weight loss, and thirst.*[12]

■ **Vitamin E** (tocopherol), an immune system stimulant and antioxidant, specifically reduces the free radicals that cause the oxidation of fats, fatty acids, and fat-soluble nutrients in the body. It is important for healthy hair and skin, reducing scarring, improving athletic performance, lessening muscle cramps, and preventing cancer, blood clots, and heart disease.[13] Vitamin E helps treat anemia, autoimmune diseases, cataracts, diabetes, fibrocystic breast conditions, herpes virus (shingles), impotence, PMS, menstrual pain, osteoarthritis, ulcers, and viruses. Vitamin E protects the body against the toxic effects of alcohol, estrogen, ozone, smoke, and other environmental toxins. *Precautions: People should not take more than 200 IU of vitamin E per day if they are also taking blood-thinning medications. People suffering from diabetes, rheumatic heart disease, or overactive thyroid should take only recommended doses of vitamin E.*

■ **Vitamin K** is necessary for proper clotting of the blood and formation and repair of bones. It promotes healthy liver function and the conversion of glucose into glycogen for storage in the liver. Vitamin K is useful for liver cirrhosis, jaundice, osteoporosis, heavy menstrual flow, painful menstruation, and nausea and vomiting during pregnancy. *Precautions: Large doses of vitamin K can cause toxic reactions, especially for a woman in her last few weeks of pregnancy. People taking blood-thinning medication should use vitamin K with care, because this vitamin supports the formation of blood clots.*

Glossary of Herbs and Other Nutrients

Herbal medicine is also known as phytotherapy, or phytomedicine (*phyto* means plant). Herbal remedies can be made from the bark, flower, fruit, leaf, root, seed, stem, or any other part of a plant that is used to make food flavorings, fragrances (aromatherapy), or medicines. Herbal formulas, if carefully and scientifically prepared, exert a profound influence on a person's physiology and body chemistry, usually without side effects.

Recommendations—Inform your health-care professional about any herbal supplements you are taking. This is especially important if you are using prescribed medications.

When buying herbal supplements for symptoms of specific health conditions, look for products that have standardized extracts. This means that the herb's active ingredient has been isolated and extracted in a standardized percentage. For example, some garlic supplements are standardized to contain 80% allicin, the active component of garlic. Standardization ensures the consistency of the supplement.

But isolating and extracting the active ingredient of an herb removes the other unknown components that might provide broader health benefits. Herbal remedies that work on many levels in the body are more effective for general health maintenance or treating underlying nutritional deficiencies. In these cases, we recommend buying herbal extracts that have undergone water distillations. Traditionally used by Chinese herbalists, these water extracts are prepared by boiling the raw herbs at low temperatures (less then 100° C)—much like preparing a tea. Boiling the herbs draws out the water-soluble nutrients, which are combined with other herbs with similar health benefits for a synergistic effect.

HERBS
can be used in many forms

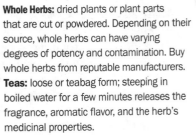

Whole Herbs: dried plants or plant parts that are cut or powdered. Depending on their source, whole herbs can have varying degrees of potency and contamination. Buy whole herbs from reputable manufacturers.

Teas: loose or teabag form; steeping in boiled water for a few minutes releases the fragrance, aromatic flavor, and the herb's medicinal properties.

Capsules and Tablets: convenient and popular form of herbs. Some herbs, such as goldenseal, have repulsive flavors that are hidden in a capsule or tablet.

Extracts and Tinctures: high concentrations of an herb that are more quickly assimilated by the body than tablets; alcohol (or glycerin) is used as a solvent to extract non-water-soluble compounds from the herb and as a preservative. Tinctures usually contain more alcohol than extracts (sometimes 70% to 80% alcohol). Herbal tinctures and extracts should look and taste like the herb or plant it was derived from.

Essential Oils: distilled from various parts of medicinal and aromatic plants, except oils of citrus fruits, which come directly from the fruit peel. Essential oils are highly concentrated and should be used sparingly for internal purposes. Dilute essential oils in water or in fatty oils if using topically, except eucalyptus and tea tree oils, which can be applied directly to the skin without concern of irritation.

Salves, Balms, and Ointments: used for muscle aches, insect bites, or wounds; usually available in a vegetable oil or petroleum jelly base.

Other nutritional supplements include food nutrients that contain natural ingredients to aid in metabolism, support specific tissues, glands, or organs, or address both general and specific health conditions. In many cases, the health claims made by the manufacturers are based on historical data; however, modern science continues to verify the effectiveness of the food nutrient's ingredients.

Acidophilus (Lactobacillus acidophilus)
"Friendly" bacteria that reside in the intestinal tract; aids digestion and the assimilation of nutrients, and assists in the production of certain enzymes, vitamins, hydrogen peroxide, and lactic and acetic acid; inhibits pathogenic (disease-causing) organisms in the intestine, including fungus and yeast; also helps reduce blood cholesterol.

Ajowan Oil (from wild celery seeds)
Antiparasitic; stimulates the digestive tract and reduces gas formation; used in Ayurvedic medicine for indigestion and abdominal pains.

Alfalfa (Medicago sativa)
Antifungal, anti-inflammatory, diuretic; balances cholesterol, blood sugar, and hormones; rich source of minerals, nutrients, vitamins, and trace minerals. *Precautions: Excessive amounts have been shown to thin the blood.*

Algae (blue-green and green; "superfood")
(See also Chlorella, Chlorophyll, "Green" Drink Powders, and Spirulina, below)
Fresh-water phytoplankton that is rich in amino acids (assimilable protein), chlorophyll, enzymes, essential fatty acids, fiber, minerals, and vitamins; the world's greatest single-food source of beta carotene (water-soluble vitamin A) and vitamin B12; helps stimulate immunity, improve digestion and assimilation of nutrients, detoxify the body, repair tissues, and prevent radiation damage and degenerative disease.

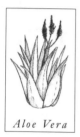

Aloe Vera (Aloe vera)
Moisturizer, skin healer, and softener. Taken internally, the juice is a digestive tonic that improves protein digestion and assimilation, reduces stomach acid, relieves and prevents constipation, and helps heal peptic ulcers. *Precautions: Pregnant women and elderly people should not drink concentrated aloe juice, although diluted juices are fine. Externally, try aloe first on a small area to rule out allergic reaction.*

Aloe Vera

Anise *(Pimpinella anisum)*
Assists digestion, prevents infection, reduces mucus, and relieves dry cough.

Arnica *(Arnica montana)*
Homeopathic analgesic, anti-inflammatory. *Precautions: Can be poisonous if taken internally; seek professional assistance.*

Artichoke *(Cynara scolymus)*
Stimulates digestive juices and bile flow, improves liver function, and promotes general detoxification of the body; used traditionally to treat digestive and liver conditions, as well as diabetes.

Astragalus *(Astragalus membranaceus)*
Adaptogen, immune system and lung tonic; increases metabolism, promotes healing, and prevents fatigue. *Precautions: Not recommended during acute phase of conditions in which high fever or pronounced swelling is present.*

Barberry *(Berberis vulgaris)*
Berberine, an alkaloid component of barberry, has strong antimicrobial properties and stimulates the production of hydrochloric acid in the stomach, as well as bile and liver secretions in general. *Precautions: Not recommended for people in debilitated, emaciated conditions or for pregnant women.*

Barley Grass
Anti-inflammatory; promotes alkalinity in digestive system; high in amino acids, chlorophyll, enzymes, bioflavonoids, vitamins B12 and C, calcium, and other minerals.

Bayberry *(Myrica spp.)*
Clears congestion, improves circulation, and reduces fever.

Bee Pollen (plant sex cells collected by bees)
Antimicrobial; high in amino acids, B vitamins, calcium, carotene, copper, essential fatty acids, iron, magnesium, manganese, potassium, protein, sodium, sterols, and vitamin C.

Bee Propolis (plant resins collected by bees)
Antibacterial, immune stimulant; traditionally used externally on bruises, cuts, and scrapes, and internally for treating allergies, inflamed mucous membranes of the mouth and throat, tonsillitis, and ulcers.

Bentonite Clay

Chelating agent (pulls out metals and toxins); useful for detoxifying the colon; a bentonite and psyllium combination works well to "scrub" the colon clean and pull out unwanted toxins and wastes.

Beta Carotene

(See Carotene, below)

Bifidus (Bifidobacteria bifidum)

"Friendly" bacteria of the intestinal tract that competes with and kills pathogenic (disease-causing) organisms; assists in creating an optimal environment in the colon for the production of B-complex vitamins and vitamin K.

Bilberry (Vaccinium myrtillus, V. arboreum)

Controls insulin, improves night vision, maintains capillary integrity, supports stability of collagen, and is rich in bioflavonoids (see below).

Bioflavonoids (plant pigments)

Antioxidant, anti-inflammatory, antimicrobial; enhances the function of vitamin C and should be taken together; helps maintain capillary, artery, and vein strength, and also helps prevent bleeding or bruising. Bioflavonoids include hesperitin, hesperidin, eriodictyol, quercetin, and rutin. Quercetin is an antiviral and antihistamine; since it helps reduce inflammation, it is useful for allergies and asthma.[14]

Birch (Betula alba)

Diuretic; decreases inflammation and pain.

Black Cohosh (Cimicifuga racemosa)

Relaxant, phytoestrogenic for balancing female reproductive tract; lowers blood pressure; helpful for menstrual cramps, dysmenorrhea (painful menstruation), uterine pain and spasm, menopause. *Precautions: Pregnant or lactating women should not use black cohosh. Women using estrogen therapy should consult a qualified health-care professional before using supplements of this herb.*

Black Walnut (Juglans nigra)

Antifungal, antiparasitic, antiviral; helps digestion.

Blessed Thistle (Cnicus benedictus, Carduus benedictus)

Bile and appetite stimulator, liver tonic; useful for indigestion or acid indigestion. *Precautions: People with active intestinal ulcers should not take blessed thistle.*

Blue Cohosh *(Caulophyllum thalictriodes)*

Uterine contraction stimulator; promotes labor and contractions during childbirth; helpful for joint pain and symptoms of PMS (premenstrual syndrome). *Precautions: Pregnant women should only use to induce labor; may increase blood pressure in some people.*

Boneset *(Eupatorium perfoliatum)*

Anti-inflammatory, decongestant, laxative.

Borage *(Borago officinalis)*

Antihypertensive; oil high in GLA (gamma-linolenic acid, an omega-6 essential fatty acid); balances glands.

Boswellia *(Boswellia serrata)*

Ayurvedic herb, anti-inflammatory; effective for inflammatory skin conditions, low back pain, osteoarthritis and rheumatoid arthritis, and muscle pain.

Bovine Cartilage (from cows)

Anti-inflammatory; accelerates wound healing.

Brewer's Yeast

(See also Yeast, below)

Contains over 50% protein, high in amino acids, B vitamins, and minerals. *Precautions: People with yeast infections or candidiasis should avoid taking yeast supplements.*

Buchu *(Agathosma crenulata)*

Anti-inflammatory, diuretic, urinary antiseptic; soothing and healing properties. *Precautions: Children under the age of two should not use buchu.*

Burdock *(Arctium lappa)*

Blood purifier and immune stimulator; supports the liver and gallbladder; also contains chemical constituents that have antibacterial, antifungal, and antitumor properties;[15] helpful for inflammatory skin conditions. *Precautions: Pregnant women should use burdock root with caution because of its stimulating effects on the uterus; can interfere with iron absorption.*

Butcher's Broom (*Ruscus aculeatus*)
Anti-inflammatory, vasoconstrictor (slows blood flow). *Precautions: People with high blood pressure should use with care.*

Calendula (*Calendula officinalis*)
Anti-inflammatory for skin, mucous lining, and other tissues.

Caprylic Acid
Found in cow and goat milk and palm and coconut oils, caprylic acid is a short-chain fatty acid known for its ability to prevent the growth of yeast (*Candida albicans*).

Carotene (alpha, beta, and gamma carotene, lutein, and lycopene)
Antioxidant, anti-infective; converted by the liver into vitamin A; supports the immune system's response during allergic reactions and prevents certain cancers. *Precautions: People who suffer from hypothyroidism should avoid beta carotene due to the possibility that their bodies cannot convert it to vitamin A.*

Cascara Sagrada (*Rhamnus purshiana*)
Colon cleanser, laxative, liver and gallbladder tonic, purgative; promotes peristalsis. *Precautions: Pregnant women or people in weakened conditions should avoid use; everyone should avoid prolonged use.*

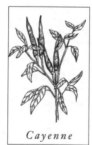
Cayenne

Catnip (*Nepeta cataria*)
Antispasmodic, mild sedative.

Cayenne (*Capsicum frutescens*)
Digestive and circulatory system aid, catalyst for combined herbs; contains the active ingredient capsaicin. *Precautions: Do not use topically on sensitive areas, mucous membranes, or near the eyes. Externally, try capsaicin cream first on a small area to rule out allergic reaction.*

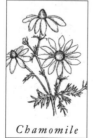
Chamomile

Chamomile (*Matricaria chamomilla*)
Digestive relaxant, nervine. *Precautions: Rare reports of allergic reactions.*

Chastetree (*Vitex agnus-castus*)
Controls and regulates the female reproductive system and menstrual cycle; strong hormone-stimulating action; reduces premenstrual syndrome (PMS) symptoms.

Chickweed *(Stellaria media)*
Source of vitamin C; helpful for treating cuts, irritations, insect bites and stings, wounds.

Chlorella *(Chlorella pyrenoidosa)*
(See also "Green" Drink Powders, below)
High chlorophyll content; contains over 50% protein; high in amino acids, B vitamins, beta carotene, carbohydrates, trace minerals, vitamins C and E.

Chlorophyll
(See also "Green" Drink Powders, below)
Detoxifier of the blood, liver, and the body in general; has healing, nourishing, and soothing effects on the intestines and mucous membranes.

Cinnamon *(Cinnamomum zeylanicum)*
Digestive aid, stimulant; improves blood flow; extracts of cinnamon have antifungal, antibacterial, and antiviral properties. *Precaution: Cinnamon should not be used in large amounts during pregnancy.*

Citrus Bioflavonoids (from citrus fruits, especially grapefruits, lemons, and oranges)
(See Bioflavonoids, above)
Antioxidant; supports and increases vitamin C actions; improves capillary health.

Clove *(Syzygium aromaticum)*
Antiparasitic, antifungal, digestive aid. *Precautions: Clove oil should not be used internally other than in the mouth without swallowing. Large quantities can be irritating to the digestive system.*

Coenzyme Q10
Also called ubiquinone, occurs naturally in all human cells; its actions are similar to vitamin E; assists cellular energy production, improves circulation (increasing oxygen delivery to tissues), supports and stimulates the immune system, and has anti-aging properties;[16] useful for diabetes, energy production, heart disease, mental deficits (Alzheimer's and memory loss), periodontal (gum) disease, weight loss, and respiratory conditions related to histamine release, such as allergies and asthma.

Comfrey (Symphytum officinale)
Anti-inflammatory; useful for healing injuries and relieving pain; used externally in compress or poultice. *Precautions: Comfrey can cause liver damage and should only be used internally under the supervision of a qualified health-care professional.*

Cornsilk (Zea mays)
Diuretic; good for urinary tract conditions in adults and children.

Cramp Bark (Viburnum opulus)
Antispasmodic, muscle relaxant. *Precautions: Pregnant women should not use except during last month of pregnancy.*

Cranberry (Vaccinium macrocarpon)
Acidifier, antibacterial; commonly used to treat urinary tract infections; source of vitamin C.

Damiana (Turnera diffusa)
Aphrodisiac, tonic for energy and the nervous and hormonal systems. *Precautions: Not recommended for people in debilitated, emaciated, or weakened states or while inflammation is present.*

Dandelion (Taraxacum officinale)
Blood cleanser, diuretic, liver tonic; improves function of the kidneys, pancreas, and stomach. *Precautions: People with gastric acidity, digestive ulcers, or gallstones should use dandelion with caution.*

Desiccated Liver
High in vitamins A, B complex, C, and D, and calcium, copper, phosphorus, and iron.

Devil's Claw (Harpagophytum procumbens)
Analgesic, anti-inflammatory, antirheumatic, diuretic, sedative.

See Appendix: Great Smokies Diagnostic Laboratory Tests, pp. 484-485, **for information about DHEA testing.**

DHEA (Dehydroepiandrosterone)
Hormone produced by the adrenal glands (and ovaries of women); a building block of the hormones estrogen and testosterone; also stimulates the immune system (increases T-cell production), prevents osteoporosis in post-menopausal women, and maintains muscle and skin tone and bone integrity. *Precautions: Before taking any supplements, have a saliva test to determine deficiencies in DHEA.*

DMSO (Dimethylsulfoxide)
Simple by-product of wood that contains sulfur; anti-inflammatory, immune stimulant, and free-radical scavenger;[17] easily absorbed into the skin.

Dong Quai (Chinese Angelica, *Angelica sinensis*)
Analgesic, anti-inflammatory, antispasmodic, blood and female tonic, hormonal regulator. *Precautions: Women who are pregnant or experiencing heavy menstrual flow should not use dong quai.*

Echinacea *(Echinacea angustifolia)*
Antibiotic, anti-inflammatory, antiviral, and immune and lymphatic regulator.[18]

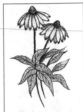

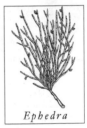

Echinacea

Elecampane *(Inula helenium)*
Expectorant; relieves bronchial irritation. *Precautions: People with high fever or acute swelling should not use elecampane.*

Ephedra (*ma huang* or *Ephedra sinica*)
Anti-inflammatory, antiviral, bronchodilator (clears lungs), stimulant. *Precautions: People who experience panic or anxiety attacks, have glaucoma or high blood pressure, or are taking MAO (monoamine oxidase) inhibitor drugs (most commonly for depression), children under the age of six, or pregnant or lactating women, should avoid ephedra.*

Ephedra

Essential Fatty Acids (EFAs)
(See also Black Currant, Borage, and Evening Primrose Oils)
EFAs are unsaturated fats required in the diet. Omega-3 and omega-6 oils are the two principal types. The primary omega-3 oil is alpha-linolenic acid (ALA), found in flaxseed (58%) and canola oils, as well as pumpkins, soybeans, and walnuts. Fish oils, such as salmon, cod, and mackerel, contain the other important omega-3 oils, DHA (docosahexaenoic acid) and EPA (eicosapentaenoic acid). Linoleic acid or cis-linoleic acid is the main omega-6 oil and is found in most plants and vegetable oils, including safflower (73%), corn, peanut, and sesame. The most therapeutic form of omega-6 oil is gamma-linolenic acid (GLA), found in black currant, borage, and evening primrose oils.

EFAs are converted in the body to prostaglandins, hormone-like substances that regulate many metabolic functions, particularly inflammatory processes. Linoleic, linolenic, and eicosapentaenoic acids have antimicrobial properties.[19] *Precautions: Heating or cooking oils will destroy the essential fatty acids in them and also cause the formation of harmful free-radical oxidants. Consume EFAs with a meal that contains some fat.*

Essiac Tea
Herbal tea originally formulated by the Ojibway Indians and later made famous as a cancer treatment by Canadian nurse Rene Caisse; contains burdock root, turkey rhubarb, sheep sorrel, and slippery elm, among other herbs.

Evening Primrose
(See Essential Fatty Acids, above)
High in gamma-linolenic acid (omega-6 essential fatty acid); analgesic, antibacterial, anti-inflammatory, antioxidant, cell energy source, precursor of prostaglandins (regulate hormones and metabolism), skin softener; improves circulation.

Eyebright *(Euphrasia officinalis)*
Eye tonic.

False Unicorn *(Chamaelirion luteum)*
Hormone balancer, ovarian adaptogen. *Precautions: People who are emaciated or are experiencing acute inflammation should not take false unicorn root.*

Fennel *(Foeniculum vulgare)*
Appetite suppressant, eyewash; calms digestive tract.

Feverfew *(Tanacetum parthenium)*
Anti-inflammatory, digestive stimulant; reduces blood vessel spasms and reestablishes proper blood vessel tone. *Precautions: Can cause mouth soreness and ulcers. Pregnant women and children under the age of two should avoid feverfew.*

Fiber (grapefruit, apple, or vegetable pectin, guar gum, psyllium husks, oat bran, and alfalfa seeds)
Fiber is the indigestible parts of plants. The main bulking agent for stools (keeps bowel movements regular), fiber helps control blood cholesterol levels, maintain balanced blood sugar, and detoxify the colon (of heavy metals and chemicals). It can also help prevent colon cancer, constipation, diverticulitis, gallstones, heart disease, hemorrhoids, obesity, ulcers, and varicose veins.[20]

Fo-Ti (He Shou Wu)
Astringent; tonic for blood, liver, and kidney.

Flax (Linum usitatissimum)
(See Essential Fatty Acids, above)
Analgesic, anti-inflammatory, antioxidant, skin softener; alkaline-forming multinutrient rich in alpha-linolenic acid, an omega-3 essential fatty acid.

Garcinia (Tamarind, Garcinia cambogia)
Appetite suppressant. *Precautions: Can cause nausea in some people.*

Garlic (Allium sativum)
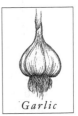
Antibiotic, antifungal, antiparasitic, antitoxin, antiviral, expectorant, blood-thinner; lowers blood pressure. *Precautions: Can cause irritation of the digestive tract. People who are weak, feeble, or emaciated should not use garlic. Because garlic has anticlotting actions, people who are taking anticoagulant drugs (coumadin) should avoid supplements of this herb.*

Garlic

Genistein, Daidzein (isoflavones from soybeans and other legumes)
Balances hormones and cholesterol.

Gentian (Gentiana lutea)
Antacid, antispasmodic, bitter tonic, mild laxative, stomach tonic.

Ginger (Zingiber officinale)
Anti-inflammatory, antimicrobial, antinausea; stimulates circulation and reduces cramping, spasms, and intestinal gas.

Ginkgo (Ginkgo biloba)
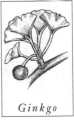
Antioxidant; increases blood flow, circulation, and oxygenation of tissues; inhibits platelet aggregation (clustering of the blood cells that facilitate clotting); reduces water retention associated with premenstrual syndrome (PMS).

Ginseng, American (Panax quinquefolius)
Ginkgo

Adaptogen, anti-fatigue; helpful for anxiety, diabetes, menopause, chronic fatigue syndrome (CFS), and hypertension or hypotension headaches. *Precautions: Should not be used by people with acute illness, fever, or swelling.*

Ginseng, Korean or Chinese *(Panax ginseng)*

Adaptogen, antioxidant, general tonic, restorative, central nervous system stimulant, immune regulator; protects against radiation. *Precautions: Should not be used by people with acute illness, fever, or swelling.*

Ginseng, Siberian *(Eleutherococcus senticosus)*

Adaptogen, adrenal gland regulator; increases resistance to fatigue and stress. *Precautions: People with high blood pressure or a high fever should not take Siberian ginseng.*

Glandular Extracts (from animals)

Glandular extract therapy is based on the idea that extracts from animal glands prompt normal functioning in the equivalent human gland, via micronutrients and polypeptides. Glandular products are usually derived from bovine sources. *Precautions: Be absolutely certain that any glandular extract is derived from organically raised animals.*

Glucosamine

Component of many of the tissues and structures of the body, including the bones, cartilage, eyes, heart, ligaments, nails, skin, and tendons; maintains joint function and stimulates joint repair.

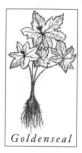

Goldenseal *(Hydrastis canadensis)*

Antibiotic, antibacterial, antifungal, antiparasitic, anti-inflammatory, nervous system stimulant, mucous membrane tonic.[21] *Precautions: Should not be used for extended periods of time (can cause decreased absorption of vitamin B12). People who have hypoglycemia (low blood sugar), high blood pressure, weak digestion, or are weak and emaciated should not use goldenseal. Some herbalists recommend that pregnant women avoid goldenseal.*

Goldenseal

Gotu Kola *(Centella asiatica)*

Anti-infective, anti-inflammatory, central nervous system stimulant; healing effect on connective tissues. *Precautions: Pregnant or lactating women should avoid gotu kola.*

Grape Seed Extract

(See Pycnogenol, below).

Grapefruit Seed Extract

Antifungal, antiseptic, multipurpose antibiotic for bacterial infections.

Gravel Root *(Collinsonia)*
Diuretic, urinary tract tonic.

"Green" Drink Powders
Contains "green" foods such as chlorella, spirulina and other blue-green algae, barley and wheat grass, and alfalfa; rich in chlorophyll, enzymes, and minerals; general detoxifiers to help clean the blood of unwanted substances.

Green-Lipped Mussel *(Perna canaliculus)*
A shellfish extract high in amino acids, enzymes, and minerals; works well in reducing the pain and inflammation of arthritic joints; generally beneficial for many organs and systems of the body, including the eyes, heart and blood vessels, the lymphatic and hormonal systems, and mucous membranes.

Green Tea *(Camellia sinensis)*
Anticarcinogen, antioxidant, bioflavonoid (synergistic with vitamin C); useful for treating gingivitis, high cholesterol, and high blood pressure.

Guarana *(Paullinia cupana)*
Stimulant (contains two to three times the caffeine of coffee), diuretic; prevents diarrhea. *Precautions: Contains caffeine and can cause anxiety, heart palpitations, insomnia, and nervousness. Pregnant women should avoid the use of guarana.*

Guggul or Gugulipid
Ayurvedic herb, anti-inflammatory, cholesterol balancer, metabolic tonic. *Precautions: Pregnant women and people with bleeding disorders should not use guggul.*

Gymnema *(Gymnema sylvestre)*
Ayurvedic herb that reduces sugar levels in urine; helpful for diabetes; helps repair damaged cells in the pancreas and increases the pancreas' ability to produce insulin.

Hawthorn *(Crataegus spp.)*
Antispasmodic, sedative; supports heart muscle and coronary blood vessels, dilates blood vessels, decreases cholesterol levels, reduces arterial plaque; useful for hypertension (high blood pressure).

Honey

Contains amino acids, B vitamins, vitamins C, D, and E, protein, and trace minerals; has antiseptic properties (bacteria will not grow easily in honey); when no other remedies are available, honey will work as a topical salve for burns, cuts, minor skin infections, and wounds.

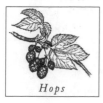

Hops

Hops *(Humulus lupulus)*

Action/Properties: antispasmodic, diuretic, and central nervous system sedative.

Horehound *(Marrubium vulgare)*

Expectorant, immune stimulant.

Horse Chestnut *(Aesculus hippocastanum)*

Anti-inflammatory, astringent; reduces vascular engorgement (distension of the blood vessels).

Horsetail (Shave Grass, *Equisetum arvense*)

Anti-inflammatory, mild diuretic; high in silica (building block of bones, cartilage, connective tissues, and skin), which is helpful for arthritis, osteoporosis, acne, and wound healing.

Hyssop *(Hyssopus officinalis)*

Antispasmodic, decongestant, nervine.

Juniper *(Juniperus communis)*

Anti-inflammatory, antimicrobial, diuretic. *Precautions: Pregnant women and people with kidney disease, nephritis, nephrosis, or inflamed kidneys should avoid the use of juniper berries.*

Kava-Kava *(Piper methysticum)*

Natural tranquilizer (central nervous system depressant), muscle relaxant, sleep aid.[22]

Kola (Cola) Nut

Antidepressant, astringent, diuretic, stimulant (high in caffeine). *Precautions: Contains caffeine which can cause anxiety, heart palpitations, insomnia, and nervouness.*

Lavender *(Lavendula angustifola)*

Antidepressant; helps relieve stress, emotional upset, nervous depression, and insomnia.

Lecithin

Derived from legumes such as soybeans, brewer's yeast, eggs, fish, grains, or wheat germ, lecithin is a fat (lipid) used by every cell in the body. It helps maintain healthy nerve and brain cells and prevent certain cardiovascular diseases (atherosclerosis, arteriosclerosis) by protecting the body from a buildup of fat in the arteries and organs. Lecithin also aids in the assimilation of nutrients.[23]

Lemon Balm *(Melissa officinalis)*

Antidepressant, antiviral, nervine.

Lemongrass *(Cymbopogon citratus)*

Astringent, tonic.

Licorice *(Glycyrrhiza glabra)*

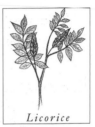

Licorice

Anti-inflammatory, expectorant; supports the endocrine (adrenal gland) system; deglycyrrhizinated (DGL) licorice is helpful for peptic ulcers. *Precautions: People with high blood pressure should take the DGL form of licorice.*

Lobelia *(Lobelia inflata)*

Systemic relaxant, expectorant, nervous system depressant. *Precautions: Large doses can produce unpleasant side effects such as nausea, sweating, and vomiting. Take small doses repeatedly throughout the day to avoid unwanted effects.*

Lutein and Zeaxanthin (carotenoid from green vegetables such as broccoli, collards, and kale)

Antioxidant; provides eye protection; helpful for macular degeneration, a common cause of blindness.

Lycopene (from red-colored fruits and vegetables, especially tomatoes and red grapefruit)

Useful for healthy prostate function; reduces the risk of prostate and other cancers.

Maitake Mushroom

Adaptogen; normalizes metabolic functions, improves immune function (activates T cells); helps prevent cancer (especially hormone-related); may be helpful in preventing arthritis, diabetes, hepatitis, high blood pressure, or obesity.

Marshmallow *(Althaea officinalis)*
Anti-inflammatory, diuretic, expectorant.

Melatonin
Pineal gland hormone; powerful antioxidant (free-radical scavenger), immune stimulant, and anticancer and antitumor agent; important for hormone production and helps regulate the body's sleeping/waking cycle.

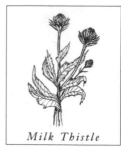

Milk Thistle

Milk Thistle *(Silybum marianum)*
Antioxidant, anti-inflammatory; contains liver-protecting bioflavonoids; tonic for the gallbladder, female organs, liver, spleen, and stomach.

Motherwort *(Leonorus cardiaca)*
Female and heart tonic, nervine. *Precautions: Pregnant women or women experiencing heavy menstrual flow should not use motherwort.*

Mullein *(Verbascum thapsus)*
Analgesic, anti-inflammatory, laxative.

Myrrh
Antimicrobial, antiseptic, disinfectant, deodorizer. *Precautions: Toxic in large doses. Pregnant women or women experiencing heavy menstrual flow should not use myrrh.*

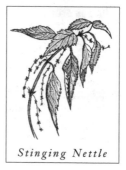

Stinging Nettle

Nettle, Stinging *(Urtica dioica)*
Anti-arthritic, anti-inflammatory, antirheumatic, expectorant; immune-system stimulant; useful for allergies, arthritis, urinary tract infections, and enlarged prostate gland.

Oatstraw, Oats, or Wild Oats *(Avena sativa)*
Antidepressant, nerve tonic; general nutritional support in prostate conditions; useful for depression and menopause symptoms.

Octacosanol (from wheat germ oil)
Increases the body's ability to utilize oxygen and the muscles' ability to store glycogen (sugar used for energy); helps increase physical endurance; useful for athletes or those with muscle pain.

Oregon Grape Root (Berberis aquifolium)

Active ingredient is berberine; liver and gallbladder tonic. *Precautions: Pregnant women and emaciated people with weak digestion should not use Oregon grape root.*

Papaya (Carica)

Appetite stimulant, digestive aid.

Parsley (Petroselinum crispum)

Diuretic, digestive regulator. *Precautions: Not recommended for dehydrated or emaciated people.*

Passionflower (Passiflora incarnata)

Antispasmodic, sedative; helpful for insomnia, anxiety, and other nervous disorders.

Pau d'Arco (Tabebuia avellandae)

Antibacterial, antifungal, blood cleanser; contains quinones which may have anti-cancer effects.

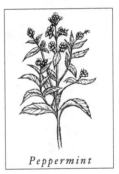

Passionflower

Peppermint (Mentha piperita)

Mild anesthetic, nervine; improves digestion. *Precautions: Excessive use of oil can irritate skin. Peppermint oil should not be used for children under the age of six.*

Plantain (Plantago major)

Antibiotic, anti-inflammatory.

Pumpkin (Cucurbita maxima)

High in zinc; seeds useful for prostate conditions and certain parasitic infections.

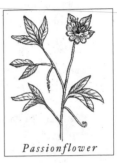

Peppermint

Pycnogenol (grape seed or pine tree bark extract)

Anti-inflammatory, antioxidant, bioflavonoid (synergistic with vitamin C); stabilizes collagen (component of connective tissue, skin, and bone), promotes circulation and oxygenation of the blood.

Pygeum (Pygeum africanum)

Anti-edema (swelling), anti-inflammatory; absorbs cholesterol; useful for prostate problems.

Red Clover *(Trifolium pratense)*
Antibiotic, antispasmodic, appetite suppressant, blood cleanser, expectorant.

Red Raspberry *(Rubus idaeus)*
Astringent, uterine tonic; prevents hemorrhaging.

Reishi Mushroom *(Ganoderma lucidum)*
Enhances the immune system and increases vitality; helpful for chronic disease, fatigue, heart disease, high blood pressure, high cholesterol, tumors, and cancer.

Rhubarb *(Rheum spp.)*
Antibiotic, antiparasitic, laxative. *Precautions: Strong laxative; combine with ginger to reduce chance of abdominal upset.*

Rose Hips *(Rosa canina)*
Astringent; high in vitamin C.

Rosemary *(Rosmarinus officinalis)*
Antibacterial, astringent, calming agent, decongestant; improves cardiovascular health; useful for arthritic or nerve pain or during convalescence.

Royal Jelly (produced by bees)
Antibiotic, stimulates immunity; high in acetylcholine, amino acids, B vitamins, vitamins A, C, D, and E, enzymes, hormones, and minerals; helpful for asthma, bone fractures, bronchitis, skin disorders, sleep disorders, and disorders of the kidney, liver, pancreas, and stomach.

Sage *(Salvia officinalis)*
Antacid, antibiotic, antidiarrheal, anti-inflammatory, antioxidant, antiseptic, central nervous system stimulant, estrogenic; reduces perspiration and night sweats; useful as a gargle for mouth and throat conditions.

Sarsaparilla *(Smilax sarsaparilla)*
Anti-inflammatory, antirheumatic, hormonal and nervous system regulator, liver protector; helpful for psoriasis and eczema.

Saw Palmetto *(Serenoa repens)*
Antiseptic (urinary), immunostimulant, expectorant, mucous mem-

brane tonic; inhibits conversion of male hormone testosterone; has proven as effective as conventional medications in treatment of enlarged prostate.[24]

Schisandra *(Wu Wei Zi)*

Adaptogen, antibacterial, antidepressant, antioxidant, detoxifier, heart tonic. *Precautions: People with acute illness, high fever, or swelling should avoid schisandra.*

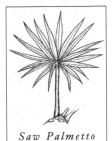

Saw Palmetto

Sea Cucumber (bêche-de-mer, *Parastichopus parvimensis*)

Marine animal related to starfish that has a long history of use in Asia as a remedy for arthritis; rich source of chondroitin (a component of cartilage often deficient in arthritis sufferers), minerals, and vitamins A, C, B1, B2, and B3; useful for osteoarthritis, rheumatoid arthritis, rheumatism, and most inflammatory, musculoskeletal conditions.

Sea Vegetables

Nutrient-dense sea vegetables include arame, bladderwrack, dulse, hijiki, kelp, kombu, nori, sea palm, and wakame; high in antioxidants, carbohydrates, minerals (especially iodine), proteins, and vitamins.

Shark Cartilage

Immune stimulant; the active ingredient of shark cartilage is a protein that prevents the abnormal growth of new blood vessels as occurs in cancerous tumors, diabetic retinopathy, or macular degeneration in the eye. *Precautions: Children and pregnant women should not use shark cartilage.*

Shiitake Mushroom

High in amino acids, B vitamins, and vitamin D; stimulates and strengthens the immune system, and is believed to stimulate the production of interferon (protein released by the immune system) in the body, which has anticancer and antitumor effects.

Skullcap *(Scutelbria lateriflora)*

Antispasmodic, calming remedy, nervine, sedative, sleep aid.

Slippery Elm *(Ulmus fulva)*

Soothing action for mucous membranes of the gastrointestinal tract; used topically for boils and abscesses. *Precautions: Not recommended for treating external ulcers.*

Spearmint *(Mentha spicata)*
Dispels intestinal gas.

Spirulina
(See also "Green" Drink Powders, above)
A form of algae; high in essential amino acids, essential fatty acids, vitamin B12, chlorophyll, iron, easily assimilable protein (70%), DNA and RNA, and a blue pigment (phyocyanin) that may be theraputic for certain forms of cancer.

Squaw Vine *(Mitchella repens)*
Astringent, diuretic, sedative; useful for insomnia; commonly used during last few weeks of pregnancy to promote labor and by nursing mothers to relieve painful nipples; also useful for heavy menstrual flow or engorged veins (hemorrhoids, varicose veins).

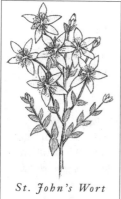

St. John's Wort

St. John's Wort *(Hypericum perforatum)*
Analgesic, antibacterial, anti-inflammatory, antidepressant, diuretic, sedative.[25] *Precautions: Can cause skin to be light-sensitive; avoid exposure to sunlight.*

Suma (Brazilian Ginseng, *Pfaffia paniculata*)
Adaptogen, analgesic, anti-inflammatory, nutrient, regenerative tonic. *Precautions: People with acute illness, high fever, or swelling should avoid suma.*

Tea Tree *(Melaleuca alternifolia)*
Antibacterial, antifungal, antiseptic, antiviral.[26]
Precautions: Dilute oil before taking internally.

Thyme *(Thymus vulgaris)*
Antimicrobial, antiseptic; soothes digestive tract.

Tocotrienol (from rice bran)
Helps control the formation of cholesterol.

Turmeric *(Curcuma longa)*
Antibacterial, anticancer, antifungal, anti-inflammatory, antioxidant; the active ingredient is curcumin. *Precautions: People with acute colic, gallstones, obstructive jaundice, or toxic liver conditions should not take large doses of turmeric.*

Uva Ursi *(Arctostaphylos uva-ursi)*
Astringent, diuretic, liver tonic, urinary tract antiseptic. *Precautions: Pregnant or lactating women should use uva ursi with extreme caution.*

Valerian *(Valeriana officinalis)*
Anticonvulsant, antispasmodic, anti-anxiety, sedative, relaxant. *Precautions: Valerian should not be combined with alcoholic beverages.*

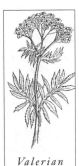

Valerian

Wheat Grass (juice or powder)
(See also "Green" Drink Powders, above)
High in chlorophyll, minerals, and vitamins; effective as a blood and liver cleanser and general detoxifier; stimulates metabolism and enzymatic activity. The chlorophyll in wheat grass helps protect the body from environmental pollutants and radiation.

White Willow *(Salix alba)*
Analgesic, anti-inflammatory, astringent.

Wild Yam *(Dioscorea villosa)*
Anti-inflammatory, antispasmodic. *Precautions: Pregnant women should avoid wild yam except to induce labor.*

Wintergreen *(Gaultheria procumbens)*
Anti-inflammatory, analgesic.

Witch Hazel *(Hamamelis virginiana)*
Astringent.

Wood Betony *(Betonica officinalis)*
Nervous system tonic, relaxant.

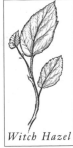

Witch Hazel

Wormwood *(Artemisia annua, Artemesia absinthium)*
Mild sedative, digestive stimulant; used in nutritional formulas to expel parasitic worms. *Precautions: For short-term use only; wormwood can be toxic if used for prolonged periods. Do not use if pregnant; can cause abortion.*

Yarrow *(Achillea millefolium)*
Anti-inflammatory, diuretic.

Yeast (Baker's, Brewer's, Tortula)

High in amino acids, B vitamins, assimilable proteins, and minerals; aids in the metabolism of sugars, provides a source of energy, relieves nervous anxiety and fatigue, supports immune function; helpful for people with suppressed immunity or who are undergoing immune-suppressive treatments (antibiotic, chemotherapy, corticosteroid, radiation). *Precautions: Live Baker's yeast should not be used as a nutritional supplement. People with yeast infections or candidiasis should avoid taking yeast supplements.*

Yellowdock *(Rumex crispus)*

Blood cleanser/purifier; systemic tonifier.

Yerba Maté *(Ilex paraguariensis)*

General tonic, diuretic, laxative, immune modulator, and nutrient; enhances the action of other herbs.

Yerba Santa *(Eriodictyon californicum)*

Bronchial dilator (opens the air passageways in the lungs), expectorant.

Yohimbe *(Pausinystalia yohimbe)*

Active ingredient from the bark of this evergreen tree is yohimbine; hormone stimulant; useful for impotence. *Precautions: Pregnant or lactating women or people with kidney disease or stomach ulcers should not use yohimbe.*

Yucca *(Yucca spp.)*

Anti-inflammatory, blood purifier, mild laxative. *Precautions: Slight laxative effect, which can cause intestinal cramping.*

In America, we have
an overabundance of food
but an underabundance of nutrition.
We rarely encounter severe
nutritional deficiencies or hear of an
American child suffering from malnutrition.
But we have all experienced
insomnia, mood swings, and
the inability to concentrate—
all signs of a deficiency in B vitamins.
The symptoms of nutritional deficiencies
encompass many of today's
common ailments: chronic infections,
digestive problems, fatigue, headaches,
premenstrual syndrome (PMS), allergies,
ADD, anxiety, and depression.

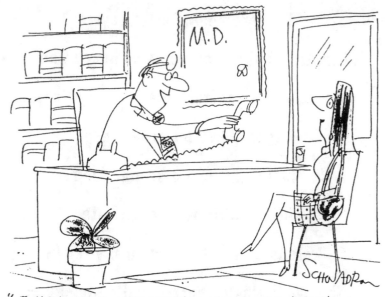

"I NOW OFFER NUTRITIONAL COUNSELING. HERE'S A
RECORDING OF MY MOM'S RECIPE FOR CHICKEN SOUP."

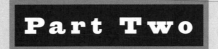

Part Two

An A-Z of Health Conditions: Nutrients and Herbal Remedies

Allergies

An allergy is the immune system's abnormal reaction to a substance that is harmless to most people. Typically, the immune system fights only dangerous invaders, such as bacteria or viruses, and ignores "normal" substances such as food. People develop allergies when the immune system has become weakened and can no longer tell the difference between harmful and harmless substances. In response to these otherwise normal substances, the immune system releases chemicals, such as histamines, resulting in many of the symptoms associated with allergies, including sneezing, stuffy nose, watery eyes, fatigue, and headaches.

Types of Allergies

There are two main categories of allergies, food and environmental.

Food Allergies—The foods most commonly associated with allergies are wheat, corn, yeast, milk and other dairy products, egg whites, tomatoes, soy, shellfish, peanuts, chocolate, and strawberries. In addition, food additives such as nitrates, sulfites, monosodium glutamate (MSG), and artificial flavoring and coloring are the source of allergies in many people.

Environmental Allergies—Environmental allergens (substances provoking an allergic response) include common airborne substances such as pollens from grass, weeds, trees, or other plants along with animal dander, dust, tobacco smoke, and chemicals, among many other potential allergens in the world around us. Cosmetics, toiletries, and even some nutritional supplements and "natural" products contain artificial flavoring and coloring, artificial fragrances (the leading cause of allergic skin reactions), petroleum products, formaldehyde (under the name quaternium) as a preservative, shellac, and talc (often contaminated with asbestos), all of which can cause allergic reactions in some people.

Although the allergy known as hay fever (or allergic rhinitis) is usually related to flower pollens in the air, it can also result from continuous exposure to other environmental allergens such as house dust, certain chemicals, and animal hair.

Symptoms of Allergies

Common symptoms of both environmental and food allergies include itchy and watery eyes, runny nose, skin itching and rashes, headaches, edema (swelling and puffiness), menstrual problems, learning disabilities, asthma, chronic respiratory and sinus infections, and rapid heart rate.[1] Other symptoms indicative of food allergies include abdominal bloating, gas, cramps, sweating, and fuzzy-headedness after eating.

Allergies can contribute to an extensive list of disorders, which include anxiety, depression, hyperactivity, insomnia, seizures, gastrointestinal disorders such as colitis, diabetes, obesity, bed-wetting, chronic bladder infections, kidney disease, and joint problems such as arthritis and bursitis.[2]

Causes of Allergies

Allergies are usually rooted in underlying problems related to the digestive system, the adrenal glands, and/or the immune system. In our practice, we have found that about 80% of our patients who have food or airborne allergies also have some degree of adrenal stress or adrenal weakness that can be linked to the allergies.

As mentioned above, weakened immunity is a primary cause in the development of allergies. There are many factors that weaken immunity, among them chronic stress, recurrent infections, and toxic overload. In the case of the latter, environmental toxins, vaccines, antibiotics, steroids, and other medications both deplete and confuse the immune system, rendering it unable to distinguish friend from foe. Allergies develop and a downward spiral ensues, because histamine, a substance produced by the body during an allergic reaction, is an immune suppressant.

Another potential cause of allergies is poor digestion, which often results from deficiencies in digestive enzymes or *acidophilus* (a beneficial intestinal bacteria), combined with an incorrect stomach pH (SEE QUICK DEFINITION). If digestive dysfunction becomes chronic, a disorder called "leaky gut syndrome" can develop. Undigested food particles pass through the intestinal wall into the bloodstream where the immune system perceives them as "for-

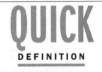

DEFINITION

The term **pH**, which means "potential hydrogen," represents a scale for the relative acidity or alkalinity of a solution. Acidity is measured as a pH of 0.1 to 6.9, alkalinity is 7.1 to 14, and neutral pH is 7.0. The numbers refer to how many hydrogen atoms are present compared to an ideal or standard solution. Normally, blood is slightly alkaline, at 7.35 to 7.45; urine pH can range from 4.8 to 8.0, but is usually somewhat acidic, with a normal reading between 5.0 and 6.0.

eign" invaders (antigens) and mobilizes to rid the body of them. Over time, the result is an allergy to the "invading" food.

Treatment of Allergies

For more about **adrenal stress**, see Stress, pp. 369-384. For **leaky gut syndrome**, see Gastrointestinal Disorders, pp. 198-217. For enzymes, see An A to Z Nutrient Guide in Part I, pp. 24-62.

See **Detoxification** in Part III, pp. 446-461. For **Immune support**, see Part III, pp. 462-483.

The first step is to avoid exposure to environmental allergens when possible and remove problem foods from the diet. By improving digestion, supplementing with the appropriate enzymes, treating infections or yeast overgrowth, identifying and reducing the stress load on the body, and supporting adrenal and immune function, we have succeeded in decreasing or eliminating allergies in many of our patients. For patients with chronic allergies, it is also often necessary to detoxify the tissues, colon, and liver.

Decreasing Allergic Reactions to Food

■ Improve the digestion of the offending foods using the appropriate plant enzyme supplements: protease digests protein, lipase digests fats, amylase digests carbohydrates, lactase digests dairy products, and disaccharidases digest sugars. As digestion improves, the reactions to the offending food will be minimized or completely eliminated.

■ Eliminate existing antigens circulating in the body by taking plant enzyme supplements between meals. Taken on an empty stomach, enzymes are absorbed into the bloodstream where they act as scavengers and "eat" the invaders.

■ Improve overall digestion and reverse leaky gut syndrome by taking nutrients such as the amino acid glutamine, the essential fatty acid GLA (gamma-linolenic acid), gamma-oryzanol (antioxidant found in grains), vitamin E, liquid chlorophyll, aloe vera, beneficial bacteria (*Lactobacillus acidophilus* and *Bifidobacteria bifidum*), and the herbs slippery elm, marshmallow root, comfrey, pau d'arco, and goldenseal. After digestion has been restored, it may be possible to gradually reintroduce into the diet foods that previously produced allergies.

Nutrients and Herbs for Allergies

For any respiratory condition, it is imperative to drink plenty of pure filtered water (six to eight 8-ounce glasses per day) and avoid smoke, exhaust, perfume, and chemical fumes.

Vitamins B6, B12 and C, quercetin, products for adrenal support, and the herbs stinging nettle, feverfew, licorice root, and ginkgo are helpful in the treatment of allergies.[3] Pycnogenol (grape seed or pine bark extract) is also used to reduce allergic reactions because of its antioxidant properties.

The Chinese herb ephedra (*ma huang* or *Ephedra sinica*) is commonly used for alleviating symptoms of hay fever and asthma. It is a respiratory stimulant and dilator (opener) of the bronchioles (a subdivision of the lung's bronchial tubes).[4]

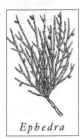

Ephedra

Products for Allergies

Activated Quercetin: Tablets. Inhibits the release of histamines and leukotrienes (inflammation-mediating substances released by mast cells) into the bloodstream.

SOURCE NATURALS, THRESHOLD ENTERPRISES, 23 Janis Way, Scotts Valley, CA 95066; tel: 800-777-5677 or 831-438-1144.

Ephedra is for short-term use only. Do not take ephedra at all if you are pregnant, have kidney problems, or suffer from high blood pressure or other cardiovascular stress.

AL-Alergy: Tablets. For immune system support when experiencing allergies; contains pantothenic acid (vitamin B5), potassium, glandular extracts (adrenal, thymus, and pancreas), vitamin C (vegetable source), citrus bioflavonoids, and rutin in a base of thyme, ginger, goldenseal root, seaweed, licorice, Oregon grape root, fenugreek, burdock, parsley, chamomile, barberry, and capsicum (from cayenne).

NATURAL ENERGY PRODUCTS, 21101 Welch Road, Snohomish, WA 98296; tel: 425-486-5956.

Aler-Key: Capsules. For the allergen-sensitive; ingredients include vitamins B2, B6, and C, quercetin, pantothenic acid, and calcium.

J.R. CARLSON LABS, INC., 15 College Drive, Arlington Heights, IL 60004-1985; tel: 800-323-4141 or 708-255-1600.

Aller Bee-Gone: Tablets. For allergies and asthma; contains glutamic acid HCl, betaine HCl, high-desert bee pollen, pepsin, potassium chloride, pyridoxine, bovine pancreas, cayenne, niacinamide, papain, alfalfa, peppermint, goldenseal root, burdock root, skullcap, slippery elm bark, marshmallow root, horseradish root, queen of the meadow, shave grass, eyebright, parsley leaf, mullein flower, blessed thistle, chickweed, white oak bark, black walnut leaf, papaya leaf, passionflower, barberry root, oatstraw, and fenugreek seed.

CC POLLEN CO., 3627 East Indian School Road, #209, Phoenix, AZ 85018-5126; tel: 800-875-0096 or 602-957-0096.

Allerelief: Capsules. Herbal formula to help relieve nasal congestion due to allergies and hay fever; helps reduce the swelling of nasal passages, shrink swollen membranes, and promote nasal and sinus drainage; contains Chinese ephedra, white willow bark, white pine bark, valerian root, goldenseal root, burdock root, marshmallow root, licorice, and bee pollen.

NATURE'S HERBS, 600 East Quality Drive, American Fork, UT 84003; tel: 800-437-2257 or 801-763-0700.

Aller Free: Capsules. Helps "dry up" congestion and allergies; ingredients include pau d'arco, mullein, red raspberry, marshmallow root, echinacea, eyebright, papaya, skunk cabbage, peppermint, and white pine.

WGI, 35008 Emerald Coast Parkway, 5th Floor, Destin, FL 32541; tel: 800-854-8353 or 850-654-4744.

Allergy: Homeopathic tablets. For temporary relief of sneezing and coughing, runny nose, watery eyes, skin rashes, and hives; helps regulate the flow of histamine, relieving minor allergies or hay fever.

HEEL/BHI, INC., 11600 Cochiti Road Southeast, Albuquerque, NM 87123-3376; tel: 800-621-7644 or 505-293-3843.

Allergy: Tablets. Supports the immune system; soothes, relaxes, and clears the nasal passages; helps protect against the effects of stress, poor digestion, and toxicity; contains pantothenic acid, potassium, glandular substances, thyme, licorice root, chamomile, catnip, fenugreek, parsley, goldenseal, barberry, Oregon grape root, burdock root, ginger, cayenne, and seaweed.

ALTERNATIVE THERAPY, INC., 1664 Fairlawn Avenue, San Jose, CA 95125; tel: 800-311-7922.

Allergy Balance: Tablets. Analgesic, antiseptic, and anti-inflammatory; for allergic bronchitis, dermatitis, and other allergies; contains clove, ginkgo, turmeric, aloe vera, and haritaki (an Ayurvedic herb).

VEDA HEALTH, INC., P.O. Box 1535, Soquel, CA 95073; tel: 888-856-8334 or 408-465-9084.

AllergyCare: Capsules. For temporary relief of upper respiratory allergies, hay fever, and nasal/sinus congestion without causing drowsiness; active ingredient is pseudoephedrine HCl, an extract of the plant ephedra (*ma huang*).

NATURE'S WAY PRODUCTS, Inc., 10 Mountain Springs Parkway, Springville, UT 84663; tel: 800-962-8873 or 801-489-1500.

Allergy Drops: Homeopathic liquid. For hay fever sufferers.
BIOENERGETICS, INC., P.O. Box 127, Sandy, OR 97055; tel: 800-334-4043 or 503-668-7478.

Allergy Formulae: Homeopathic liquid. Relieves runny nose, itchy/watery eyes, nausea, congestion, redness, hives, headache, and sneezing; safe for children.
LIDDELL, LABORATORIES, 1036 Country Club Drive, Moraga, CA 94556; tel: 800-460-7733 or 925-377-3000.

Allerid: Homeopathic lozenges. Alleviates frequent sneezing, runny nose, nasal blockage, itchiness in the throat and eyes, spasmodic wheezing, headaches, tearing, and general fatigue that characterize hay fever; does not interfere with any other medicine.
SUPHERB LTD., P.O. Box 1135, Nahariya 22100, Israel; tel: 800-409-HERB (4372).

Allerin and Allerin Plus: Capsules. For temporary relief of allergy, hay fever, common cold, and sinusitis symptoms; suitable for children. Allerin contains 60 mg of pseudoephedrine and other herbs. Allerin Plus contains 30 mg of pseudoephedrine plus vitamins C and E, quercetin, Chinese ephedra, and turmeric.
NATURE'S HERBS, 600 East Quality Drive, American Fork, UT 84003; tel: 800-437-2257 or 801-763-0700.

Aller-Stop: Capsules. Nasal decongestant for seasonal allergies; ingredients include ephedra, bay leaf, eucalyptus leaf, fenugreek seed, grindelia, and goldenseal root.
RIDGECREST HERBALS, 1151 South Redwood Road #106, Salt Lake City, UT 84104-3729; tel: 800-242-4649 or 801-978-9633.

BHI Hayfever: Homeopathic nasal spray. For relief of typical hay fever symptoms.
HEEL/BHI, INC., 11600 Cochiti Road Southeast, Albuquerque, NM 87123-3376; tel: 800-621-7644 or 505-293-3843.

BHI Sinus: Homeopathic tablets. For temporary relief of sinusitis and rhinitis, sinus pressure and headaches, and nasal/sinus congestion, sneezing, and runny nose.
HEEL/BHI, INC., 11600 Cochiti Road Southeast, Albuquerque, NM 87123-3376; tel: 800-621-7644 or 505-293-3843.

Broad Spectrum Enzymes: Chewable tablets or vegicaps. Enzyme replacement formula for people who eat cooked, processed food; when ingested with food, digestion can begin before the body's own enzymes go to work, reducing stress in the lower stomach and intestines and demand on the pancreas for digestive enzymes; contains protease, lipase, amylase, and cellulase. *Authors' note: To help reduce food allergies.*

ENZYMES INC., 8500 Northwest River Park Drive #223, Parkville, MO 64152; tel: 800-647-6377 or 816-746-6461.

Congest-Ease: Capsules. For relief of sinus congestion and sinus pressure without drowsiness.

NATURE'S HERBS, 600 East Quality Drive, American Fork, UT 84003; tel: 800-437-2257 or 801-763-0700.

CSE-3 (Cell Signal Enhancer): Homeopathic liquid. Assists in the relief of allergies.

BIOMED COMM, INC., 2 Nickerson Street, Suite 102, Seattle, WA 98109; tel: 888-637-3516 or 206-284-3433.

Dairy Enzyme Formula: Capsules. Contains concentrated plant enzymes to aid in the digestion of dairy proteins, milk sugar, carbohydrates, and fat. *Authors' note: For allergy to dairy products.*

PREVAIL CORP., 2204-8 Northwest Birdsdale, Gresham, OR 97030; tel: 800-248-0885 or 503-667-5527.

Decongest Herbal Formula: Capsules. Herbal decongestant containing only 4 mg of ephedrine (an active component of the plant ephedra) per capsule, reducing the potential for side effects from ephedra; helps relieve sinus congestion caused by hay fever, colds, and sinus infection; provides anti-inflammatory, astringent, and cooling properties.

ZAND HERBAL FORMULAS, 1722 14th Street #230, Boulder, CO 80302; tel: 800-800-0405 or 303-786-8558.

HAS Fast-Acting Formula: Capsules. For temporary relief of nasal congestion in hay fever, allergies, sinusitis, or colds; ingredients include plant extract of pseudoephedrine (active component of ephedra) in an herbal base of Brigham tea, marshmallow root, burdock root, cayenne, goldenseal root, lobelia, parsley, cleavers, and rosemary.

NATURE'S WAY PRODUCTS, INC., 10 Mountain Springs Parkway, Springville, UT 84663; tel: 800-962-8873 or 801-489-1500.

Hay Fever by Jade: Tablets. Herbal decongestant to help reduce swollen nasal membranes, drain nasal and sinus passages, relieve itching and headache, and open the lungs.
EAST EARTH HERB, INC., P.O. Box 2802, Eugene, OR 97402; tel: 800-827-HERB (4372) or 541-687-0155.

Hay Fever Formulae: Homeopathic liquid. Relieves symptoms associated with hay fever, including runny/itchy nose, burning/watery eyes, spasmodic sneezing accompanied by acrid discharge, and severe frontal headache; safe for children.
LIDDELL LABORATORIES, 1036 Country Club Drive, Moraga, CA 94556; tel: 800-460-7733 or 925-631-0257.

Hay Relief: Caplets or liquid. Herbal blend to strengthen the body's resistance to seasonal airborne irritants.
RAINBOW LIGHT, P.O. Box 600, Santa Cruz, CA 95061; tel: 800-635-1233 or 408-429-9089.

Hyland's Hayfever: Homeopathic tablets. For relief of sneezing, irritated eyes and runny nose due to seasonal allergies or hay fever.
P & S LABS, 210 West 131st Street, Los Angeles, CA 90061; tel: 800-624-9659 or 310-768-0700.

Lung: Tablets. For respiratory health; contains NAG (N-acetyl-glucosamine, a component of the lungs' mucosal lining), which helps repair mucous membranes; NAC (N-acetyl-cysteine), which pulls heavy metals from the lungs' lining; and antioxidants (vitamins A, C, and E, beta carotene, and glutathione), which help prevent free radical damage.
OPTIMAL NUTRIENTS, 1163 Chess Drive #F, Foster City, CA 94404; tel: 800-966-8874 or 650-525-0112.

MSM (Methylsulfonylmethane): Capsules, eye and ear drops, lotion, or powder. Contains sulfur, which is a major component of the human body and a building material for healthy, flexible cells. *Authors' note: Using MSM lotion topically can reduce the symptoms of skin allergies.*
RICH DISTRIBUTING, P.O. Box 33830, Portland, OR 97292; tel: 877-245-5742 or 503-761-7450.

Plant Enzymes: Capsules. Combination of seven plant-source digestive enzymes, friendly bacteria, pantothenic acid, and papain (protein digestant) to help break down fat, protein, plant matter, sugars, and milk, and encourage proper digestion of food; helpful for food intolerance, gas, bloating, heartburn, maldigestion, and elimination of wastes. *Authors' note: To help reduce food allergies.*

NUPRO, 735-L Park Street, Castle Rock, CO 80104; tel: 303-660-0562 or 800-704-8910.

Respiratory Nutrient Support: Tablets. Helps strengthen the lungs and increase the oxygen-carrying capacity of the body; for people with asthma, allergies, hay fever, sinus problems, and cold symptoms.

BIO NATIVUS, P.O. Box 3281, Ogden, UT 84401; tel: 888-628-4887 or 801-732-1294.

Respirtone: Liquid. Warming herbal formula to help support the health, maintenance, and recovery of the respiratory tract.

RAINBOW LIGHT, P.O. Box 600, Santa Cruz, CA 95061; tel: 800-635-1233 or 408-429-9089.

Sabadil: Homeopathic tablets. For temporary relief of symptoms of hay fever or other upper respiratory allergies, including itchy and runny nose, sneezing, and itchy and watery eyes.

BOIRON, 6 Campus Boulevard, Building A, Newtown Square, PA 19073; tel: 800-264-7661 or 610-325-7464.

Sinease: Capsules. Helps the body in dealing with airborne irritants; contains the plant enzymes amylase and protease along with ephedra extract.

PREVAIL CORP., 2204-8 Northwest Birdsdale, Gresham, OR 97030; tel: 800-248-0885 or 503-667-5527.

Sinus: Homeopathic liquid. Recommended for nasal decongestion, frontal headache, and painful swollen sinuses.

BIOENERGETICS, INC., P.O. Box 127, Sandy, OR 97055; tel: 800-334-4043 or 503-668-7478.

Sinusalia: Homeopathic tablets. For temporary relief of congestion and pain due to inflammation of the sinuses.

BOIRON, 6 Campus Boulevard, Building A, Newtown Square, PA 19073; tel: 800-264-7661 or 610-325-7464.

Vapor Balm Salve. Deep breathing formula; contains menthol and essential oils of camphor, peppermint, clove, wintergreen, and lavender.

NATURE'S APOTHECARY, P.O. Box 17970, Boulder, CO 80308; tel: 800-999-7422 or 303-664-1600.

Anemia

Anemia is a reduction in the normal number of red blood cells and/or a decrease in the concentration of hemoglobin, the iron-bearing component, in red blood cells. Since hemoglobin's function is to carry oxygen, anemia results in a lowered oxygen content in the blood. Iron deficiency is one of the other disorders associated with anemia.

Symptoms and Causes of Anemia

Symptoms of anemia include headaches, palpitations, fatigue, weakness, vertigo, slow healing, gastrointestinal problems, ulcers, mood swings, irritability, depression, decreased libido, paleness of the eyelids, lips, or nails, and, in women, cessation of the menstrual period.

Common causes of anemia include iron, vitamin B12, and folic acid deficiencies; extreme blood loss from excessive menstruation or other causes; hormonal disorders; liver damage; thyroid disorders; surgery; peptic ulcers; bone marrow disease; radiation treatment; repeated infections; *Candida albicans* (yeast) infection; autoimmune conditions; and alcoholism. Before using nutritional therapies for treating anemia, it is important to determine the cause(s) of the condition.

Nutrients and Herbs for Anemia

■ **Vitamin A:** for poor hemoglobin formation.[5]

■ **Vitamin B12**: the sublingual (absorbed under the tongue) form of B12 is more quickly absorbed by the body than supplements that pass through the stomach.

■ **Vitamin C:** enhances absorption of iron.[6]

■ **Iron:** a deficiency of this mineral needed to make hemoglobin results in difficulty forming enough healthy red blood cells. Double-blind studies have demonstrated the beneficial effects of iron supplementation on anemia.[7] One of the best formulas we have found that enables proper iron assimilation is Floradix, a liquid iron supplement.

■ **"Green" drink powders:** including chlorella, spirulina and other blue-green algae, barley and wheat grass, and alfalfa. Green drink powders are rich in chlorophyll, enzymes, and minerals; they are general detoxifiers to help clean the blood of unwanted substances.

■ **Yellowdock:** an herb high in elemental iron.[8] We have successfully raised an anemic's iron levels with formulas containing yellowdock.

Products for Anemia

Broken Cell Chlorella: Tablets. Contains chlorella, a microscopic green freshwater plant that has a concentrated supply of vitamins, minerals, proteins, and fatty acids; contains chlorophyll, which supports the bloodstream, bowels, kidneys, and liver, and helps support cellular growth and metabolic balance; also supports the immune system and absorbs toxins and heavy metals.

SOLAR GREENS, NUTRACEUTICAL CORP., P.O. Box 681869, Park City, UT 84068; tel: 800-669-8877.

Chlorella: Tablets. Contains concentrated chlorophyll, or "green energy," combined with rich levels of blood-building iron, folic acid, and vitamin B12. Recent Japanese research demonstrates that chlorella also offers a protective shield against toxic influences.

NEW CHAPTER, 22 High Street, Brattleboro, VT 05301; tel: 800-543-7279 or 802-257-9345.

Chlorophyll Caps. Chlorophyll derived from organically grown alfalfa.

NATURE'S PLUS, 548 Broadhollow Road, Melville, NY 11747-3708; tel: 800-645-9500 or 516-293-0030.

Floradix Iron Plus Herbs: Liquid. Contains organic iron, extracts of herbs and wheat germ, fruits, vitamins, cultured yeast, ocean kelp, and rose hips; easily absorbed, does not cause constipation. Also available without yeast, added sugar, or honey in the product Floravital Iron Plus Herbs.

FLORA INC., 805 East Badger Road, Lynden, WA 98264; tel: 800-446-2110 or 360-354-2110.

Gentle Iron (Iron Bisglycinate): Vegicaps. Contains a chelated (combined with an amino acid to improve assimilation) form of iron that is nonconstipating, nonirritating, and easily absorbed.

SOLGAR VITAMIN & HERB COMPANY, INC., 500 Willow Tree Road, Leonia, NJ 07605; tel: 800-645-2246 or 201-944-2311.

Sun Energy: Capsules or powder. Contains organically grown grasses, micro-algaes, vegetables, and Chinese energetics; maintains and restores health, vitality, and immunity, and cleanses, detoxifies, and nourishes the body on a cellular level.

R GARDEN, 3881 Enzyme Lane, Kettle Falls, WA 99141; tel: 800-700-7767 or 425-271-0539.

Anxiety is defined as feelings of apprehension, uncertainty, dread, and/or fear, often without apparent stimulus.

Symptoms and Causes of Anxiety

Symptoms include increased heart rate, sweating, and tremors, and acute attacks of panic.

Adrenal gland exhaustion is often an underlying cause of anxiety and, unfortunately, creates a vicious cycle by decreasing one's ability to deal with stress, which produces more anxiety.

Nutrients and Herbs for Anxiety

A deficiency in calcium and magnesium can produce an anxiety syndrome.[9] Common symptoms of calcium/magnesium deficiencies include tension without good cause, irritated moods, sudden or angry responses to normal stimuli, frustration, fear, fear of social activities, indecision, inattention, failure to recall, despondency, and pessimism. Supplementing often reverses the condition.

■ **To support the adrenal glands:** vitamin B complex, spirulina or other blue-green algae, and adaptogenic (assisting the body in adapting to stress) herb formulas, which often contain ginseng, are helpful. *Panax ginseng*, in particular, has a nutritive or tonic effect on the adrenal glands, improving blood flow to the brain and reducing the stress associated with mental/emotional issues.[10]

Stabilium, a product containing *Garum armoricum* (a fish, salt, and herb preparation), is an adaptogen which can also help balance mood, improve sleep, and increase energy and stamina.[11] GABA (gamma-aminobutyric acid), an amino acid, can also affect mood by increasing levels of the brain neurotransmitter serotonin (a mood regulator).

■ **To calm the nervous system:** balm, like various members of the mint family, relaxes the nervous system and is often used for insomnia, headaches, and muscle tension, all of which can heighten anxiety.[12]

Valerian root, an herbal tranquilizer and muscle relaxant, is another proven agent for calming the nervous system.[13] It helps balance mood swings and is not habit-forming. Valerian-hops combination formulas are good daytime sedatives

For more about **adrenal support**, see Stress, pp. 369-384.

because they don't cause drowsiness.

Passionflower also helps reduce anxiety, high blood pressure, nervous tension, and muscle tension, and encourages deep, restful sleep.

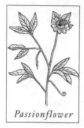
Passionflower

Extracts of the kava-kava plant, an herbal tranquilizer native to Polynesia, can lower anxiety levels and alleviate panic disorder and general tension in as quickly as a week.[14]

St. John's wort, a highly popular remedy for depression, has proven effective for anxiety and mood swings as well. St. John's Wort Supreme (formerly Phyto-Proz Supreme) is a product we have used with success in the treatment of anxiety.

Products for Anxiety

Amino-Mag 200: Tablets. Contains elemental magnesium as an amino acid chelate (magnesium glycinate/lysinate combination), which can be absorbed intact without gastrointestinal side effects.

AMNI, 2247 National Avenue, Hayward, CA 94540-5012; tel: 800-437-8888 or 510-783-6969.

Balanced B-100: Tablets. B vitamins work together to convert food into energy and are necessary for a healthy nervous system.

NATURE MADE LLC, NATURE'S RESOURCE, P.O. Box 9606, Mission Hills, CA 91346-9606; tel: 800-314-HERB (4372) or 800-423-2405.

Beyond St. John's Wort: Tablets. Contains active compound hypericin, kava-kava, magnesium, royal jelly concentrate, calcium, vitamin B12, thiamine, and L-tyrosine. St. John's wort can provide nutritive support to help maintain a healthy central nervous system.

KAL, NUTRACEUTICAL CORP., P.O. Box 681869, Park City, UT 84068; tel: 800-669-8877.

BHI Calming: Homeopathic tablets. For temporary relief of insomnia, restlessness, anxiety, and symptoms of PMS.

HEEL/BHI, INC., 11600 Cochiti Road Southeast, Albuquerque, NM 87123-3376; tel: 800-621-7644 or 505-293-3843.

Calcium Plus: Tablets. To support the skeletal and muscular systems; contains calcium, magnesium, vital co-nutrients, superfoods, and seven Chinese herbs for skeletal health.

RAINBOW LIGHT, P.O. Box 600, Santa Cruz, CA 95061; tel: 800-635-1233 or 408-429-9089.

Calm: Tablets. Calming herbal blend containing kava-kava, chamomile, catnip, valerian root, hops, and passionflower.
AMERIFIT, 166 Highland Park Drive, Bloomfield, CT 06002; tel: 800-990-FIRM (3476) or 860-242-3476.

Calms: Tablets. Composed of four botanicals (passionflower, hops, wild oats, and chamomile) long used by the homeopathic medical profession to soothe and quiet irritated nerves and edginess without sedatives or tranquilizers; no side effects or drug hangover.
P & S LABS, 210 West 131st Street, Los Angeles, CA 90061; tel: 800-624-9659 or 310-768-0700.

Calms Forté: Tablets. Contains the same four botanicals as Calms (see above) plus five biochemic phosphates in three times the potency; helps feed and strengthen the nerves of the body to withstand everyday stress and strain.
P & S LABS, 210 West 131st Street, Los Angeles, CA 90061; tel: 800-624-9659 or 310-768-0700.

Eleuthero Chamomile: Capsules or liquid. Herbal adaptogen in a primary base of eleuthero root (Siberian ginseng), with the calming herbs chamomile, valerian, passionflower, skullcap, and oatstraw.
FRONTIER COOPERATIVE HERBS, 3021 78th Street, Norway, IA 52318; tel: 800-669-3275 or 319-227-7996.

EuroCalm Valerian Special Formula: Capsules. Contains valerian extract with a guaranteed potency of 0.8% valeric acid, chamomile, passionflower, and hawthorn; valerian root helps provide nutritive support for restful sleep.
SOLARAY, NUTRACEUTICAL CORP., P.O. Box 681869, Park City, UT 84068; tel: 800 669-8877.

5 HTP SeroTonic: Capsules. Contains 5-HTP, St. John's wort (*Hypericum perforatum*), pyridoxal-5-phosphate, and the co-factors magnesium hydroxide, inositol hexanicotinate (a form of niacin), and calcium citrate. Scientists have discovered that conditions of anxiety, depression, carbohydrate cravings (with resultant weight gain), sleeplessness, obsessions, and compulsions are all connected to reduced levels of serotonin in the brain. A metabolic precursor of serotonin, the amino acid 5-HTP can increase production and availability of serotonin.

LIFEENHANCEMENT PRODUCTS INC., P.O. Box 751390, Petaluma, CA 94975-1390; tel: 800-543-3873 or 707-762-6144.

GABA: Capsules. Alternative to valium and other tranquilizers without fear of addiction; helps prevent anxiety and stress-related messages from reaching the motor centers of the brain by filling its receptor site; also helps promote better sleep; ingredients include 500 mg of GABA (gamma-aminobutyric acid).

INFINITY HEALTH, 1519 Contra Costa Boulevard, Pleasant Hill, CA 94523; tel: 800-733-9293 or 925-676-8982.

Gelsemium: Homeopathic remedy. Helpful in stage fright, nervous dread, apprehension of dental work or surgery, headache, and flu.

STANDARD HOMEOPATHIC CO., 201 West 131st Street, Los Angeles, CA 90061; tel: 800-624-9659 or 310-768-0700.

Herbal Calm: Capsules. Dietary supplement of the soothing natural herbs valerian, passionflower, skullcap, hops, and kava-kava. Caution: May cause drowsiness.

NATURE'S HERBS, 600 East Quality Drive, American Fork, UT 84003; tel: 800-437-2257 or 801-763-0700.

Herbal Relax: Liquid. Contains kava-kava, passionflower, hops, schisandra, skullcap, oatseed, milk thistle, ginger, hawthorn, rose hips, and red clover in a base of purified water, brown rice syrup, honey, natural flavor, and 18% USP alcohol.

NATURE'S APOTHECARY, P.O. Box 17970, Boulder, CO 80308; tel: 800-999-7422 or 303-664-1600.

Herbal Tranquillity Complex: Vegicaps. Herbal combination for the support and maintenance of the body's normal relaxation process.

SOLGAR VITAMIN & HERB COMPANY, INC., 500 Willow Tree Road, Leonia, NJ 07605; tel: 800-645-2246 or 201-944-2311.

Hypericalm: Capsules. Nutritional support containing St. John's wort extract for healthy mental and nervous system function.

ENZYMATIC THERAPY, 825 Challenger Drive, Green Bay, WI 54311-8328; tel: 800-558-7372 or 920-469-1313.

Liquid Calcium Rx Calcium 1000 Complex: Softgels. Contains six sources of calcium, two sources of magnesium, herbs, vitamins, and minerals for optimum bioavailability.

PHYTO-THERAPY, INC., OPTIMUM HEALTH, 483 West Middle Turnpike, Manchester, CT 06040; tel: 800-228-1507 or 860-647-9729.

Mood Balance: Tablets. For daily anxiety, stress, and irritability; contains standardized St. John's wort and valerian extracts; calming compounds such as lemon balm, kava-kava root extract, taurine, and GABA (gamma-aminobutyric acid); also contains amino acids used to synthesize neurotransmitters, chemical messengers that support mental acuity and memory.

SOURCE NATURALS, Threshold Enterprises, 23 Janis Way, Scotts Valley, CA 95066; tel: 800-777-5677 or 831-438-1144.

Mood Swing Support: Capsules. Contains St. John's wort, which provides support for mild anxiety and depressed moods.

NUTRITION NOW, 501 Southeast Columbia Shore Boulevard #350, Vancouver, WA 98661; tel: 800-929-0418 or 360-737-6800.

Relax: Caplets or liquid. Herbal blend, containing valerian and California poppy, that promotes relaxation and ease of mind during the day, without inducing drowsiness.

RAINBOW LIGHT, P.O. Box 600, Santa Cruz, CA 95061; tel: 800-635-1233 or 408-429-9089.

St. John's Positive Thoughts: Tablets. Contains St. John's wort, valerian, kava-kava, and lemon balm with key amino acids, vitamins, and minerals; designed to soothe and uplift one's mood.

SOURCE NATURALS, THRESHOLD ENTERPRISES, 23 Janis Way, Scotts Valley, CA 95066; tel: 800-777-5677 or 831-438-1144.

St. John's Special Formula: Capsules. Contains St. John's wort extract (hypericin), kava-kava, L-tyrosine, DL-phenylalanine, and *Ginkgo biloba*.

SOLARAY, NUTRACEUTICAL CORP., P.O. Box 681869, Park City, UT 84068; tel: 800-669-8877.

St. John's Wort Formula: Capsules. Contains St. John's wort and herbal energy tonics, adaptogens, and nervines to support the body's effort to overcome stress, chronic fatigue, and weak immunity as well as tyrosine, magnesium, malic acid, and vitamin B6 to support neurotransmitter function and energy levels.

ZAND HERBAL FORMULAS, 1722 14th Street #230, Boulder, CO 80302; tel: 800-800-0405 or 303-786-8558.

St. John's Wort • Kava Compound: Liquid. Mild relaxing sedative, anti-spasmodic, and muscle relaxant; indicated in depression and despondency, and associated anxiety, nervous agitation, stress, restlessness, and sleeplessness; ingredients include St. John's wort flower and bud, kava-kava lateral root, skullcap flowering herb, and prickly ash bark.

HERB PHARM, 20260 Williams Highway, Williams, OR 97544; tel: 800-348-4372 or 541-846-6262.

St. John's Wort-Kava Compound: Tablets. Blend of Chinese and western herbs to promote mental well-being.

PLANETARY FORMULAS, 23 Janis Way, Scotts Valley, CA 95066; tel: 800-606-6226.

St. John's Wort • Melissa SuperComplex: Liquid. Herbal blend containing St. John's wort, lemon balm, and wild indigo.

RAINBOW LIGHT, P.O. Box 600, Santa Cruz, CA 95061; tel: 800-625-1233 or 408-429-9089.

St. John's Wort Supreme: Liquid. Herbal extracts with antidepressant properties that can be used in conjunction with other doctor-prescribed therapies in cases of mild depression or when being weaned off of antidepressant drugs; can also be used for symptoms related to chronic fatigue, recurrent viral infections (herpes, Epstein-Barr, and hepatitis C), compromised immune systems, or for cancer patients after chemotherapy; contains kava-kava root, St. John's wort flower buds, passionflower, schisandra berry, wild oats, calamus root, Siberian ginseng, nettle seed, prickly ash bark, and gotu kola leaf and root.

GAIA HERBS, INC., 108 Island Ford Road, Brevard, NC 28712; tel: 800-831-7780 or 828-884-4242.

Stabilium (Garum armoricum): Softgels. *Garum armoricum*, a fish and salt preparation discovered by the ancient Celts, has been used since the time of the Roman Empire and traditionally used for its high nutritive value. An adaptogen and antidepressant, garum helps balance mood, correct sleep disturbances, and increase energy and stamina.

ALLERGY RESEARCH GROUP/NUTRICOLOGY, P.O. Box 55907, Hayward, CA 94544; tel: 800-545-9960 or 510-487-8526.

Stress-D: Capsules. Herbal formula to help calm the central nervous system and help the body adapt to stress and fatigue; contains nutrients known to support the adrenal glands and central nervous system, including Siberian ginseng, American ginseng, magnesium, vitamin

C, kava-kava root, passionflower, chamomile, and vitamins B1, B2, B3, B5, B6, and B12.

BioDynamax, 6525 Gunpark Drive #150-507, Boulder, CO 80301; tel: 800-926-7525 or 303-530-4665.

TranQaCalm: Tablets. Contains herbs for support of nervous system and a balance of minerals and digestive enzymes.

Bio Nativus, P.O. Box 3281, Ogden, UT 84401; tel: 888-628-4887 or 801-732-1294.

Valerian • Passionflower Compound: Liquid. Gentle, non-narcotic sedative, which is indicated in nervous excitement and hysteria, mental depression due to worry or imagined wrongs, nervous headache, insomnia, and in nervousness associated with menopause.

Herb Pharm, 20260 Williams Highway, Williams, OR 97544; tel: 800-348-4372 or 541-846-6262.

Arthritis

Arthritis, the inflammation of a joint and its surrounding tissues, affects tendons, ligaments, and cartilage. The areas of the body most often afflicted with arthritis are the neck, back and spine, shoulders, elbows, wrists, fingers, hips, knees, ankles, and toes.

Symptoms and Causes of Arthritis

Symptoms of arthritis range from slight pain, stiffness, limited motion, and swelling in affected joints to crippling and disability.

Arthritis is caused by many factors, among them nutritional deficiencies, joint instability, imbalanced body chemistry (acid pH–SEE QUICK DEFINITION), hormonal and glandular imbalances, allergic reactions, autoimmune reactions, and stress. Other contributing factors include extended use of arthritis drugs, dietary practices (such as low consumption of vegetables and high consumption of mucus-producing foods such as dairy), genetic predisposition, calcium depletion, and osteoporosis.[15]

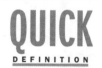

DEFINITION

The term **pH**, which means "potential hydrogen," represents a scale for the relative acidity or alkalinity of a solution. Acidity is measured as a pH of 0.1 to 6.9, alkalinity is 7.1 to 14, and neutral pH is 7.0. The numbers refer to how many hydrogen atoms are present compared to an ideal or standard solution. Normally, blood is slightly alkaline, at 7.35 to 7.45; urine pH can range from 4.8 to 8.0, but is usually somewhat acidic, with a normal reading between 5.0 and 6.0.

Types of Arthritis

The three most common forms of arthritis are osteoarthritis, rheumatoid arthritis, and gout.

Osteoarthritis—Also known as degenerative joint disease (DJD), osteoarthritis is the degeneration of the large, weight-bearing joints, often associated with aging, in which small bony growths, calcium spurs, and occasional soft cysts appear on bones and in the joints. As the disease progresses, the joint cartilage deteriorates, eventually interfering with movement. Common symptoms include joint stiffness upon rising in the morning or after periods of rest, pain that worsens with joint use, local tenderness, soft tissue swelling, creaking and cracking of joints during movement, bony swelling, and restricted mobility. Causes of osteoarthritis include lack of exercise, poor diet, and hormonal imbalances or deficiencies.[16]

Rheumatoid Arthritis—This form of arthritis is less common than osteoarthritis, but often results in crippling disabilities in both young and old. Rheumatoid arthritis (RA) incapacitates the synovial tissue (the membranes, which line joints and secrete the lubricating fluid enabling bones to move painlessly against other bones). As a result, joints—most commonly the small joints of the hands—become swollen, tender, and deformed. Over time, RA can spread to other parts of the body. RA is classified as an autoimmune disease, meaning the body attacks its own tissue. Symptoms of RA include night sweats, depression, fatigue, weakness, low-grade fever, and joint stiffness and pain. Among the causes of RA are food allergies and the related problem of intestinal permeability (leaky gut syndrome), nutritional deficiencies, and infection by microorganisms.[17]

Gout—This painful condition is caused by a buildup of uric acid in the bloodstream. The acid then crystallizes in joints and surrounding tissues, producing sharp, needle-like joint pain, loss of joint mobility, chills, and fever. In a majority of people, gout begins in the first joint of the big toe, causing intense pain, especially at night. Health problems related to or caused by gout include constipation, indigestion, headaches, depression, skin conditions, and a higher risk of heart and kidney problems. Initial gout attacks are usually preceded by a specific event such as surgery or other trauma, excessive alcohol ingestion, excessive consumption of protein-rich foods such as meat or refined sugars, or taking certain drugs.[18]

Acid-Forming Foods

Alcohol, cocoa, coffee, and caffeinated teas; meat, dairy and other animal proteins; sugar and all products that contain sugar; some fruit (especially cranberries, plums and prunes); many fats and oils; some nuts and seeds (cashew, peanut, pecan, walnut, filbert, and Brazil nut); cheese; white flour and baked products, pasta, wheat, corn, and oats; and many beans and legumes.

Alkaline-Forming Foods

Fresh vegetables, except tomatoes; avocados and most fruit; some nuts and seeds (particularly almond, chestnut, coconut, flax, pumpkin, sesame, and sunflower seeds); herbal teas (dandelion, ginseng); soy products; and aloe vera and green foods (chlorella, barley, wheat grass, alfalfa).

Treatment of Arthritis

In arthritis, as in other degenerative conditions, each individual responds to a different degree to supplements, herbal formulas, and homeopathic remedies known to be useful for arthritis. However, the following guidelines have proven helpful to the majority of people we have assisted with nutritional therapies for arthritis.

■ Reduce or eliminate acidity: In our experience, arthritic patients commonly have a urine pH that is acidic (lower than 6.3), which increases the potential for developing inflammatory conditions. Acidity can be reduced by: improving overall digestion so there is less fermentation, putrefaction, and acid created throughout the gastrointestinal tract; cleansing the liver and colon; and decreasing intake of acid-forming foods and increasing intake of alkaline-producing foods in the diet (see sidebar, p. 85).

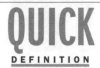

■ Obtain iron from plant sources and foods high in elemental iron instead of synthetic or processed supplements. Food sources of iron include blackstrap molasses, cauliflower, peas, broccoli, lima beans, and the herb yellowdock. We have found that some patients who take supplemental iron medications or elemental iron products experience increased pain and joint destruction and swelling.

■ Increase intake of essential fatty acids (EFAs—SEE QUICK DEFINITION).[19] A lipase enzyme supplement is also recommended to ensure that the body can break down and utilize these dietary oils, which reduce inflammation.

■ Increase intake of antioxidant nutrients, such as vitamins A, C, and E, beta carotene, and SOD (superoxide dismutase), to help eliminate and prevent the formation of free radicals which cause degeneration of the joints and aging in the tissues.

Nutrients and Herbs for Arthritis

To Rebuild Cartilage, Connective Tissue, and Bone— Glucosamine sulfate, NAG (N-acetyl-glucosamine), and shark and bovine cartilage replace joint "ground substances" that form the matrix of connective tissue, cartilage, and bone, helping to regenerate joint tissues. Horsetail contains high amounts of easily assimilable silica. Silicon (made from silica) is necessary for collagen formation in cartilage, bones, and connective tissue.[20] (Natural silicon, also found in unrefined grains and root vegetables among other dietary sources, is distinct from the synthetic silicone used in prostheses and breast implants.) Alfalfa, long used as a musculoskeletal tonic, is nutrient-packed and an excellent source of chlorophyll, which has been shown to stimulate the growth of new tissues in wounds. It is also an antirheumatic, which reduces inflammation, pain, and swelling in joints.[21]

To Reduce Inflammation—Pycnogenol and wild yam have anti-inflammatory, anti-arthritic, antirheumatic, and antispasmodic properties. Sea cucumber (bêche-de-mer) has specific anti-inflammatory compounds found to be effective with arthritic and joint conditions. Yarrow is an antiarthritic and antispasmodic herb that has a long tradition of use for arthritis and other joint diseases.[22]

To Relieve Pain—Cetyl myristoleate (CM), a fatty acid ester (a fatty acid combined with an alcohol molecule), has shown in clinical trials to decrease stiffness and pain and increase the flexibility and range of motion in both osteoarthritis and rheumatoid arthritis.[23] Devil's claw, capsicum (from cayenne pepper), white willow bark, *Boswellia serrata*, feverfew, yucca, cat's claw, and protease enzyme formulas are analgesics (pain relievers).

Products for Arthritis

Advanced Enzyme System: Vegicaps. Formula of plant-source enzymes for breaking down protein, fiber, fats, and carbohydrates (including sugar); ingredients include green papaya, apple pectin, sea vegetables, ginger, and peppermint.

RAINBOW LIGHT, P.O. Box 600, Santa Cruz, CA 95061; tel: 800-635-1233 or 408-429-9089.

Anti-Flam Caps. Anti-inflammatory herbal formula containing white willow bark.

CRYSTAL STAR HERBAL NUTRITION, 4069 Wedgeway Court, Earth City, MO 63045; tel: 800-736-6015 or 314-739-7551.

ArthArrest: Capsules. Eliminates pain and pressure related to bone and joint problems; ingredients include devil's claw, alfalfa seed, burdock root, and prickly ash bark.

RIDGECREST HERBALS, 1151 South Redwood Road #106, Salt Lake City, UT 84104-3729; tel: 800-242-4649 or 801-978-9633.

Arth-Prin: Capsules. Relieves aches and pains of arthritis and rheumatism, and helps reduce fever; ingredients include magnesium salicylate, white willow, horsetail, yucca, valerian, and wintergreen.

RIDGECREST HERBALS, 1151 South Redwood Road #106, Salt Lake City, UT 84104-3729; tel: 800-242-4649 or 801-978-9633.

Arth-Pro: Capsules. Promotes optimal joint, ligament, and cartilage function; contains bovine tracheal cartilage, glucosamines, antioxidants, and wild yam complex.

PHOENIX BIOLOGICS, 2794 Loker Avenue West #104, Carlsbad, CA 92008; tel: 800-947-8482 or 760-631-7729.

ArthRed: Powder. Contains hydrolyzed collagen from bovine cartilage (research demonstrates its benefits for connective tissue) and 19 amino acids, which are the building blocks for joint cartilage.

SOURCE NATURALS, THRESHOLD ENTERPRISES, 23 Janis Way, Scotts Valley, CA 95066; tel: 800-777-5677 or 831-438-1144.

Arthritic by Jade: Tablets. Chinese herbal formula; for relief of pain from sore, stiff, and swollen joints and muscles; also helps improve impaired flexibility.

EAST EARTH HERB INC., P.O. Box 2802, Eugene, OR 97402; tel: 800-827-HERB (4372) or 541-687-0155.

Arthritis Formula: Homeopathic liquid. Relieves aches, pains, and stiffness of arthritis, rheumatism, and sciatica (lower back pain).

ENZYMATIC THERAPY, 825 Challenger Drive, Green Bay, WI 54311-8328; tel: 800-558-7372 or 920-469-1313.

Arth-Support: Tablets. Daily multiple vitamin and mineral supplement with a blend of nutrients to promote healthy joints and relief from inflammation.

HVL INC., 600 Boyce Road, Pittsburgh, PA 15205; tel: 800-245-4441.

Atril: Phyto-homeopathic lozenges. Relieves pain, minor swelling, rigidity, and stiffness of acute arthritis, and flare-ups of pain and swelling of chronic arthritis; effective for rheumatoid and osteoarthritis.

SUPHERB LTD., P.O. Box 1135, Nahariya 22100, Israel; tel: 800-409-HERB (4372).

Baby Boomer Bone and Joint: Tablets. Helps support healthy joints and strong bones; contains glucosamine (one of the most promising natural substances of joint support), calcium, phosphorus, folic acid, curcumin, and vitamin C.

AMERIFIT, 166 Highland Park Drive, Bloomfield, CT 06002; tel: 800-990-FIRM (3476) or 860-242-3476.

Balance Plus: Softgels. Contains a blend of the essential fatty acids omega-3 (from cold-water marine fish), omega-6 (from borage seed oil), and omega-9 (from olive oil).

AMNI, 2247 National Avenue, Hayward, CA 94540-5012; tel: 800-437-8888 or 510-783-6969.

BHI Arthritis: Homeopathic tablets. For temporary relief of swollen and painful joints, muscle stiffness, and rheumatic symptoms.

HEEL/BHI, INC., 11600 Cochiti Road Southeast, Albuquerque, NM 87123-3376; tel: 800-621-7644 or 505-293-3843.

BHI Traumed: Homeopathic ointment. For temporary relief of mild to moderate pain associated with inflammatory, exudative (oozing of fluids), and degenerative processes due to arthritic conditions, acute trauma, or repetitive and overuse injuries.

HEEL/BHI, INC., 11600 Cochiti Road Southeast, Albuquerque, NM 87123-3376; tel: 800-621-7644 or 505-293-3843.

BioE Myalgia: Homeopathic liquid. For temporary relief of muscles and joint pain, tenderness, and weakness.

BIOENERGETICS, INC., P.O. Box 127, Sandy, OR 97055; tel: 800-334-4043 or 503-668-7478.

Bone Builder: Chewable tablets. Ingredients include MCHC (microcrystalline hydroxyapatite, the core matrix substance of bones), vitamin D and the essential minerals magnesium, zinc, copper, and manganese for additional bone support.

ETHICAL NUTRIENTS, 971 Calle Negocio, San Clemente, CA 92673; tel: 800-668-8743 or 949-366-0818.

Bone Builder With Boron: Tablets. Contains MCHC (microcrystalline hydroxyapatite, the core matrix substance of bones) and boron, a trace mineral that may play a role in calcium metabolism and in maintaining bone health.

ETHICAL NUTRIENTS, 971 Calle Negocio, San Clemente, CA 92673; tel: 800-668-8743 or 949-366-0818.

Bone Density Factors With Boron: Tablets. Contains 1,000 mg of calcium from hydroxyapatite, calcium citrate, and citrate malate, plus vitamins and minerals as a nutritional aid for periodontal and skeletal support; according to clinical trials, hydroxyapatite is an effective form of calcium to re-calcify bone.

COUNTRY LIFE, 101 Corporate Drive, Hauppauge, NY 11788; tel: 800-645-5768 or 516-231-1031.

Boswellin Cream. Contains capsaicin (from cayenne) and methyl salicylate (from wintergreen) in a soothing base of *Boswellia serrata* (standardized for boswellic acids) and vitamin E; for temporary relief of minor muscle and joint aches and pains associated with arthritis. Greaseless, stainless, with a pleasant aroma.

NATURE'S HERBS, 600 East Quality Drive, American Fork, UT 84003; tel: 800-437-2257 or 801-763-0700.

Bromelain Joint Ease: Capsules. Contains bromelain, quercetin, vitamin C, and SOD (superoxide dismutase) precursors. Bromelain and vitamin C lessen minor bruising; quercetin and SOD reduce painful inflammatory responses.

NATURE'S LIFE, 7180 Lampson Avenue, Garden Grove, CA 92841-3914; tel: 800-854-6837 or 714-379-6500.

Cat's Claw: Tablets. Contains concentrated cat's claw (three times the active ingredient of an identically weighted dosage).

PERUVIAN RAINFOREST BOTANICALS, NUTRAMEDIX, 212 North U.S. Highway 1 #17, Tequesta, FL 33469; tel: 800-730-3130 or 561-745-2917.

Cell Guard: Capsules. Combination of SOD (superoxide dismutase), glutathione peroxidase, and catalase, which acts to promote maximum cellular protection and health.

BIOTEC FOODS, 5152 Borsa Avenue, Suite 101, Huntington Beach, CA 92649; tel: 800-788-1084 or 714-899-3477.

Cetyl Myristoleate: Softgels. Medium-chain fatty acid in concentrated form from vegetable sources.

FUTUREBIOTICS, 145 Ricefield Lane, Hauppauge, NY 11788; tel: 800-FOR-LIFE (367-5433) or 516-273-6300.

CM Plus Protocol for Arthritis: Capsules and lotion. Mixture of key fatty acid esters (derivatives of essential fatty acids) including cetyl myristoleate, which has anti-inflammatory and lubricant qualities for arthritis problems; also contains glucosamine, sea cucumber, hydrolyzed bovine cartilage, and MSM (methylsulfonylmethane, a source of organic sulfur and cartilage-rebuilder); also includes a topical lotion of mixed fatty acid esters to support cartilage rebuilding.

KLABIN MARKETING, 2067 Broadway #700, New York, NY 10023; tel: 800-933-9440 or 212-877-3632.

Cold Pressed Hempseed Oil. Hempseed oil contains the ideal 3:1 ratio of omega-6 to omega-3 essential fatty acids; can be used as a condiment and recipe ingredient.

HEMPOLA, 3405 American Drive #5, Mississauga, Ontario, Canada L4V1T6; tel: 800-240-9215.

CS 500 Chondroitin Sulfate: Capsules. Contains 95% chondroitin sulfate from bovine tracheal cartilage to promote joint flexibility and circulation and stimulate the production of chondroitin sulfates (the building blocks of cartilage, connective tissue, and arterial walls).

PHOENIX BIOLOGICS, 2794 Loker Avenue West #104, Carlsbad, CA 92008; tel: 800-947-8482 or 760-631-7729.

Devil's Claw: Liquid. Herbal extract containing devil's claw harvested from the Kalihari Desert and Namibian Steppes of Africa.

NATURE'S HERBS, 600 East Quality Drive, American Fork, UT 84003; tel: 800-437-2257 or 801-763-0700.

Essential Fatty Acid Complex: Softgels. Contains evening primrose and flax seed oils, vitamin E, and plant antioxidants from rosemary and sage. The essential fatty acids linoleic acid and alpha linolenic acid found in evening primrose and flax seed oils are converted to eicosanoids in all human cells. Eicosanoids control a variety of body functions including pain, inflammation, blood pressure, and skin softness.

SCHIFF, WEIDER NUTRITION GROUP, 2002 South 5070 West, Salt Lake City, UT 84104; tel: 800-439-8042 or 801-975-5000.

Essential Oils Formula: Softgels. Contains flax seed, borage, and fish oils, which are sources of essential fatty acids; also contains vitamin E.

ATKINS NUTRITIONALS, INC., 185 Oser Avenue, Hauppauge, NY 11788; tel: 800-628-5467 or 516-951-7171; or CANADIAN AMERICAN RESOURCES, 327 West Fayette Street, Suite 211, Syracuse, NY 13202; tel: 315-476-4944.

Evening Primrose Oil: Capsules or liquid. Good source of omega-6 essential fatty acids necessary for optimal health, maintaining cell structure, and producing energy. Contains about 72% (1.1 g) omega-6 or linoleic acid and about 9% (135 mg) gamma-linolenic acid (GLA, a derivative of omega-6), which helps improve circulation and hormonal balance.

SPECTRUM NATURALS, 133 Copeland Street, Petaluma, CA 94952; tel: 800-995-2705 or 707-778-8900.

Flex: Tablets. For tissue structure and connective tissue support and formation; contains manganese and zinc (important for proper formation of connective tissue), pantothenic and folic acid (B vitamins that enable the body to deal with stress and lessen inflammation), NAG (N-acetyl-glucosamine) and glucosamine sulfate (the base components of the tissue structure forming joint, ligaments, and tendons), vitamin C (aids in body's utilization of NAG and glucosamine sulfate and helps form collagen found in connective tissue), calcium, horsetail, magnesium, and potassium.

OPTIMAL NUTRIENTS, 1163 Chess Drive #F, Foster City, CA 94404; tel: 800-966-8874 or 415-525-0112.

GlucosaMend: Tablets. Contains glucosamine sulfate and NAG (N-acetyl-glucosamine) with nutrients designed to enhance the body's innate joint and tissue repair processes.

SOURCE NATURALS, THRESHOLD ENTERPRISES, 23 Janis Way, Scotts Valley, CA 95066; tel: 800-777-5677 or 831-438-1144.

GS-500 Glucosamine Sulfate: Capsules. Glucosamine sulfate is the form of supplemental glucosamine (naturally present in joint cartilage) recommended by researchers.

ENZYMATIC THERAPY, 825 Challenger Drive, Green Bay, WI 54311-8328; tel: 800-558-7372 or 920-469-1313.

Herbal Aloe Force: Juice or topical gel. Ingredients include processed aloe vera juice containing vitamins, minerals, enzymes, amino acids, essential fatty acids, growth factors, glycoproteins, sterols, bioflavonoids, and polysaccharides (complex sugars), plus ionized colloidal silver and herbal extracts (cat's claw, chamomile, burdock root, hawthorn berry, astragalus root, sheep sorrel, pau d'arco bark, slippery elm bark, and rhubarb root).

HERBAL ANSWERS, INC., P.O. Box 1110, Saratoga Springs, NY 12866; tel: 888-256-3367 or 518-581-1968.

Hyland's Arthritis Pain Formula: Homeopathic remedy. For relief of symptoms of pain in joints associated with over-exertion. P & S LABS, 210 West 131st Street, Los Angeles, CA 90061; tel: 800-624-9659 or 310-768-0700.

InflamActin: Capsules. Supports the body's normal adaptogenic function; contains the Ayurvedic herbs boswellia and turmeric and nutrients bromelain, DLPA (DL-phenylalanine), and vitamin C. NATURE'S PLUS, 548 Broadhollow Road, Melville, NY 11747-3708; tel: 800-645-9500 or 516-293-0030.

InflamActin: Cream. For muscular aches, pains, soreness, or stiffness; contains boswellin, turmeric, and gorgonian extracts; "lipoceutical" delivery system (botanical ingredients in a liposome sphere) allows for greater effectiveness and long-lasting results. NATURE'S PLUS, 548 Broadhollow Road, Melville, NY 11747-3708; tel: 800-645-9500 or 516-293-0030.

Inflam-Aid: Capsules. Contains vitamins C and E, standardized ginger root, quercetin, selenium, and white willow, turmeric, and licorice root extracts in a base of bilberry, odorless garlic, and white willow. NATURE'S HERBS, 600 East Quality Drive, American Fork, UT 84003; tel: 800-437-2257 or 801-763-0700.

Joint-Ease Pain: Capsules. Relieves chronic and arthritic pain; contains white willow bark, cherry bark, shave grass, yucca, licorice root, yellowdock, cayenne, and glucosamine sulfate. WGI, 35008 Emerald Coast Parkway, 5th Floor, Destin, FL 32541; tel: 800-854-8353 or 850-654-4744.

Joint Factors: Capsules. Contains glucosamine sulfate with vitamins A, C, and E, manganese, zinc, and copper. TWIN LABS, 150 Motor Parkway, Hauppauge, NY 11788; tel: 800-645-5626.

Joint Health Formula: Capsules. Ingredients include two forms of glucosamine, as well as *Boswellia serrata*, turmeric, and cayenne, which help support proper inflammatory response as well as tissue recovery in the body. BIODYNAMAX, 6525 Gunpark Drive #150-507, Boulder, CO 80301; tel: 800-926-7525 or 303-530-4665.

Joint • Ligament • Tendon: Tablets. Herbal combination that helps support the body's natural balance and maintain healthy connective tissue.

VEDA HEALTH, INC., P.O. Box 1535, Soquel, CA 95073; tel: 888-856-8334 or 408-465-9084.

Joint Lubrication: Softgels. Supports normal joint function through essential fatty acids and powerful antioxidants; contains evening primrose, borage, black currant, and flaxseed oils, vitamin E, and rosemary extract.

ALTERNATIVE THERAPY, INC., 1664 Fairlawn Avenue, San Jose, CA 95125; tel: 800-311-7922.

Jointment: Tablets. Intensive joint and ligament therapy that helps provide pain-free joint performance.

UNIVERSAL, 3 Terminal Road, New Brunswick, NJ 08901; tel: 800-872-0101 or 732-545-3130.

Joint Modulators: Tablets. Contains the cartilage-protective agents glucosamine sulfate and bovine cartilage, which have been shown to support the health and repair of joint and cartilage tissue.

SOLGAR VITAMIN & HERB CO. INC., 500 Willow Tree Road, Leonia, NJ 07605; tel: 800-645-2246 or 201-944-2311.

Joint-Power: Capsules. Herbal, mineral, and vitamin supplement for joints; contains glucosamine sulfate, vitamin C, vitamin E, manganese, zinc, copper, turmeric extract, *Boswellia serrata* extract, bromelain, and selenium.

NATURE'S HERBS, 600 East Quality Drive, American Fork, UT 84003; tel: 800-437-2257 or 801-763-0700.

Joint Support: Capsules. Contains nutrient building blocks, which the body uses to help rebuild cartilage and joint fluid, as well as herbs that provide soothing and anti-inflammatory properties; ingredients include glucosamine sulfate, sea cucumber, feverfew, white willow, *Boswellia serrata*, yucca, cat's claw, and bromelain.

ALTERNATIVE THERAPY, INC., 1664 Fairlawn Avenue, San Jose, CA 95125; tel: 800-311-7922.

Liga-Tend (Formula III): Tablets. Combination of L-proline, glycine, and mucopolysaccharide (cements cells together and lubricates joints and bursae) complex, together with vitamins, minerals, and enzymes for the maintenance of ligaments and tendons.

COUNTRY LIFE, 101 Corporate Drive, Hauppauge, NY 11788; tel: 800-645-5768 or 516-231-1031.

Mobil-Ease: Capsules. For people with reduced joint function and mobility; contains glucosamine sulfate, *Boswellia serrata*, white willow bark, and pure plant enzymes to help the body break down and absorb key nutrients.

PREVAIL CORP., 2204-8 Northwest Birdsdale, Gresham, OR 97030; tel: 800-248-0885 or 503-667-5527.

MSM (Methylsulfonylmethane): Capsules, eye and ear drops, lotion, or powder. Contains sulfur, which is a major component of the human body. Diet is normally a source of sulfur, but food processing has resulted in a depletion of sulfur from foods. MSM provides the body with building materials for healthy, flexible cells.

RICH DISTRIBUTING, P.O. Box 33830, Portland, OR 97292; tel: 877-245-5742 or 503-761-7450.

Multiplete: Tablets. Joint care component including glucosamine, turmeric, white willow bark, boron, calcium, magnesium, and vitamin C; also green tea, echinacea, grape skin, garlic, peppermint leaves, ginseng root, licorice root, cranberry, schisandra, rosemary, astragalus, sarsaparilla, soy, hops, valerian root, and passionflower.

SYNERGY PLUS, IVC, 500 Halls Mill Road, Freehold, NJ 07728; tel: 800-666-8482.

Noni Hawaiian Morinda Citrifolia by Earth's Bounty: Capsules. For easing joint pain, cellular regeneration, and boosting immune system; Noni plant grows best in mineral-rich Hawaiian volcanic ash.

MATRIX HEALTH PRODUCTS, 8400 Magnolia Avenue, Suite N, Santee, CA 92071; tel: 800-736-5609 or 619-448-7550.

Orthopedic Rejuvenation System: Tablets. Blend of essential minerals combined with herbs to benefit joint health.

BIO NATIVUS, P.O. Box 3281, Ogden, UT 84401; tel: 888-628-4887 or 801-732-1294.

Pain Free: Caplets. Ingredients include glucosamine complex and chondroitin sulfate to help support and maintain joints.

SCHIFF, WEIDER NUTRITION GROUP, 2002 South 5070 West, Salt Lake City, UT 84104; tel: 800-439-8042 or 801-975-5000.

Rhus Toxicodendron: Homeopathic remedy. Helps sprains and strains, sore muscles, rheumatic pains, sciatica, influenza, and restlessness.

STANDARD HOMEOPATHIC CO., 201 West 131st Street, Los Angeles, CA 90061; tel: 800-624-9659 or 310-768-0700.

Shark Cartilage: Capsules. Contains mucopolysaccharides (cement cells together and lubricate joints and bursae) and proteins that have strong therapeutic potential.

FUTUREBIOTICS, 145 Ricefield Lane, Hauppauge, NY 11788; tel: 800-FOR-LIFE (367-5433) or 516-273-6300.

SOD/CAT Superoxide Dismutase and Catalase: Tablets. Helps eliminate the inflammation and free radicals associated with arthritis.

BIOMED COMM, INC., 2 Nickerson Street, Suite 102, Seattle, WA 98109; tel: 888-637-3516 or 206-284-3433.

Tiger Balm: Ointment. Helps relieve arthritis, strained muscles, backaches, sore shoulders, knotted calves, tightened thighs, and aching ankles.

PRINCE OF PEACE ENTERPRISES, INC., 3450 Third Street #3G, San Francisco, CA 94124; tel: 800-PEACE2U (732-2328).

Vita Carte Bovine Cartilage: Capsules. 100% pure bovine cartilage, derived from range-grown, certified hormone-free cattle; research has proven that bovine tracheal cartilage is effective in treating arthritis by selectively stimulating the body's immune system.

PHOENIX BIOLOGICS, 2794 Loker Avenue West #104, Carlsbad, CA 92008; tel: 800-947-8482 or 760-631-7729.

Yucca Devil's Claw: Capsules or liquid. Traditional herbs for joint health. Caution: Do not use during pregnancy.

FRONTIER COOPERATIVE HERBS, 3021 78th Street, Norway, IA 52318; tel: 800-669-3275 or 319-227-7996.

ZEEL: Homeopathic liquid, ointment, or tablets. Stimulates normal cartilage and joint function; for osteoarthritis, spondyloarthritis, and improvement of cartilage and connective tissue function.

HEEL/BHI, INC., 11600 Cochiti Road Southeast, Albuquerque, NM 87123-3376; tel: 800-621-7644 or 505-293-3843.

Asthma

The respiratory condition called asthma manifests in the form of an attack characterized by narrowing of the bronchial passages along with an excessive excretion of mucus. The result is impaired breathing. The symptoms often accelerate rapidly, to the terror of the asthmatic who cannot draw a breath.

Symptoms and Causes of Asthma

An asthma attack usually begins with a non-mucus-producing cough, followed by a rapidly progressing difficulty in breathing, and an audible wheeze.

A number of environmental agents can precipitate an asthma attack; these include pollen, dust, mold, animal dander, feathers, detergents, petrochemicals, air pollution, and smoke. Foods to which the person is allergic can also trigger an attack, as can aspirin, infections, exercise, and exposure to cold air.

Common dietary factors in asthma include excessive sugar consumption, pasteurized dairy products, and fried foods. A deficiency of magnesium, which is a natural muscle relaxant, may also play a role in asthma.[24] Adrenal imbalance or exhaustion, hypoglycemia (low blood sugar), and poor blood circulation are other factors linked to this respiratory condition.

Treatment of Asthma

With the advent of steroid-based inhalers in the 1990s as the primary conventional treatment, asthmatics now breathe easier. While these synthetic prescription hormones temporarily relieve inflammation in the lungs and bronchial passages, there can be a large price to pay for long-term use. Side effects include high blood pressure, weight gain, suppressed adrenal gland function, osteoporosis, high blood sugar, glaucoma, cataracts, and impaired immunity resulting in decreased ability to fight off infections.[25]

The safest approach to reducing or eliminating asthma attacks, is to avoid known irritants or initiators, to create a personal environment containing purified (filtered) air, and to build a strong respiratory tract and balanced immune system which will not overreact to external agents.

Nutrients and Herbs for Asthma

CAUTION

Ephedra is for short-term use only. Do not take ephedra at all if you are pregnant, have kidney problems, or suffer from high blood pressure or other cardiovascular stress.

■ **Magnesium, vitamins B6 and C:** may be deficient in asthmatics.[26]

■ **Quercetin:** antihistaminic bioflavonoid (antioxidant plant pigment); recommended if the asthmatic condition is linked to airborne or food allergens.

■ **Ephedra *(ma huang)*:** Chinese herb commonly used for alleviating symptoms of asthma and hay fever; a respiratory stimulant and dilator (opener) of the bronchioles (subdivisions of the lung's bronchial tubes).[27]

■ **Khella *(Ammi visnaga)*:** extract of this Mediterranean plant can be a useful tonic in the prevention of asthma attacks.[28]

■ **Lobelia:** helps reduce the symptoms associated with asthma, bronchitis, and pneumonia by stimulating the adrenal glands to release hormones that cause the bronchiole muscles of the lungs to relax. Lobelia is also a good expectorant, promoting the breakdown and ejection of mucus from the lungs and respiratory tract.[29]

■ ***Tylophora asthmatica*:** Ayurvedic herb used to treat asthma and other respiratory tract problems.[30] We find Tylophora works well for many people as a bronchial dilator. As with ephedra, it should not be employed on a long-term basis.

Products for Asthma

Alkyrol: Capsules. Purified and standardized shark liver oil, which numerous clinical studies have proven to be an immune stimulant; helps reduce symptoms of asthma and psoriasis, prevent colds and other infections, and lessen the side effects of chemotherapy and radiation treatments.

SCANDINAVIAN NATURAL HEALTH & BEAUTY PRODUCTS, INC., 13 North 7th Street, Perkasie, PA 18944; tel: 800-688-2276 or 215-453-2505.

Asthmaclear: Capsules. Provides temporary relief from shortness of breath, tightness of chest, and wheezing due to bronchial asthma; ingredients include Chinese ephedra (*ma huang*), cinnamon, asarum, ginger root, pinella, schizandra, paeonia, and licorice (*Glycyrrhiza glabra*) root.

RIDGECREST HERBALS, 1151 South Redwood Road #106, Salt Lake City, UT 84104-3729; tel: 800-242-4649 or 801-978-9633.

Astragalus Formula Deep Toning Formula: Liquid or tablets. Herbal tonics to nourish and strengthen the immune system, energy, and lungs; speeds recovery and increases energy after colds, flu, or other illness; lung tonic for people with a history of chronic respiratory problems.

ZAND HERBAL FORMULAS, 1722 14th Street #230, Boulder, CO 80302; tel: 800 800-0405 or 303-786-8558.

BHI Asthma: Homeopathic tablets. For temporary relief of common asthmatic symptoms.

HEEL/BHI, INC., 11600 Cochiti Road Southeast, Albuquerque, NM 87123-3376; tel: 800-621-7644 or 505-293-3843.

Breathe-Aid Formula: Capsules. For the temporary relief of shortness of breath, tightness of chest, and wheezing due to bronchial asthma.

NATURE'S WAY PRODUCTS, INC., 10 Mountain Springs Parkway, Springville, UT 84663; tel: 800- 962-8873 or 801-489-1500.

BronCare: Capsules. Bronchodilator for temporary relief of wheezing, tightness of chest, and shortness of breath due to bronchial asthma; contains the clinically proven active ingredients ephedrine HCl and guaifensein; does not induce drowsiness.

NATURE'S WAY PRODUCTS, INC., 10 Mountain Springs Parkway, Springville UT 84663; tel: 800- 962-8873 or 801-489-1500.

Bronc-Ease: Capsules. Helps the body to relieve shortness of breath, tightness of chest, and wheezing due to bronchial asthma; contains ephedra extract in a base of white pine bark, horehound, valerian, slippery elm, odorless garlic, elecampane, fenugreek, marshmallow, thyme, and mullein.

NATURE'S HERBS, 600 East Quality Drive, American Fork, UT 84003; tel: 800-437-2257 or 801-763-0700.

ClearLungs: Capsules. Helps clear the lungs of heavy mucus buildup, restoring free breathing; also aids in relieving shortness of breath, tightness of chest, and wheezing due to bronchial congestion; ingredients include Chinese ephedra herb, scute, platycodon, hoelen, citrus, *dong quai*, morus root, fritillaria, ophiopogon, asparagus, gardenia, schizandra, licorice, and almond.

RIDGECREST HERBALS, 1151 South Redwood Road #106, Salt Lake City, UT 84104-3729; tel: 800 242-4649 or 801-978-9633.

Lung: Tablets. Formula for respiratory health containing NAG (N-acetyl-glucosamine, a component of the mucosal lining of the lungs), which helps repair mucous membranes; NAC (N-acetyl-cysteine), which acts as a magnet to pull heavy metals from the lung's lining; and antioxidants (vitamins A, C, and E, beta carotene, and glutathione), which help prevent free radical damage to the lungs from toxic contaminants such as cigarette smoke and car exhaust.

OPTIMAL NUTRIENTS, 1163 Chess Drive #F, Foster City, CA 94404; tel: 800 966-8874 or 650-525-0112.

Respiratory Nutrient Support: Tablets. Helps strengthen the lungs, increase the oxygen-carrying capacity of the body, and keep the breathing passages open; aids in asthma, allergies, hay fever, sinus problems, cold symptoms, and air pollution problems.

BIO NATIVUS, P.O. Box 3281, Ogden, UT 84401; tel: 888-628-4887 or 801-732-1294.

RespirMax: Liquid. Herbal formula for nutritional support of a healthy respiratory system.

NATURAL MAX, NUTRACEUTICAL, P.O. Box 681869, Park City, UT 84068; tel: 800-669-8877.

Respirtone: Liquid. Warming herbal formula to help support the health, maintenance, and recovery of the respiratory tract.

RAINBOW LIGHT, P.O. Box 600, Santa Cruz, CA 95061; tel: 800-635-1233 or or 408-429-9089.

Backache

Pain in the back can be related to muscle or ligament strain or structural misalignment leading to nerve interference, or it can be a symptom of underlying organic imbalance or disease.

Symptoms and Causes of Backache

Symptoms of backache include spinal pain, back muscle pain, and impairment of even simple movements such as bending.

Common causes include poor posture, poor lifting habits, improper shoes, sleeping on an overly soft mattress, vertebral (spinal) misalignment, kidney or bladder disorders, female pelvic disorders, arthritis, bone disease, spinal disc problems, or scoliosis (abnormal curvature of the spine). Stress and being overweight are also contributing factors.

If spinal misalignment is causing localized inflammation and pressure to the point of affecting the related spinal nerve, pain and symptoms, such as numbness and tingling, muscle weakness, or organ dysfunction in the organ related to that specific nerve, will result. In this case or if you experience numbness, persistent pain, or radiating pain in the arms or legs, we recommend consulting a chiropractic doctor. They are trained in interpreting X rays and CT (computerized tomography, formerly CAT) scans and most have working relationships with orthopedic surgeons and neurologists, if such a referral is necessary.

Nutrients and Herbs for Backache

Since bone is composed of protein, collagen, and minerals, and muscle fiber is mainly protein with large quantities of minerals comprising the fluid inside muscle, it is logical that nutritional deficiencies in these basic building blocks will compromise the health and function of both bone and muscle. When deficiencies are contributing to your back pain, nutritional supplements are an essential treatment component.

■ **For acute and chronic back pain:** willow bark, feverfew, rosemary, and the enzyme protease are useful to ease inflammation. For additional support, include a multivitamin, multimineral, and amino acid complex. We do not recommend the use of aspirin and other nonsteroidal anti-inflammatory drugs (NSAIDs), such as Advil, Motrin, and Naprosyn, for arthritic conditions. They may alleviate pain temporarily, however, clinical studies show that long-term use of NSAIDs may actually accelerate joint destruction and the progression of arthritis.[31]

■ **For degenerated cartilage (osteoarthritis):** glucosamine sulfate and glucosamine HCL are the building blocks of cartilage and connective tissue, which maintain strong and flexible joints.[32] Other useful supplements and herbs include NAG (N-acetyl-glu-cosamine), bovine and shark cartilage, and antioxidants such as pycnogenol, coenzyme Q10, devil's claw, cat's claw, and vitamins C and E.

See **Arthritis**, pp. 84-96.

■ **For acute and chronic muscle spasm:** calcium, magnesium, and potassium supplements, as well as home-opathic topical creams containing calendula, arnica, and ivy extracts can relieve spasm.

■ **For acute and chronic inflammation:** protease enzymes (if no ulcer or gastritis is present), bromelain (enzyme compound from pineapple), mucopolysaccharides (such as bovine and shark cartilage), evening primrose oil, and the herbs yucca root, *Boswellia serrata*, and wild yam can help ease inflammation.

Products for Backache

Advanced Enzyme System: Vegicaps. Formula of plant-source enzymes for breaking down protein, fiber, fats, and carbohydrates (including sugar); ingredients include green papaya, apple pectin, sea vegetables, ginger, and peppermint.

RAINBOW LIGHT, P.O. Box 600, Santa Cruz, CA 95061; tel: 800-635-1233 or 408-429-9089.

Amino-Mag 200: Tablets. Contains elemental magnesium as an amino acid chelate (magnesium glycinate/lysinate combination), which can be easily absorbed without gastrointestinal side effects.

AMNI, 2247 National Avenue, Hayward, CA 94540-5012; tel: 800-437-8888 or 510-783-6969.

Anti-Flam Caps: Capsules. Anti-inflammatory herbal formula with white willow bark.

CRYSTAL STAR HERBAL NUTRITION, 4069 Wedgeway Court, Earth City, MO 63045; tel: 800-736-6015 or 314-739-7551.

Back-Prin: Capsules. (Alternative to Doan's Pills, DeWitt's Pills.) Provides relief of minor muscular back pain; ingredients include magnesium salicylate, white willow, calcium lactate, valerian, bromelain, manganese chelate, and lupulin (hops).

RIDGECREST HERBALS, 1151 South Redwood Road #106, Salt Lake City, UT 84104-3729; tel: 800-242-4649 or 801-978-9633.

BioE Myalgia: Homeopathic liquid. For temporary relief of muscle and joint pain, tenderness, and weakness.

BIOENERGETICS, INC., P.O. Box 127, Sandy, OR 97055; tel: 800-334-4043 or 503-668-7478.

Boswellin Cream. Ingredients include capsaicin (from cayenne) and methyl salicylate (from wintergreen) in a base of *Boswellia serrata* (standardized for boswellic acids) and vitamin E; for temporary relief of minor aches and pains of muscles and joints. Greaseless, stainless, with a pleasant aroma.

NATURE'S HERBS, 600 East Quality Drive, American Fork, UT 84003; tel: 800-437-2257 or 801-763-0700.

CSE-2 (PDGF BB) Cell Signal Enhancer: Homeopathic liquid. Contains homeopathic PDGF (platelet-derived growth factor BB) for temporary relief of minor muscle aches and pains; aids in faster recovery from strenuous exercise.

BIOMED COMM, INC., 2 Nickerson Street, Suite 102, Seattle, WA 98109; tel: 888-637-3516 or 206-284-3433.

Hyland's Low Back Pain: Homeopathic caplets or tablets. For relief of lower back pain due to strain, cold, or exposure.

P & S LABS, 210 West 131st Street, Los Angeles, CA 90061; tel: 800-624-9659 or 310-768-0700.

InflamActin: Cream. For muscle aches, pains, soreness, or stiffness; contains boswellin, turmeric, and gorgonian extracts in a liposome sphere for greater effectiveness and long-lasting results.

NATURE'S PLUS, 548 Broadhollow Road, Melville, NY 11747-3708; tel: 800-645-9500 or 516-293-0030.

Rhus Toxicodendron: Homeopathic remedy. Helps sprains, strains, sore muscles, rheumatic pains, sciatica (lower back pain), influenza, and restlessness.

STANDARD HOMEOPATHIC CO., 201 West 131st Street, Los Angeles, CA 90061; tel: 800-624-9659 or 310-768-0700.

Sciatica: Homeopathic lozenges. Reduces pain, burning sensation, and discomfort of sciatica in the lower back and leg; without the side effects of conventional treatments, does not interfere with any other medicine.

SUPHERB LTD., P.O. Box 1135, Nahariya 22100, Israel; tel: 800-409-HERB (4372).

Tiger Balm: Ointment. Helps relieve backaches, strained muscles, sore shoulders, knotted calves, tightened thighs, and aching ankles.

PRINCE OF PEACE ENTERPRISES, INC., 3450 Third Street #3G, San Francisco, CA 94124; tel: 800-PEACE2U (732-2328) or 510-887-1899.

Traumed: Homeopathic liquid or ointment. For the temporary relief of pain, discomfort, inflammation of various origins, and other symptoms of minor sprains, strains, bruises, and sports injuries.

HEEL/BHI, INC., 11600 Cochiti Road Southeast, Albuquerque, NM 87123-3376; tel: 800-621-7644 or 505-293-3843.

Bacterial Infections

There are many types of bacterial infections. *Staphylococcus* (informally called staph) and *Streptoccocus* (strep) are two of the more well-known. The manifestations of an infection are many. For example, staph can cause pneumonia, and different strains of strep can variously produce septic sore throat, scarlet fever, rheumatic fever, arthritis, and inflammation, among other disorders.

Symptoms and Causes of Bacterial Infections

Symptoms of bacterial infections generally include fever, increased perspiration, localized pain and swelling, acidic urine pH (acid-alkaline balance in the body), raised white blood cell count, and mucus congestion. While viruses affect the whole body, bacterial infections are usually localized in a given area; if left untreated or recurrent, they can become systemic.

Bacterial infections gain a hold in the body when the immune system is not functioning optimally. Numerous factors weaken immunity, from toxic overload, chronic disease, and nutritional deficiencies to stress and depression.

Be Careful With Antibiotics

When used appropriately, antibiotics are effective for serious or life-threatening bacterial infections. Their indiscriminate use, however, is ill-advised. First, although they are often prescribed for such conditions, antibiotics do not work against viruses or inflammatory conditions. Second, they kill not only harmful bacteria, but also beneficial bacteria in the gastrointestinal tract, which can lead to digestive and intestinal problems (notably *Candida albicans* yeast overgrowth) if not remedied. Third, indiscriminate use of antibiotics has produced multiple-drug-resistant bacterial strains and may ultimately render antibiotics ineffective against life-threatening infections.

If you suspect you have a bacterial infection, ask your doctor to take a culture of saliva or tissues or fluids from the infected area. If it is a bacterial infection, samples of different antibiotics can be placed in bacteria culture to determine which will be the most effective in killing that specific bacteria; this is called a sensitivity test. If you do take antibiotics, be sure to supplement with *acidophilus* (see below) during and after the course of treatment.

Nutrients and Herbs for Bacterial Infections

Research has established a connection between bacterial infections and the efficacy of supplementation with and/or deficiencies in the following nutrients:[33]

■ **Vitamin A:** deficiency is associated with impaired immune function and diminished immune response.

■ **Vitamin B complex:** deficiency in B vitamins (particularly folic acid and vitamins B2, B5, and B6) can compromise immune function and leave the body more vulnerable to infection.

■ **Vitamin C:** supplementation can reduce severity, duration, and possibly the incidence of bacterial infections.

■ **Vitamin E:** supplementation has been shown to enhance immune response and increase resistance to infection.

■ **Iron**: deficiency increases the susceptibility to infections.

■ **Selenium:** an important antioxidant, selenium is used by the body specifically to fight bacterial infections.

■ **Zinc and copper:** correct intake of zinc and copper contributes to the health of the immune system and reduces the incidence of infection.

■ **Colloidal silver:** mineral compound with antibacterial and immune-stimulating properties; can be used topically or internally for a wide variety of infections.

■ *Acidophilus*: this beneficial bacterium normally found in the intestines has an antibacterial effect on infections in the gastrointestinal tract. Acidophyllin, the antibacterial component of *acidophilus*, has been shown to suppress the growth of 27 kinds of bacteria.[34]

■ **Essential fatty acids (EFAs):** found in the oil of linseed, evening primrose, and certain fish, among other sources; have antibacterial properties.

■ **Bromelain**: an enzyme compound found in pineapples; an anti-inflammatory that has been shown to be as effective as antibiotics in treating pneumonia, bronchitis, kidney infection, and staph infection of the skin.[35]

■ **Berberine:** an alkaloid component of certain plants, notably goldenseal, Oregon grape, and barberry, berberine is a strong antimicrobial.[36]

■ **Cranberry and blueberry:** juices and extracts of these berries can be useful in preventing and treating urinary tract infections (UTIs) because they contain substances which deter *E. coli* bacteria (the source of many UTIs) from attaching to the walls of the bladder and other parts of the urinary tract.[37]

■ **Echinacea:** has a broad spectrum of beneficial effects on the immune system, and has proven effective in treating infections in general, including colds, flu, upper respiratory infections, and urinary tract and genital infections.[38]

■ **Garlic:** well-established antimicrobial properties in both fresh and extract form; may also be an immune stimulant.

■ **Goldenseal:** one of nature's most potent antibiotics that also stimulates immune response. Its effects have been demonstrated against harmful bacteria including *E. coli*.[39] Goldenseal should not be used continuously; like pharmaceutical antibiotics, it kills the beneficial gastrointestinal flora along with the pathogenic (disease-causing), increasing the possibility of *Candida albicans* (yeast-like fungus) or other harmful overgrowth. For this reason, we recommend that, as with antibiotics, people take *acidophilus* during and after a course of goldenseal and that they do not take either antibiotics or goldenseal for more than a four-week course, unless under specific doctor's recommendation. Goldenseal stimulates uterine contractions, so it should not be taken by pregnant women.

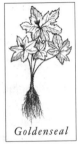

Goldenseal

■ **Grapefruit seed extract:** multipurpose antibiotic for bacterial infections; can be applied topically or taken orally.[40]

■ **Olive leaf extract:** with antibacterial and antiviral properties; useful for a range of infections.[41]

■ **Tea tree oil:** antiseptic that assists in fighting a broad range of infectious microorganisms and is one of the best topical skin disinfectants, helpful for acne and other skin infections.[42]

Products for Bacterial Infections

ACES Gold: Tablets. Antioxidant formula that contains coenzyme Q10, vitamins A, C, and E (to boost immune function), and glutathione peroxidase support (selenium, glutathione, and N-acetyl-cysteine), superoxide dismutase support (zinc, copper, and manganese), alpha-lipoic acid, citrus bioflavonoids, quercetin bioflavonoid, and odorless garlic (antimicrobial properties).

J.R. CARLSON LABS, INC., 15 College Drive, Arlington Heights, IL 60004-1985; tel: 800-323-4141 or 708-255-1600.

Anti-Bio Caps: Capsules or liquid. Herbal formula that has antiviral, antibacterial, and antiseptic properties; ingredients include echinacea, goldenseal, capsicum, marshmallow, black walnut hulls, elecampane, propolis, myrrh gum, turmeric, and potassium chloride.

CRYSTAL STAR HERBAL NUTRITION, 4069 Wedgeway Court, Earth City, MO 63045; tel: 800-736-6015 or 314-739-7551.

Begone: Liquid. Herbal remedy for bacterial, yeast, fungal, and viral control; contains concentrated glycerine extract of echinacea, lovage root, and myrrh gum with herbal dilution and flower essences.

OLYMPIC BOTANICALS, 231 Otto Street, Port Townsend, WA 98368; tel: 800-310-6924 or 360-385-9468.

BioBoost: Capsules. Contains the herbs echinacea and goldenseal with antioxidant vitamins and minerals to support the body's own defenses.

BIODYNAMAX, 6525 Gunpark Drive #150-507, Boulder, CO 80301; tel: 800-926-7525 or 303-530-4665.

Biocidin: Tablets. Herbal antimicrobial for intestinal dysbiosis (imbalance in intestinal flora) in which bacterial, fungal, or parasitic pathogens have been identified. *In vitro* testing by Great Smokies Diagnostic Laboratories has shown that all strains of bacteria and yeast show high levels of sensitivity to this combination of medicinal plants.

According to Dr. Martin Lee, Ph.D., Laboratory Director at Great Smokies, "The herbal mixture Biocidin has been the most broadly acting and powerful natural or nonprescriptive substance evaluated. In separate experiments, we have found that Biocidin was a potent inhibitor of growth for *Candida albicans*, as well as other *Candida* species." When used for an extended period of time, the cold nature of the herbs in Biocidin may weaken digestive energy, causing nausea or loss of appetite; in this case, appropriate tonic formulations can be chosen.

For more on **Great Smokies Diagnostic Laboratory tests**, see Appendix, pp. 484-485.

See **Biotonic** in Gastrointestinal Disorders product listing, p. 204.

BIO-BOTANICAL RESEARCH, INC., 144 Pioneer Road, Corralitos, CA 95076; distributed by WELLNESS HEALTH PHARMACY, tel: 800-227-2627 or 205-879-6551.

Buffered Vitamin C Powder or Beet Source "Buffered Vitamin C": Capsules or powder. Contains ascorbic acid, derived from a non-corn source and buffered with the carbonates of potassium, calcium, and magnesium; some severely ill, allergic, or hypersensitive people are able to tolerate this product if unable to tolerate other vitamin C products.

ALLERGY RESEARCH GROUP/NUTRICOLOGY, P.O. Box 55907, Hayward, CA 94544; tel: 800-545-9960 or 510-487-8526.

C Complex Plus: Tablets. Vitamin C rids the body of toxins as it travels through the bloodstream; contains vitamin C (vegetable source) and vitamin A (fish liver oil) in a base of seaweed, capsicum (cayenne), goldenseal root, yerba santa, and lemon bioflavonoids.

NATURAL ENERGY PRODUCTS, 21101 Welch Road, Snohomish, WA 98296; tel: 425-486-5956.

Echatin Plus: Capsules. Formula blends concentrated extracts of astragalus root, ligustrum berry, schisandra berry, shiitake and reishi mushroom, echinacea, and licorice root for support of immune system and prevention of colds.

NF FORMULAS, INC., 9755 Southwest Commerce Circle C-5, Wilsonville, OR 97070; tel: 800-547-4891 or 503-682-9755.

Echinacea Astragalus: Capsules or liquid. Enhances the body's resistance to infection.

FRONTIER COOPERATIVE HERBS, 3021 78th Street, Norway, IA 52318; tel: 800-669-3275 or 319-227-7996.

Echinacea Glycerites: Liquid. Naturally sweet alternative to the traditional bitter-tasting echinacea liquid supplements.

PLANETARY FORMULAS, 23 Janis Way, Scotts Valley, CA 95066; tel: 800-606-6226.

Echinacea Goldenseal: Capsules or liquid. Provides resistance during cold and flu season.

FRONTIER COOPERATIVE HERBS, 3021 78th Street, Norway, IA 52318; tel: 800-669-3275 or 319-227-7996.

Echinacea • Goldenseal Compound: Liquid. Remedy for colds and flu accompanied by nasal congestion and other respiratory symptoms; can also be used as a strengthening, preventative tonic for those susceptible to colds and flu; ingredients include echinacea root, goldenseal rhizome and roots, osha root, spilanthes flowering herb and root, yerba santa leaf, horseradish root, elder flower, yarrow flower, watercress herb, and wild indigo root.

HERB PHARM, 20260 Williams Highway, Williams, OR 97544; tel: 800-348-4372 or 541-846-6262.

Echinashield: Liquid or chewable tablets. Contains echinacea, vitamins A, B6, and C, and zinc, available in assorted flavors.

NF FORMULAS, INC., 9755 Southwest Commerce Circle C-5, Wilsonville, OR 97070; tel: 800-547-4891 or 503-682-9755.

E.H.B.: Capsules. Blend of echinacea, goldenseal, and berberis (which have been standardized to ensure potency of active ingredients) with herbs and vitamins, including vitamin C, beta carotene, and zinc.

NF FORMULAS, INC., 9755 Southwest Commerce Circle C-5, Wilsonville, OR 97070; tel: 800-547-4891 or 503-682-9755.

Garlic, Echinacea, Goldenseal Plus: Tablets. Contains standardized echinacea extract, echinacea herbal blend, goldenseal, garlic, and other valuable herbs for immune support.

FUTUREBIOTICS, 145 Ricefield Lane, Hauppauge, NY 11788; tel: 800-FOR-LIFE (367-5433) or 516-273-6300.

GSE Liquid Concentrate (Grapefruit Seed Extract): Capsules, liquid, or tablets. Use internally as a dental, nasal, ear, and vaginal rinse, and throat gargle or externally as a facial cleanser, skin rinse, nail and scalp treatment, and all-purpose cleaner (for toothbrushes, vegetables, fruits, meats, dishes, utensils, and cutting boards).

NUTRIBIOTIC, NUTRITION RESOURCES, Inc., P.O. Box 238, Lakeport, CA 95453; tel: 800-225-4345 or 707-263-0411.

Herbal Aloe Force: Juice or topical gel. Processed aloe vera juice containing vitamins, minerals, enzymes, amino acids, essential fatty acids, growth factors, glycoproteins, sterols, bioflavonoids, and polysaccharides (complex sugars), plus ionized colloidal silver and herbal extracts (cat's claw, chamomile, burdock root, hawthorn berry, astragalus root, sheep sorrell, pau d'arco bark, slippery elm bark, and rhubarb root).

HERBAL ANSWERS, INC., P.O. Box 1110, Saratoga Springs, NY 12866; tel: 888-256-3367 or 518-581-1968.

Immune-Neem by Farmacopia: Capsules or tea. Contains neem leaf (a mainstay of the Ayurvedic health system of India; laboratory studies have shown its antibacterial, antifungal, and antiviral activities), ginger, stevia, peppermint, lemon grass, cinnamon, licorice, and natural flavors.

BOTANICAL PRODUCTS INTERNATIONAL, P.O. Box 174, Hakalau, HI 96710; tel: 808-963-6771.

Katsu Herbal Garlic Complex: Tablets. Concentrated extract of garlic, coix, and rice bran, with shark cartilage and vitamin C; garlic is well-known for its ability to inhibit bacteria, fungi, yeast (including *Candida*) and parasites (protozoa and worms); promotes immune functions; lowers cholesterol; reduces platelet aggregation; and aids digestion.

KENSHIN TRADING CORP., P.O. Box 7511, Torrance, CA 90504; tel: 800-766-1313 or 310-212-3199.

Olive Leaf Extract: Capsules. Contains extract of olive leaf with a minimum of 17% of the active compound oleuropein.

SOLARAY, Nutraceutical Corp., P.O. Box 681869, Park City, UT 84068; tel: 800-669-8877.

Oregamax: Capsules. Contains crushed wild oregano, rhus cariaria, garlic, and onion; wild oregano contains the active ingredients carvacrol (antimicrobial), bioflavonoids (antiseptic), and terpenes (anti-inflammatory).

PURITY PRODUCTS, 1804 Plaza Avenue, New Hyde Park, NY 11040; tel: 800-769-7873.

Oxy-Caps by Earth's Bounty: Capsules. Releases molecular oxygen once it comes in contact with the stomach's hydrochloric acid; increased levels of oxygen can help the body work more efficiently and neutralize anaerobic bacteria.

MATRIX HEALTH PRODUCTS, 8400 Magnolia Avenue, Suite N, Santee, CA 92071; tel: 800-736-5609 or 619-448-7550.

Oxy-Max by Earth's Bounty: Liquid. High-potency supplement that provides electrolytes of stabilized oxygen, a form readily assimilated and utilized by the body. A shortage of oxygen in the body leaves it susceptible to bacterial, fungal, and viral infections, as well as a loss of mental acuity.

MATRIX HEALTH PRODUCTS, 8400 Magnolia Avenue, Suite N, Santee, CA 92071; tel: 800-736-5609 or 619-448-7550.

Proflora: Liquid. Encourages the growth of beneficial flora in the intestinal tract, inhibits the proliferation of pathogenic or abnormal flora, and soothes irritated intestinal lining; recommended during and after the use of antipathogenic supplements or antibiotics.

BIO-BOTANICAL RESEARCH, INC., 144 Pioneer Road, Corralitos, CA 95076; distributed by WELLNESS HEALTH PHARMACY, 2800 South 18th Street, Homewood, AL 35209; tel: 800-227-2627 or 205-879-6551.

Royal Scandinavian Colloidal Silver 500 ppm: Liquid. Highest-quality silver with a fine particle size to ensure maximum permeability through body tissues; can be used internally or as a sinus flush; *acidophilus* should be used after administration.

BIO-NUTRITIONAL FORMULAS, 106 East Jericho Turnpike, Mineola, NY 11501; tel: 800-950-8484.

Silver: Liquid. Electroprocessed and chemical-free; ingredients include deionized water and colloidal silver, which is tasteless, nontoxic, and contains no artificial ingredients, preservatives, or additives.

FUTUREBIOTICS, 145 Ricefield Lane, Hauppauge, NY 11788; tel: 800-FOR-LIFE (367-5433) or 516-273-6300.

SP-21 Echinacea-Goldenseal Blend: Capsules. Contains echinacea root, goldenseal root, myrrh gum, garlic, licorice root, vervain, butternut bark, and kelp with a homeopathically prepared mineral formula.

SOLARAY, NUTRACEUTICAL CORP., P.O. Box 681869, Park City, UT 84068; tel: 800-669-8877.

100% Pure Tea Tree Oil. Antiseptic first aid for minor cuts, burns, abrasions, bites, and stings.

THURSDAY PLANTATION, INC., NATURE'S PLUS, 548 Broadhollow Road, Melville, NY 11747-3708; tel: 800-645-9500 or 516-293-0030.

Tea Tree Antiseptic Cream. Herbal antiseptic for minor skin irritations and relief of sunburn, windburn, minor burns, or chafing.

THURSDAY PLANTATION, INC., NATURE'S PLUS, 548 Broadhollow Road, Melville, NY 11747-3708; tel: 800-645-9500 or 516-293-0030.

Wild West Manuka Honey: Ointment. Helpful as a topical ointment when treating scrapes, cuts, boils, and athlete's foot.

WGI, 35008 Emerald Coast Parkway, 5th Floor, Destin, FL 32541; tel: 800-854-8353 or 850-654-4744.

Bronchitis, a respiratory condition, is characterized by inflammation and irritation of the lungs' bronchial tubes, with symptoms ranging from chills, fever, and coughing to difficulty breathing and chest pain.

Types and Causes of Bronchitis

Bronchitis is classified as acute, chronic, or acute irritative.

Acute Bronchitis—A short-term infection, acute bronchitis occurs most frequently in the winter and often follows a cold, flu, or other viral infection. Malnutrition, fatigue, and air pollution are contributing factors.[43]

Chronic Bronchitis—Long-term or recurrent infection, chronic bronchitis may be associated with chronic sinus or lung infections or, in children, enlarged tonsils and adenoids (overgrowth of the lymphatic tissue in the pharynx, or throat). Common causes include a diet of mucus- and acid-forming foods, drugs that suppress the immune system, lack of exercise, poor circulation, fatigue, and diminished immunity.[44]

For a list of **acid-forming foods**, see Arthritis, p. 85.

Acute Irritative Bronchitis—This form of bronchitis is caused by environmental irritants such as smog, tobacco and other smoke, mineral and vegetable dusts, and fumes from ammonia, chlorine, sulfur dioxide, and other chemicals.[45]

Nutrients and Herbs for Bronchitis

For infections involving the respiratory tract, we often recommend colloidal silver, goldenseal, echinacea, garlic, and pau d'arco, which act as antibiotics, destroying fungi, viruses, and bacteria , while supporting the immune system. We also recommend beta carotene and bioflavonoids (quercetin, rutin, and hesperidin).

■ **Water:** for any respiratory condition, drink plenty of filtered water (six to eight 8-ounce glasses per day) and avoid smoke, exhaust, perfume, and chemical fumes.

■ **Vitamins A and C:** help reduce inflammation.

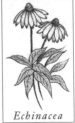

Echinacea

■ **Bromelain:** an enzyme compound derived from pineapple, helps relieve the chronic cough associated with bronchitis. It also decreases the stickiness of mucus and saliva in the respiratory tract, which increases the ability to breathe.

■ **Ephedra (*ma huang*):** has been used for the treatment of bronchitis, edema, and the common cold. Ephedra can raise blood pressure and produce insomnia and anxiety in some people; use with caution and only in recommended doses.

CAUTION

Ephedra is for short-term use only. Do not take ephedra at all if you are pregnant, have kidney problems, or suffer from high blood pressure or other cardiovascular stress.

■ **Ginkgo:** helps decrease the constriction of the bronchioles (subdivision of the lungs' bronchial tubes).

■ **Lobelia:** helps reduce the symptoms associated with bronchitis, asthma, and pneumonia. Lobelia's primary effect is to stimulate the adrenal glands to release hormones, causing the bronchiole muscles of the lungs to relax. Lobelia is also an expectorant, promoting the breakdown and ejection of mucus from the lungs and respiratory tract.

■ **Marshmallow root:** contains mucilage, which is excellent for treating irritated airways.

■ **Mullein oil:** another good bronchial dilator (opener), reduces bronchial congestion, clears bronchial tubes, and reduces cough.

■ **Olive leaf extract:** antibacterial and antiviral proven useful for bronchitis, colds, flu, and pneumonia, among other conditions.[46]

■ **Siberian ginseng:** reduces inflammation in bronchial passages.

■ **Thyme:** relieves bronchial spasms and symptoms of bronchitis.

Products for Bronchitis

Astragalus Formula Deep Toning Formula: Liquid or tablets. Herbal tonic to nourish and strengthen the immune system, energy, and lungs; increases recovery and energy after colds, flu, and illness; lung tonic for people with a history of chronic respiratory problems.

ZAND HERBAL FORMULAS, 1722 14th Street #230, Boulder, CO 80302; tel: 800-800-0405 or 303-786-8558.

ClearLungs: Capsules. Helps clear the lungs of heavy mucus buildup, restoring free breathing; aids in relieving shortness of breath, tightness of chest, and wheezing due to bronchial congestion; contains Chinese ephedra, scute, platycodon, hoelen, citrus, *dong quai*, morus root, fritillaria, asparagus, gardenia, schisandra, licorice, and almond.

RIDGECREST HERBALS, 1151 South Redwood Road #106, Salt Lake City, UT 84104-3729; tel: 800-242-4649 or 801-978-9633.

Congestaway: Oil. Contains pure eucalyptus, dandelion and olive oils, and flower essences for relief of coughs due to bronchitis, sinusitis, colds, viruses, and lymphatic congestion; can be used as a vaporizer oil or for massaging and bathing feet, hands, and body.

OLYMPIC BOTANICALS, 231 Otto Street, Port Townsend, WA 98368; tel: 800-310-6924 or 360-385-9468.

Cough & Bronchial (B & T's): Homeopathic syrup. Soothes throat and bronchial irritation, relieves coughs caused by cold and flu viruses or air pollution (inhaled gases and dusts), loosens stubborn phlegm, thins bronchial secretions, and helps clear the lungs of mucus and drain the bronchial tubes.

BOERICKE & TAFEL, INC., 2381 Circadian Way, Santa Rosa, CA 95407; tel: 800-876-9505 or 707-571-8202.

Herbal Resistance: Liquid. Contains osha root, lomatium, and echinacea for strengthening respiratory functions.

NOW, 550 Mitchell Road, Glendale Heights, IL 60139; tel: 800-283-3500.

Hyland's Bronchial Cough: Tablets. For relief of cough due to colds; helps coughs with mucus and a sensation of tickling in the throat.

P & S LABS, 210 West 131st Street, Los Angeles, CA 90061; tel: 800-624-9659 or 310-768-0700.

Lung: Tablets. Contains NAG (N-acetyl-glucosamine, a component of the mucosal lining of the lungs), which helps repair mucous membranes; NAC (N-acetyl-cysteine), which acts as a magnet to pull heavy metals from the lung's lining; and antioxidants (vitamins A, C, and E, beta carotene, and glutathione), which help prevent free radical damage to the lungs from toxic contaminants such as cigarette smoke and car exhaust.

OPTIMAL NUTRIENTS, 1163 Chess Drive #F, Foster City, CA 94404; tel: 800-966-8874 or 650-525-0112.

Lymphomyosot: Homeopathic liquid or tablets. For temporary relief of symptoms bronchitis, colds, flu, and edema (swelling of tissues or glands).

HEEL/BHI, INC., 11600 Cochiti Road Southeast, Albuquerque, NM 87123-3376; tel: 800-621-7644 or 505-293-3843.

Carpal Tunnel Syndrome

Carpal tunnel syndrome is a nerve inflammation in the wrist producing numbness, tingling, and swelling in the wrist and hand. Chronic muscle weakness and atrophy can develop if the condition persists.

Causes of Carpal Tunnel Syndrome

Common causes of carpal tunnel syndrome include overuse (repetitive motion) of the wrist and hand, vitamin B6 deficiency (prolonged use of birth control pills can produce this deficiency), magnesium and other cell mineral deficiencies, and hormonal imbalances during pregnancy. As misalignment in the cervical (neck) vertebrae produces symptoms similar to carpal tunnel, misdiagnosis can occur; consultation with a chiropractor can rule out this possibility.

Nutrients and Herbs for Carpal Tunnel Syndrome

■ **Supplements:** vitamins A, B complex (especially increased B6 intake), C, and E, beta carotene, bromelain, coenzyme Q10, essential fatty acids (primrose oil), kelp, manganese, multimineral and multivitamin complex, protease enzyme formula, pycnogenol, and zinc.

■ **Herbs:** aloe vera, butcher's broom, corn silk, devil's claw, cayenne (capsicum), ginkgo, gravel root, marshmallow, skullcap, turmeric (curcumin), wintergreen oil, yarrow, and yucca.

Products for Carpal Tunnel Syndrome

Actives InflamActin: Capsules. Dietary supplement to support the body's normal adaptogenic (stress-handling) function. Contains boswellia, turmeric, bromelain, DLPA (DL-phenylalanine), and vitamin C.

NATURE'S PLUS, 548 Broadhollow Road, Melville, NY 11747-3708; tel: 800-645-9500 or 516-293-0030.

Balanced B-100: Tablets. Contains a combination of B vitamins that work together to convert food into energy and are necessary for normal functioning of the nervous system.

NATURE MADE LLC, NATURE'S RESOURCE, P.O. Box 9606, Mission Hills, CA 91346-9606; tel: 800-314-HERB (4372) or 800-423-2405.

B-Complex-50: Capsules. Contains all of the B-complex vitamins, which are needed for numerous metabolic functions, including energy production, detoxification, nerve transmission, blood formation, synthesis of proteins and fats, production of steroid hormones, maintenance of blood sugar levels and appetite, and toning of the muscles.

HEALTH PRODUCTS DISTRIBUTORS, INC., 23847 Peaceful Ridge Road, Smithsburg, MD 21783; tel: 800-228-4265 or 301-416-0500.

Carpaltun: Tablets. Contains vitamin B6 and its active coenzyme form (pyridoxal-5-phosphate), bromelain, and serratia peptidase, a proteolytic enzyme which has anti-inflammatory properties.

ECOLOGICAL FORMULAS, 1061-B Shary Circle, Concord, CA 94518; tel: 800-888-4585 or 925-827-2636.

Cold Pressed Hempseed Oil. Hempseed oil contains the ideal 3:1 ratio of omega-6 to omega-3 essential fatty acids; can be used as condiment and recipe ingredient.

HEMPOLA, 3405 American Drive #5, Mississauga, Ontario, Canada L4V1T6; tel: 800-240-9215.

Max Omega: Oil. Contains black currant seed oil, which is the most complete source of essential fatty acids; contains linoleic acid (LA, an omega-6 essential fatty acid) and, unlike primrose or borage oil, alpha linolenic acid (ALA, an omega-3 essential fatty acid). Also, unlike flaxseed, black currant seed oil contains 18% gamma-linolenic acid (GLA), twice the amount in primrose oil.

BIO-NUTRITIONAL FORMULAS, 106 East Jericho Turnpike, Mineola, NY 11501; tel: 800-950-8484.

Ultra Antioxidant Plus: Softgels. Contains pycnogenol, coenzyme Q10, SOD (superoxide dismutase), glutathione, zinc, beta carotene, vitamins C and E, and selenium to neutralize free radical production. Clinical data has shown the damaging effects of free radicals and single oxygen on cells and body systems.

PHILLIPS NUTRITIONALS, 27071 Cabot Road #122, Laguna Hills, CA 92653; tel: 800-514-5115 or 702-898-8141.

Children's Health Problems

To ensure a child's overall health and to identify all the contributing factors in even common childhood ailments, it is important to consider allergies (often hidden), sugar consumption, and the use of pharmaceutical drugs.

Children and Food Allergies

Many common childhood illnesses and conditions, including bed-wetting, chronic upper respiratory infections, asthma, and hyperactivity/attention deficit disorder, are potentially connected to food allergies.[47] Animal dander, molds, dusts, smoke (especially second-hand tobacco smoke), pollen, and environmental pollutants also can contribute to allergic reactions and respiratory tract inflammation in children.

See **Allergies**, pp. 66-74.

The protocol we follow when treating allergic children is the same as for allergic adults: that is, to improve their digestion, nutritionally bolster their immune system, and remove as many allergens as possible from their diet. The most common food allergens are sugar, wheat, dairy (especially cow's milk), corn, citrus, chocolate, peanut butter, and food additives such as artificial colors, flavorings, and preservatives.

When eliminating offending foods from your children's diet, be strict but reasonable: try to find natural snacks (vegetables, rice cakes, popcorn, and nonwheat, nondairy treats containing no sugar) to replace restricted foods; assist your children in becoming responsible for their health; and, if possible, have them participate in charting their symptoms on a scale of 0 (no symptoms) to 10 (worst symptoms), so they can monitor their own progress. Always create a baseline chart of how bad the allergies were to start with and refer back to that list when the symptoms improve and children want sugar snacks again.

Children and Sugar

Many children are picky eaters who have developed a desire for (addiction to) sweets and processed foods. If you don't think your kids are addicted to sugar, try eliminating it completely from their diet for a few days and see if they have any withdrawal symptoms such as anxiety, tension, mood swings, behavioral changes, and hypoglycemia (low blood sugar). Addicted people (both children and adults) get intense cravings for candy and often have compulsive or habitual-use patterns such as "sneaking" their sugar products of choice. Excess sugar in the diet has been shown to upset mineral balance in the body and reduce immune function.[48]

Children and Pharmaceutical Drugs

On any given day in the United States, over five million children use a prescription medication, whether it's an inhaler for asthma or a drug for ear infection, depression, hyperactivity/attention deficit disorder (ADD), or other condition. Unfortunately, the testing of these medications was done mainly on adults—less than 20% of the tests are performed on children—and once a drug has been approved by the FDA for use on adults, physicians are free to prescribe it to anyone.[49]

Along with lack of testing, overuse of certain drugs, particularly antibiotics, is an area of concern in children's health. In fact, one study found that 44% of children suffering from a common cold were given antibiotics by their pediatricians.[50] The majority of colds are caused by viruses, against which antibiotics are ineffective.

Often parents request antibiotics "just in case." This is a dangerous practice. Antibiotics are not for prevention, but should only be used when a bacterial infection is present. Overuse of antibiotics weakens immunity and leads to drug-resistant bacteria.

If you suspect your child has a bacterial infection, ask your doctor to take a culture of saliva or tissues or fluids from the infected area. If it is a bacterial infection, samples of different antibiotics can be placed in the bacteria culture to determine which will be the most effective in killing that specific bacteria; this is called a sensitivity test. If you do elect to give your child antibiotics, be sure to reintroduce "friendly" bacteria such as *acidophilus* during and especially after the course of treatment.

Common Children's Health Problems

Anemia—Childhood anemia (lowered red blood cell count and/or decrease in hemoglobin concentration) often occurs in very young children and teenage girls and is primarily caused by iron deficiency.

Childhood Depression—Symptoms of depression include excessive grief, despair, anger, worry, and/or guilt, extreme fatigue, disturbance of normal sleep patterns and appetite, and withdrawal from normal activity. These characteristics distinguish depression from the normal mood swings of childhood and adolescence.

Childhood Essential Fatty Acid (EFA) Deficiency—EFAs (unsaturated fatty acids that the body cannot manufacture but must get from the diet or nutritional supplements) are essential for children's growth and cell and tissue health. EFA deficiency can result in skin problems, poor wound-healing, and increased rates of infection.

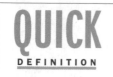

Colic—The spasm-type stomach pains and attendant crying and irritability of colic is often related to poor digestion resulting from a deficiency of digestive enzymes, a low intestinal population of the beneficial bacteria *acidophilus*, or an imbalance in digestive pH (SEE QUICK DEFINITION). Other causes include overfeeding, swallowing air, emotional upset, and sensitivity or allergic reaction to something in the mother's milk (caused by something the mother ate).

Ear Infection (Otitis Media)—Infections usually occur after a cold or other illness when the eustachian tube (the tube that allows the equalization of pressure between the middle ear and back of the throat) becomes blocked, causing pus buildup, pressure, inflammation, and pain in the ear. We often find the underlying cause of ear infections is some type of food allergy. The constant activation of the immune system to defend the body from a food it regards as a "foreign" invader weakens immunity and leaves the body more susceptible to infection.

Fever—Conventional medicine recommends fever-reducing medications such as Tylenol or aspirin. The alternative medical view is that the body creates fever for a reason: to kill bacteria and viruses. Thus, purposely lowering the fever to make the child more comfortable may actually prolong the illness. Instead of Tylenol (or other chemical treatments), we recommend homeopathic or herbal remedies for fever and its related symptoms. These types of remedies are safe, inexpensive, and free of side effects. If high fever persists, consult your health-care practitioner.

Hyperactivity/Attention Deficit Disorder (ADD)—A growing number of children in the United States are being given an ADD diagnosis (the current term for what used to be simply termed hyperactivity) and receiving medication (such as Ritalin) due to their inattentiveness, short attention span, distractability, failure to follow directions or finish tasks, forgetfulness, fidgeting, excessive talking or moving about, and lack of impulse control. Hyperactivity may be caused by learning disabilities, an unstable home life, food allergies (especially wheat, sugar, and dairy) or reactions to food additives, excessive sugar (or sweetener) consumption, lead poisoning, and even the need for eye glasses.[51] Simply removing sugar and sweeteners such as corn syrup from the diet can have a dramatic impact on the behavior of many children diagnosed with ADD.

Measles—A highly contagious viral infection characterized by sneezing, runny nose, cough, fever, red eyes that are sensitive to light, and white spots in the mouth and throat. These symptoms are followed by a rash that begins on the face and neck then spreads to the rest of the body.

Stomachache—Pain in the stomach is often related to poor diet or indigestion. The foods most often linked to stomachache are sugar, salt, fats, and food additives such as artificial colors, flavors, and preservatives. Food allergies can also produce stomach pain.

Nutrients and Herbs for Children's Health

■ **For immune system support:** deficiencies of almost any of the vitamins or minerals, most importantly vitamins A and C, iron, and zinc, will negatively affect the performance of a developing immune system.

■ **For healthy bones, teeth, hair, and nails:** the minerals calcium, boron, silica, and vanadium are key.

■ **For tissue protection:** the antioxidant vitamins A, C, and E, beta carotene, selenium, vitamin B5, and the amino acid taurine promote tissue health.

■ **For airborne/environmental allergies:** vitamin C with bioflavonoids, beta carotene, vitamin B complex, and quercetin can all be helpful in alleviating allergies.

■ **For anemia:** iron is critical to red blood cell production and is best absorbed by the body from a plant-based source, such as the herb yellowdock, which has a high iron content. When taken in supplemental form, vitamin C should be combined with the iron for best absorption. Other nutrients required for production of red blood cells are folic acid and vitamins B1, B6, and B12.

■ **For burns, cuts, stings, and bites:** tea tree oil is an effective antibacterial, antiviral, and antifungal agent.

■ **For bruises:** vitamin C with bioflavonoids should be given to children who bruise easily.

■ **For colic:** liquid extract of chamomile in warm water eases intestinal cramping and has a mild sedative effect that helps the baby go to sleep. Digestive enzymes mixed into a wet paste and applied to the mother's nipple before breast-feeding can also be effective for colicky babies.

■ **For constipation:** increasing fiber in the diet, raising the intake of pure, filtered water, and using liquid aloe vera as a gentle laxative are good preventive and treatment measures for constipation.

■ **For growing pains or nighttime leg pains and cramps:** calcium, magnesium, and vitamin E can help with muscle aches and growing pains.

■ **For headaches:** calcium and magnesium and the herb feverfew can be effective in headache relief.

■ **For hyperactivity and ADD:** deficiencies of vitamin B6, chromium, copper, and zinc are often present in hyperactive children and supplementation may alleviate the condition. By helping correct blood sugar metabolism and adrenal gland function, Siberian ginseng is also useful for ADD. Valerian root, a well-known herbal sedative, has the unique capacity to calm and at the same time increase concentration; research has demonstrated its successful application to hyperactivity in children.[52] Passionflower and chamomile are other useful calming agents.

■ **For infections and fever:** echinacea and goldenseal (short-term use only), berberine, odorless garlic, and olive leaf extract support the immune system and are appropriate for children with infections or fever; we recommend grapefruit seed extract or tea tree oil for topical infections.

■ **For sleeplessness:** calcium and magnesium, hops, skullcap, passionflower, and valerian root extract can all help promote sleep. Valerian is a good sleep aid sedative, especially when anxiety or nervousness is a cause of the insomnia.

■ **For sore throats:** zinc lozenges can relieve a sore throat, but should be used sparingly as excessive zinc intake can produce a zinc-copper imbalance.

■ **For stomachache and indigestion:** digestive enzymes, ginger, and chamomile can ease stomach pain and indigestion.

■ **For viruses:** echinacea and goldenseal (short-term use only), cat's claw, garlic, and yarrow are all useful antivirals.

Products for Children's Health

Acneteen: Phyto-homeopathic gel. Helps soothe inflamed skin and heal pimples; ingredients include acneteen in a base of marigold, Australian tea tree oil, and echinacea; does not interfere with any other medicine.

SUPHERB LTD., P.O. Box 1135, Nahariya 22100, Israel; tel: 800-409-HERB (4372).

Aconitum Napellus: Homeopathic remedy. Helpful for earache, colic, fright, injury, fear of dental treatment or surgery, headache, and painful urination.

STANDARD HOMEOPATHIC CO., 201 West 131st, Los Angeles, CA 90061; tel: 800-624-9659 or 310-768-0700.

AMNI Kids: Chewable wafers. Contains essential nutrients for children; available in animal-shaped wafers.

AMNI, 2247 National Avenue, Hayward, CA 94540-5012; tel: 800-437-8888 or 510-783-6969.

Arnicalm: Homeopathic remedy. For bumps and bruises.

BOIRON, 6 Campus Boulevard, Building A, Newtown Square, PA 19073; tel: 800-264-7661 or 610-325-7464.

Baby Care Kit: Liquid, oil, and salve. Includes the multi-herbal combinations of Calming Formula and Lullaby Land Formula to promote relaxation, calendula oil for healthy skin, and an all-purpose salve.

NATURE'S APOTHECARY, P.O. Box 17970, Boulder, CO 80308; tel: 800-999-7422 or 303-664-1600.

Baby Gum: Phyto-homeopathic gel. Soothes the pain of teething, reduces swelling and local irritation, and eases restlessness day or night; ingredients include German chamomile and plantain; does not interfere with any other medicine.

SUPHERB LTD., P.O. Box 1135, Nahariya 22100, Israel; tel: 800-409-HERB (4372).

Baby Plex: Liquid. Each drop (1 ml) contains between 100% and 125% of the U.S. RDA (Recommended Daily Allowance) of vitamins for infants; sugar-free.

NATURE'S PLUS, 548 Broadhollow Road, Melville, NY 11747-3708; tel: 800-645-9500 or 516-293-0030.

Bed Wetting: Tablets. Homeopathic remedy for bed-wetting.

P & S LABS, 210 West 131st Street, Los Angeles, CA 90061; tel: 800-624-9659 or 310-768-0700.

Belladonna: Homeopathic remedy. Helpful for fever, headache, earache, toothache, sore throat, and colic.

STANDARD HOMEOPATHIC CO., 201 West 131st, Los Angeles, CA 90061; tel: 800-624-9659 or 310-768-0700.

Building Blocks Children's Chewable Multivitamin: Tablets. Balanced, complete daily multivitamin and multimineral supplement; contains extra trace minerals for children's growth and is easily ingested by ages four and older.

NF FORMULAS, INC., 9755 Southwest Commerce Circle C-5, Wilsonville, OR 97070; tel: 800-547-4891 or 503-682-9755.

Calcarea Phosphorica: Homeopathic remedy. Helpful for teething difficulties, "growing pains," and headaches.

STANDARD HOMEOPATHIC CO., 201 West 131st, Los Angeles, CA 90061; tel: 800-624-9659 or 310-768-0700.

Calm Child: Liquid or tablets. Blend of herbs to soothe children, particularly in moments of restlessness, anxiety, or stress.

PLANETARY FORMULAS, 23 Janis Way, Scotts Valley, CA 95066; tel: 800-606-6226.

Calming Formulae: Homeopathic liquid. Helps relieve hyperactivity, apprehension, and nightmares resulting from physiological imbalance.

LIDDELL LABORATORIES, 1036 Country Club Drive, Moraga, CA 94556; tel: 800-460-7733 or 925-377-3000.

Camilia: Homeopathic liquid. For teething babies.

BOIRON, 6 Campus Boulevard, Building A, Newtown Square, PA 19073; tel: 800-264-7661 or 610-325-7464.

Chamomilla: Homeopathic remedy. Helpful for pain, fever, earache, toothache, teething difficulties, colic, and temper.

STANDARD HOMEOPATHIC CO., 201 West 131st, Los Angeles, CA 90061; tel: 800-624-9659 or 310-768-0700.

Chamomile Calm: Liquid. Herbal extract that supports healthy functioning of the nervous system (recommended for older children or children suffering from nightmares); ingredients include skullcap herb, chamomile flowers, valerian root, fennel seed, hops, and catnip herb.

HERBS FOR CHILDREN, 151 Evergreen Drive, Suite D, Bozeman, MT 59715; tel: 406-587-0180.

Cherry Bark Blend: Liquid. Herbal extract that supports the respiratory system and mucous membranes of the throat; ingredients include thyme leaf, cherry bark, mullein leaf, peppermint leaf, orange peel, hops, horehound herb, pleurisy root, and Oregon grape root.

HERBS FOR CHILDREN, 151 Evergreen Drive, Suite D, Bozeman, MT 59715; tel: 406-587-0180.

Chestal for Children: Liquid. Alcohol-free and sucrose-free cough relief for children; doesn't cause drowsiness or side effects.

BOIRON, 6 Campus Boulevard, Building A, Newtown Square, PA 19073; tel: 800-264-7661 or 610-325-7464.

Chewable Orange Vitamin C: Tablets. Contains vitamin C (ascorbic acid), rose hips, natural orange flavor and sweeteners.

AMERICAN HEALTH, 4320 Veterans Memorial Highway, Holbrook, NY 11741; tel: 800-445-7137.

Chewy Bears Acidophilus Probiotic Supplement: Chewable wafers. Ingredients include *Lactobacillus acidophilus*, *L. rhamnosus*, *L. plantarum*, *L. sporogenes*, *Bifidobacterium longum*, and FOS (fructo-oligosaccharide, which feeds friendly microflora) in a base containing concentrates of raspberries, grapes, pears, cherries, black currants, and fructose.

AMERICAN HEALTH, 4320 Veterans Memorial Highway, Holbrook, NY 11741; tel: 800-445-7137.

Chewy Bears Chewable Calcium: Chewable wafers. Ingredients include calcium (as carbonate and citrate) and lactase (an enzyme to digest the lactose in goat milk included) in a base of malted goat milk, fructose, fruit juice solids, dried honey, vegetable gums, and pectin.

AMERICAN HEALTH, 4320 Veterans Memorial Highway, Holbrook, NY 11741; tel: 800-445-7137.

Chewy Bears Citrus Free Vitamin C: Chewable wafers. For children who have an intolerance for citric acid; ingredients include vitamin C (buffered) and a base containing black currant juice, apricots, peaches, rose hips, acerola, and fructose.

AMERICAN HEALTH, 4320 Veterans Memorial Highway, Holbrook, NY 11741; tel: 800-445-7137

Chewy Bears Multi-Vitamins with Calcium: Chewable wafers. Multivitamin formula contains no iron, phosphorous, fish or animal derivatives, or citrus. For children who cannot tolerate the acid in citrus fruits.

AMERICAN HEALTH, 4320 Veterans Memorial Highway, Holbrook, NY 11741; tel: 800-445-7137.

Children's Chewable: Capsules. Multivitamin and mineral supplement that provides a full range of B-complex vitamins (for proper energy production, growth, and development), the antioxidant vitamins A, C, and E (for protection from free-radical oxidation), and a full mineral complex (for healthy bone development and tissue functions).

SOLARAY, NUTRACEUTICAL CORP., P.O. Box 681869, Park City, UT 84068; tel: 800-669-8877.

Children's Defense Formula: Capsules. Dietary supplement to combat colds, flu, and infections; also promotes normal healing; contains a blend of essential nutrients, herbs, glandular extracts, and plant enzymes, which help young bodies to break down and absorb nutrients.

PREVAIL CORP., 2204-8 Northwest Birdsdale, Gresham, OR 97030; tel: 800-248-0885 or 503-667-5527.

Children's Digestive Formula: Capsules. Mealtime supplement with plant enzymes to help break down foods so that children can better absorb nutrients.

PREVAIL CORP., 2204-8 Northwest Birdsdale, Gresham, OR 97030; tel: 800-248-0885 or 503-667-5527.

Children's Liquid Multivitamin (Kindervital). Contains calcium, vitamins A, C, D, E, and the B vitamins, plus derivatives from herb and fruit extracts; easily absorbed by the child's body.

FLORA INC., 805 East Badger Road, Lynden, WA 98264; tel: 800-446-2110 or 360-354-2110.

Children's Multi-Vitamin and Minerals: Capsules. Ingredients include vitamins, minerals, plant enzymes to promote absorption of other nutrients; especially developed for children ages 4-14.

PREVAIL CORP., 2204-8 Northwest Birdsdale, Gresham, OR 97030; tel: 800-248-0885 or 503-667-5527.

Children's Probiotic: Powder. Dairy-free blend for children; delivers healthy bacteria to the upper intestinal tract.

NF FORMULAS, INC., 9755 Southwest Commerce Circle C-5, Wilsonville, OR 97070; tel: 800-547-4891 or 503-682-9755.

Children's Tasty Chewable: Tablets. Vitamin and mineral combination that provides a balanced formula for children.

NATURE'S PLUS, 548 Broadhollow Road, Melville, NY 11747-3708; tel: 800-645-9500 or 516-293-0030.

Children's Vita-Gels: Softgels. Multivitamin/multimineral formula.

NATURE'S PLUS, 548 Broadhollow Road, Melville, NY 11747-3708; tel: 800-645-9500 or 516-293-0030.

Cocyntal: Homeopathic liquid. For babies with colic.

BOIRON, 6 Campus Boulevard, Building A, Newtown Square, PA 19073; tel: 800-264-7661 or 610-325-7464.

Colic: Tablets. Soothes and quiets babies with mild indigestion and sudden gas pains.

P & S LABS, 210 West 131st Street, Los Angeles, CA 90061; tel: 800-624-9659 or 310-768-0700.

Cough Calm: Syrup. Ingredients include organic alfalfa, honey, and vegetable glycerine; inappropriate for children under the age of one due to the honey content.

NATURE'S APOTHECARY, P.O. Box 17970, Boulder, CO 80308; tel: 800-999-7422 or 303-664-1600.

Cough Syrup with Honey. Cough remedy for children using safe, natural ingredients in a honey syrup.

P & S LABS, 210 West 131st Street, Los Angeles, CA 90061; tel: 800-624-9659 or 310-768-0700.

C-Plus Cold: Tablets. Contains three homeopathic botanicals and a potassium compound, which relieves sneezing or sniffling; formulated for ages one through six.

P & S LABS, 210 West 131st Street, Los Angeles, CA 90061; tel: 800-624-9659 or 310-768-0700.

Cradle Cap Oil: Oil or salve. Herbal extracts that support a baby's healthy scalp and prevents cradle cap; ingredients include almond oil, chamomile and calendula flowers, burdock root, and vitamin E oil.

HERBS FOR CHILDREN, 151 Evergreen Drive, Suite D, Bozeman, MT 59715; tel: 406-587-0180.

Defense Syrup for Kids. Ingredients include organic alfalfa, honey, and vegetable glycerine; inappropriate for children under age one due to the honey content.

NATURE'S APOTHECARY, P.O. Box 17970, Boulder, CO 80308; tel: 800-999-7422 or 303-664-1600.

Dino-Echinacea: Liquid or chewable tablets. Designed to boost the immune system and get children through the cold and flu season.

NUTRITION NOW, 501 Southeast Columbia Shore Boulevard #350, Vancouver, WA 98661; tel: 800-929-0418 or 360-737-6800.

Eardrops. Contains 1% grapefruit extract in a base of tea tree oil and vegetable glycerine.

NUTRIBIOTIC, NUTRITION RESOURCES, INC., P.O. Box 238, Lakeport, CA 95453; tel: 800-225-4345 or 707-263-0411.

Echinacea/Astragalus Blend: Liquid. Supports the healthy functioning of the immune system; ingredients include the herbs *Echinacea purpurea* root, astragalus root, peppermint leaf, cleavers, lemon balm, and burdock root.

HERBS FOR CHILDREN, 151 Evergreen Drive, Suite D, Bozeman, MT 59715; tel: 406-587-0180.

Echinacea/Eyebright Blend: Liquid. Supports the immune system and sinus organs; ingredients include the herbs peppermint leaf, *Echinacea purpurea* root, eyebright, Oregon grape root, boneset, and garden sage leaf.

HERBS FOR CHILDREN, 151 Evergreen Drive, Suite D, Bozeman, MT 59715; tel: 406-587-0180.

Echinacea Ginger Wonder Syrup. Ingredients include echinacea, ginger, and honey for colds and flu.

NEW CHAPTER, 22 High Street, Brattleboro, VT 05301; tel: 800-543-7279 or 802-257-9345.

Echinacea Glycerites: Liquid. Naturally sweet alternative to the traditional bitter-tasting echinacea liquid supplements.

PLANETARY FORMULAS, 23 Janis Way, Scotts Valley, CA 95066; tel: 800-606-6226.

Echinacea/Golden Root Blend: Liquid. Herbal extract that supports the body's ability to resist pathogens; contains echinacea root, Oregon grape root; available in natural blackberry or orange flavors.

HERBS FOR CHILDREN, 151 Evergreen Drive, Suite D, Bozeman, MT 59715; tel: 406 587-0180.

Echinacea Jr. Liquid. Moderate-potency echinacea formula for kids; contains organically grown echinacea flowers, leaves, and roots in a base of glycerine, honey, and orange oil; safe for children over the age of one.

RAINBOW LIGHT, P.O. Box 600, Santa Cruz, CA 95061; tel: 800-635-1233 or 408-429-9089.

Floradix Iron Plus Herbs: Liquid. Contains organic iron, extracts of herbs, fruits, vitamins, cultured yeast, ocean kelp, extracts of wheat germ, and rose hips; easily and completely absorbed, does not cause constipation. Also available without yeast or added sugar or honey as the product Floravital Iron Plus Herbs.

FLORA INC., 805 East Badger Road, Lynden, WA 98264; tel: 800-446-2110 or 360-354-2110.

Gum-omile Oil: Oil or salve. Herbal extract that supports healthy functioning of gums during teething; ingredients include almond oil, willow bark, chamomile flowers, clove bud oil, and vitamin E oil.

HERBS FOR CHILDREN, 151 Evergreen Drive, Suite D, Bozeman, MT 59715; tel: 406-587-0180.

Han's Natural Honey Loquat Syrup. Chinese herbal beverage containing loquat, a sweet tasting fruit, in a base of honey; provides cool and soothing sensation for sore and irritated throats; alcohol-free.

PRINCE OF PEACE ENTERPRISES, INC., 3450 Third Street #3G, San Francisco, CA 94124; tel: 800-PEACE2U (732-2328).

Herbal Cough Expectorant: Liquid. Helps with symptoms of colds and flu, such as coughs and sore throats; ingredients include clover honey, solid extract white pine, slippery elm bark, and the oils of eucalyptus, camphor, and anise.

PHILLIPS NUTRITIONALS, 27071 Cabot Road #122, Laguna Hills, CA 92653; tel: 800-514-5115 or 702-898-8141.

Horehound Blend: Liquid. Herbal extract that supports the respiratory system and linings of the lungs; ingredients include mullein leaf, astragalus root, horehound herb, garden sage leaf, orange peel, Oregon grape root, and ginger root.

HERBS FOR CHILDREN, 151 Evergreen Drive, Suite D, Bozeman, MT 59715; tel: 406-587-0180.

Maxi Baby-C: Liquid. Safe, non-irritating formula for babies who need extra vitamin C; natural cherry flavor.

COUNTRY LIFE, 101 Corporate Drive, Hauppauge, NY 11788; tel: 800-645-5768 or 516-231-1031.

Maxi Bears Vitamins and Mineral Formula: Gummy chewable tablets. Multivitamin for children; sweetened with fruit juices from oranges, cherries, lemons, and berries.

COUNTRY LIFE, 101 Corporate Drive, Hauppauge, NY 11788; tel: 800-645-5768 or 516-231-1031.

Minty Ginger: Liquid. Herbal extract for digestive support; ingredients include peppermint leaf, fennel seed, chamomile flowers, papaya leaf, ginger root, and orange peel.

HERBS FOR CHILDREN, 151 Evergreen Drive, Suite D, Bozeman, MT 59715; tel: 406-587-0180.

NatureSoothe Sore Throat Syrup. For relief of sore throat pain and irritation due to coughs, hoarseness, or dryness; ingredients include slippery elm (*Ulmus rubra*) inner bark, loquat (*Eriobotrya japonica*) leaves, licorice, ginger, peppermint, and fritillaria bulb (a bulbous lily plant) in a honey base.

PRINCE OF PEACE ENTERPRISES, INC., 3450 Third Street #3G, San Francisco, CA 94124; tel: 800-PEACE2U (732-2328).

NutriStars: Chewable tablets. Comprehensive blend of vitamins and minerals, antioxidants, FOS (fructo-oligosaccharides), plant-source enzymes, supporting herbs, vegetable concentrates, and superfoods for kids of all ages.

KLABIN MARKETING, 2067 Broadway #700, New York, NY 10023; tel: 800-933-9440 or 212-877-3632.

Pedi-Active A.D.D.: Chewable tablets or sublingual spray. Contains the brain nutrients phosphatidyl serine, DMAE (an amino acid from soybeans), and activated soy phosphatides, such as phosphatidyl choline.

NATURE'S PLUS, 548 Broadhollow Road, Melville, NY 11747-3708; tel: 800-645-9500 or 516-293-0030.

Primadophilus Junior: Capsules or powder. Contains a minimum potency of 5.2 billion *Bifidobacterium* and *Lactobacillus* microorganisms per gram (1 billion per capsule) at the time of manufacture; easy-to-swallow, for ages 6-12.
NATURE'S WAY PRODUCTS, INC., 10 Mountain Springs Parkway, Springville UT 84663; tel: 800-962-8873 or 801-489-1500.

Pulsatilla: Homeopathic remedy. Helpful for moodiness, colds, cough, earache, bedwetting, chicken pox, indigestion, and styes in upper eyelid.
STANDARD HOMEOPATHIC CO., 201 West 131st, Los Angeles, CA 90061; tel: 800-624-9659 or 310-768-0700.

Quietussin: Syrup. Expectorant and antitussive (anti-cough) to help reduce coughs and mucous congestion and soothe throat irritation; also aids wet and dry coughs in children aged two and older; contains Chinese herbs fritillaria bulb and loquat, with vitamin C and natural cherry flavor in honey-syrup base.
ZAND HERBAL FORMULAS, 1722 14th Street #230, Boulder, CO 80302; tel: 800-800-0405 or 303-786-8558.

Quintessence Garliphants: Capsules. Multiple vitamin with organic garlic and FOS (fructo-oligosaccharides); provides 100% of the recommended daily value of vitamins A, B6, B12, C, D, and E, thiamin, riboflavin, niacinamide, folic acid, biotin, and pantothenic acid; no added iron.
PURE-GAR, 21411 Prairie Street, Chatsworth, CA 91311; tel: 800-537-7695 or 818 739-6046.

SAF for Kids: Capsules. Contains vitamins, minerals, herbs, and amino acids for a healthy child.
NATROL, INC., 21411 Prairie Street, Chatsworth, CA 91311; tel: 818-739-6000.

SleepRelax by Farmacopia: Capsules. Contains pure kava-kava herbal extract, traditionally used in the Pacific Islands for calming restless or anxious children and inducing sleep.
BOTANICAL PRODUCTS INTERNATIONAL, P.O. Box 174, Hakalau, HI 96710; tel: 808-963-6771.

Super Kids Throat Spray. Herbal extract for healthy functioning of the throat and respiratory membranes; ingredients include *Echinacea purpurea* root, rose hips, licorice root, thyme leaf, and essential oil of peppermint and eucalyptus.

HERBS FOR CHILDREN, 151 Evergreen Drive, Suite D, Bozeman, MT 59715; tel: 406-587-0180.

Tall Tree: Chewable tablets. Daily multiple supplement containing vitamins and minerals with natural orange and pineapple flavors, sweetened with fructose and honey.

COUNTRY LIFE, 101 Corporate Drive, Hauppauge, NY 11788; tel: 800-645-5768 or 516-231-1031.

Teething: Homeopathic tablets. Relieves the restlessness, peevish whining, and irritability associated with teething.

P & S LABS, 210 West 131st Street, Los Angeles, CA 90061; tel: 800-624-9659 or 310-768-0700.

Uncle Val: Liquid. Supports the healthy functioning of the nervous system; recommended for older children or for nighttime use; ingredients include skullcap herb, chamomile flowers, valerian root, fennel seed, hops, and catnip herb.

HERBS FOR CHILDREN, 151 Evergreen Drive, Suite D, Bozeman, MT 59715; tel: 406-587-0180.

Valerian and Chamomile Plus Calcium: Softgels. Contains standardized extracts of valerian and chamomile, which have a calming effect, plus calcium.

J.R. CARLSON LABS, INC., 15 College Drive, Arlington Heights, IL 60004-1985; tel: 800-323-4141 or 708-255-1600.

Willow/Garlic Ear Oil: Oil or salve. Supports the healthy functioning of the ears; ingredients include olive oil, fresh garlic cloves, calendula flowers, willow bark, usnea lichen, and vitamin E oil.

HERBS FOR CHILDREN, 151 Evergreen Drive, Suite D, Bozeman, MT 59715; tel: 406-587-0180.

Cholesterol, Elevated

High cholesterol as an increased risk for heart disease refers to the ratio between the two kinds of cholesterol: low-density lipoprotein or LDL and high-density lipoprotein or HDL (SEE QUICK DEFINITION). A high ratio of LDLs, which initiate the formation of plaque on arterial walls, to HDLs, which help rid the body of excess cholesterol, is what contributes to heart disease, because plaque buildup interferes with blood circulation. High cholesterol is also a causal factor in gallstones, impotence, mental impairment, and colon, prostate, and breast cancers.[53]

Causes of Elevated Cholesterol

Contrary to conventional wisdom, dietary fats are not universal culprits in raising cholesterol. It is the type of fat consumed that is the issue—the kinds to avoid are saturated fats and trans-fatty acids. A high intake of saturated fats from animal sources is associated with high LDL cholesterol. Consumption of trans-fatty acids (a hydrogenated oil found in margarine, most frying oils, and other processed foods) can also contribute to cholesterol problems by blocking the normal digestion pathways of essential fatty acids.[54]

Nutrients and Herbs for Elevated Cholesterol

■ **Vitamin C and niacin:** known to elevate HDL levels; niacin also works to lower LDL levels.[55]

■ **Inositol hexaniacinate:** a form of niacin (vitamin B3) which can lower cholesterol more effectively than standard niacin and without the flushing associated with that supplement.[56]

■ **Beta-sitosterol:** nutrient-containing plant sterol (substance related to fats) which decreases absorption of cholesterol in the intestines; a dose of 3 g daily can reduce cholesterol absorption by 50%.[57]

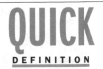

DEFINITION

Lipoproteins occur in two principal forms: low- and high-density. Low-density lipoproteins (LDLs), which are made from protein and fat molecules, circulate in the blood and act as the primary carriers of cholesterol to the cells of the body. An elevated level of LDL, often called "bad" cholesterol, contributes to atherosclerosis (a buildup of plaque deposits on the inner walls of the arteries). High-density lipoproteins (HDLs) readily absorb cholesterol and related compounds in the blood and transport them to the liver for elimination. HDL, or "good" cholesterol, may also be able to take cholesterol from plaque deposits on the artery walls, thus helping to reverse the process of atherosclerosis. A higher ratio of HDL to LDL cholesterol in the blood is associated with a reduced risk of cardiovascular disease.

See **Heart Disease**,
pp. 230-237.

For more about
cholesterol, see
*Alternative Medicine
Guide to Heart
Disease* (Future
Medicine Publishing,
1998; ISBN 1-
887299-10-6); to
order, call
800-333-HEAL.

■ **Enzymes:** lipase digests and breaks down fat and cholesterol.

■ **Fiber:** assists in decreasing cholesterol absorption from food and lowering cholesterol levels; sources of fiber include grapefruit, apple, or vegetable pectin, guar gum, psyllium husks, oat bran, and alfalfa seeds.[58]

■ **Lecithin (phosphatidyl choline):** lowers cholesterol and breaks down fat.

■ **Garlic:** lowers cholesterol and blood pressure.

■ **Gugulipid:** an Ayurvedic (traditional Indian) medicine which can reduce LDL levels while raising HDL levels.[59]

Products for Elevated Cholesterol

Celium Premium and Celium Premium Orange: Powder. Provide daily dose of soluble fiber (psyllium) to aid regularity and to help lower LDL "bad" cholesterol levels by up to 20%.

SIERRA HEALTH PRODUCTS, INC., 7949 Woodley Avenue, Van Nuys, CA 91406; tel: 818-375-5029.

Cholessterol: Tablets. Helps lower LDL cholesterol levels and inhibit the body's ability to absorb dietary fat and cholesterol; contains beta-sitosterol (derived from soy or rice) and pectin (derived from apple and citrus rinds), which binds to the fat in the gut and prevents it from passing through the wall of the intestines. According to clinical studies, patients using this product lowered their cholesterol more than 15% without altering their diet.

WGI, 35008 Emerald Coast Parkway, 5th Floor, Destin, FL 32541; tel: 800-854-8353 or 850-654-4744.

CholestaKit: Capsules. CholestaKit Formula I helps bind dietary fats and cholesterol and excrete them from the body and Formula II helps break down plaque in the arteries.

SIERRA HEALTH PRODUCTS, INC., 7949 Woodley Avenue, Van Nuys, CA 91406; tel: 818-375-5029.

Cholestrex: Tablets. Blend of vitamins, minerals and other nutrients that have been shown in scientific studies to lower total serum and LDL cholesterol and increase beneficial HDL cholesterol.

SOURCE NATURALS, THRESHOLD ENTERPRISES, 23 Janis Way, Scotts Valley, CA 95066; tel: 800-777-5677 or 831-438-1144.

Choles-Trol Control Rx System: Softgels. Contains herbal extracts, Ayurvedic herbs, fiber, minerals, and other ingredients that help regulate cholesterol levels and promote health.

PHYTO-THERAPY, INC., OPTIMUM HEALTH, 483 West Middle Turnpike, Manchester, CT 06040; tel: 800-228-1507 or 860-647-9729.

Fiber Support Barley Fiber with Beta Glucans: Capsules. Soluble dietary fibers such as beta glucans are important nutrients for maintaining healthy levels of cholesterol in the blood and boosting the immune system; also contains tocotrienols, an antioxidant related to vitamin E.

OPTIMAL NUTRIENTS, 1163 Chess Drive #F, Foster City, CA 94404; tel: 800-966-8874 or 650-525-0112.

KYOLIC-EPA: Softgels. Contains omega-3 fatty acids from Pacific sardines and Kyolic Aged Garlic Extract; recent studies have suggested that the omega-3 essential fatty acids have an effect in lowering blood pressure and cholesterol, decreasing the tendency for blood to clot, reducing triglycerides, and helping prevent tumor development and metastasis (the spreading of a tumor from its original site to distant sites).

WAKUNAGA OF AMERICA, 23501 Madero, Mission Viejo, CA 92691; tel: 800-421-2998 or 949-855-2776.

Lipex: Powder. Supports metabolism of fat and cholesterol; contains lecithin, carrageenan, niacin, vitamin B6, and guar gum.

AMNI, 2247 National Avenue, Hayward, CA 94540-5012; tel: 800-437-8888 or 510-783-6969.

Lipid #18: Tablets. Contains inositol hexaniacinate, a new and better-tolerated form of niacin (a B vitamin); also includes garlic, chromium picolinate, and pantethine (precursor to co-enzyme A).

ATKINS NUTRITIONALS, INC., 185 Oser Avenue, Hauppauge, NY 11788; tel: 800-628-5467 or 516-951-7171; or CANADIAN AMERICAN RESOURCES, 327 West Fayette Street, Suite 211, Syracuse, NY 13202; tel: 315-476-4944.

Triphala: Tablets. Internal cleanser to strengthen and tone the gastrointestinal system; for preventative maintenance or for a concentrated cleansing program; provides nutritional support for elevated cholesterol.

PLANETARY FORMULAS, 23 Janis Way, Scotts Valley, CA 95066; tel: 800-606-6226.

Chronic Fatigue Syndrome

Chronic fatigue syndrome (CFS) is an umbrella term for a multiple-symptom disorder characterized most commonly by the sudden onset of extreme, debilitating fatigue, pain in the muscles and joints, headaches, and poor concentration. The fatigue is not alleviated by rest and results in a substantial reduction in previous levels of daily activity. CFS is often cyclical, with periods of relative health followed by debilitation. Other symptoms include depression, anxiety, digestive disorders, memory loss, allergies, recurring infections, and low-grade fever.

Causes of Chronic Fatigue Syndrome (CFS)

There is no single cause of chronic fatigue syndrome; rather, multiple factors combine to overwhelm the immune system and produce the breakdown known as CFS. Prominent among these factors are: concurrent infections, one of which may or may not be Epstein-Barr virus (EBV); candidiasis (overgrowth of the *Candida* yeast in the intestines); an underactive thyroid gland; stress; toxic overload; nutritional deficiencies; allergies; and extensive use of antibiotics, hydrocortisone, or vaccinations.[60]

See also **Fatigue**, pp. 175-183. For information on **testing for toxicity**, see Appendix: Great Smokies Diagnostic Laboratory Tests, pp. 484-485.

See *Alternative Medicine Guide to Chronic Fatigue, Fibromyalgia, and Environmental Illness* (Future Medicine Publishing, 1998); ISBN 1-87299-11-4); to order, call 800-333-HEAL.

Treating CFS

Successful treatment of chronic fatigue syndrome includes: eliminating underlying pathogens (bacteria, viruses, parasites), detoxifying the body, boosting metabolism, rebuilding the immune system, and improving diet and nutrition.[61]

Nutrients and Herbs for CFS

■ **Amino acids:** under immune challenges such as a viral or bacterial infections, you may need three to four times the usual requirement of amino acids (protein building blocks), which are necessary for tissue repair, immune system support, and delivering calcium and magnesium to cells. Amino acids are readily digested and assimilated, and do not stress the kidneys as heavy proteins can. The product AminoMune is useful in cases of EBV or CFS.

■ **Olive leaf extract:** antimicrobial used successfully in cases of Epstein-Barr virus, mononucleosis, herpes, candidiasis, and *Staphylococcus* infection.[62] Multiple underlying infections are often present in CFS.

Products for CFS

Adaptogem: Caplets. Combination of adaptogenic herbs traditionally recognized for their ability to help the body adapt to physical and emotional change; particularly recommended after stress, overwork, and overconsumption of sugar and caffeine.

See **Immune Support** in Part III, pp. 462-483.

RAINBOW LIGHT, P.O. Box 600, Santa Cruz, CA 95061; tel: 800-635-1233 or 408-429-9089.

Adrenal Glandular Plus: Tablets. Supports adrenal function; combines bovine adrenal glandular extract and B vitamins involved in hormone production and regulation.

ETHICAL NUTRIENTS, 971 Calle Negocio, San Clemente, CA 92673; tel: 800-668-8743 or 949-366-0818.

ADR-NL: Capsules. Contains mullein leaves, licorice root, gotu kola, cayenne, ginger root, Siberian ginseng root, and hawthorn berries.

NATURE'S WAY PRODUCTS, INC., 10 Mountain Springs Parkway, Springville, UT 84663; tel: 800-962-8873 or 801-489-1500.

Advanced Stress System: Tablets. Contains B-complex vitamins, botanical extracts, and antioxidants to support the body in handling all kinds of stressors, particularly free-radical attack.

RAINBOW LIGHT, P.O. Box 600, Santa Cruz, CA 95061; tel: 800-635-1233 or 408-429-9089.

Amino Acids: Capsules, powder, or tablets. Contains the L form of amino acids naturally occurring in plants and animals.

NOW, 550 Mitchell Road, Glendale Heights, IL 60139; tel: 800-283-3500 or 630-545-9098.

AminoHealth: Capsules. Balanced complex of 18 isolated, L-crystalline amino acids for use during times of stress.

NUTRI-SOURCE, 3290 Cessna Drive, Cameron Park, CA 95682; tel: 800-293-1683 or 530-676-8838.

AminoMune: Capsules. Contains arginine-free, balanced complex of 18 isolated L-crystalline amino acids and the amino acid L-lysine; for viral infections or underlying viral conditions.

NUTRI-SOURCE, 3290 Cessna Drive, Cameron Park, CA 95682; tel: 800-293-1683 or 530-676-8838.

B-Complex-50: Capsules. Anti-stress formulation of yeast-free B-complex vitamins with biologically active coenzyme forms.

HEALTH PRODUCTS DISTRIBUTORS, INC., 23847 Peaceful Ridge Road, Smithsburg, MD 21783; tel: 800-228-4265 or 301-416-0500.

BioPro Thymic Protein A: Sublingual powder. Activates and increases the number of T4 cells (white blood cells vital for immunity) and allows the body to fight off infections; useful in CFS and any illness involving weakened immunity; contains purified, intact thymus protein.

KLABIN MARKETING, 2067 Broadway #700, New York, NY 10023; tel: 800-933-9440 or 212-877-3632.

B-12 Dots: Sublingual tablets. Contains vitamin B12 (cyanocobalamin), known as the "energy" vitamin.

TWIN LABS, 150 Motor Parkway, Hauppauge, NY 11788; tel: 800-645-5626.

Body Balance: Liquid. Contains vitamins, macro minerals, trace minerals and elements, amino acids, and enzymes from sea vegetation, pure aloe vera, black cherry essence, and raw honey; designed for direct absorption on the cellular level.

LIFE FORCE, INTL., 2731 Via Orange Way #106, Spring Valley, CA 91978; tel: 800-531-4877.

Concentrated Mineral Drop Complex: Liquid. Contains complete, soluble, liquid ionic minerals and trace minerals in the proper balance needed for overall health and the functioning of the body's electrical system.

BIO NATIVUS, P.O. Box 3281, Ogden, UT 84401; tel: 888-628-4887 or 801-732-1294.

Daily Fatigue: Capsules. Vitamin, mineral, and herbal CFS formula.

NATURE'S HERBS, 600 East Quality Drive, American Fork, UT 84003; tel: 800-437-2257 or 801-763-0700.

Enada NADH: Tablets. NADH (coenzyme vitamin B3) is involved in production of cellular energy. Users report increased energy and sense of well-being. NADH is necessary for the synthesis of neurotransmitters (chemical messengers in the brain), which may explain its beneficial effects on mood and mental function.

SCHIFF, WEIDER NUTRITION GROUP, 2002 South 5070 West, Salt Lake City, UT 84104; tel: 800-439-8042 or 801-975-5000.

EnerMax: Liquid. Dietary supplement to support normal energy levels in the body; contains vitamin B12, herbs, and metabolic activators.

NATURAL MAX, NUTRACEUTICAL CORP., P.O. Box 681869, Park City, UT 84068; tel: 800 669-8877.

Ginsana: Capsules. Herbal supplement to improve the way the body uses oxygen, which, in turn, enhances overall physical endurance and well-being. Contains G115, a standardized ginseng extract; not an artificial stimulant and does not contain caffeine.

BOEHRINGER INGELHEIM PHARMACEUTICALS, INC., 900 Ridgebury Road, Ridgefield, CT 06877; tel: 800-243-0127 or 203-798-9988.

Ginsenique: Homeopathic liquid. Increases energy and mental alertness. Contains ginseng, alfalfa, echinacea, oats, and homeopathic dilutions of menyanthese and cyclamen (for headaches due to fatigue) and the mineral *Kali phosporicum* (for mental and physical strain).

BOIRON, 6 Campus Boulevard, Building A, Newtown Square, PA 19073; tel: 800-264-7661 or 610-325-7464.

Herbal Energy Liquid. Ingredients include Korean and Siberian ginseng root, ginger rhizome, oatstraw, milk, schisandra berry, milk thistle seed, hawthorn berry, licorice rhizome, and rose hips fruit, in a base of purified water, brown rice syrup, and natural honey.

NATURE'S APOTHECARY, P.O. Box 17970, Boulder, CO 80308; tel: 800-999-7422 or 303-664-1600.

High Performance Stress Relief: Tablets. Helps the body adapt and relax during times of stress; replaces nutrients that may be depleted when stress challenges adrenal function and increases oxidative free radical damage; contains calming, nourishing herbs with the essential vitamins and minerals.

BIO NATIVUS, P.O. Box 3281, Ogden, UT 84401; tel: 888-628-4887 or 801-732-1294.

Nine Ginsengs by Jade: Liquid or tablets. Chinese herbal tonic to help boost vitality, promote mental alertness and emotional tranquillity, and help circulate and balance energy.

EAST EARTH HERB INC., P.O. Box 2802, Eugene, OR 97402; tel: 800-827-HERB (4372) or 541-687-0155.

Olive Leaf Extract: Capsules. Contains extract of olive leaf with a minimum of 17% of the active compound oleuropein.

SOLARAY, NUTRACEUTICAL CORP., P.O. Box 681869, Park City, UT 84068; tel: 800-669-8877.

For other products for **depression,** see Depression, pp. 155-159.

St. John's Wort Formula: Capsules. For mild to moderate depression, especially when related to chronic fatigue and stress. Contains St. John's wort and herbal energy tonics, adaptogens, nervines (which act on the nervous system), tyrosine, magnesium, malic acid, and vitamin B6 to support positive brain neurotransmitter function and improve low energy.

ZAND HERBAL FORMULAS, 1722 14th Street #230, Boulder, CO 80302; tel: 800-800-0405 or 303-786-8558.

Stabilium (*Garum armoricum*): Softgels. *Garum armoricum*, a fish and salt preparation discovered by the ancient Celts, has been used since the time of the Roman Empire. An adaptogen and antidepressant, garum helps increase energy and stamina, balance mood, and correct sleep disturbances.

ALLERGY RESEARCH GROUP/NUTRICOLOGY, P.O. Box 55907, Hayward, CA 94544; tel: 800-545-9960 or 510-487-8526.

Stress B-Complex: Capsules. Contains vitamins B1, B2, B6, B12, and C, niacinamide, pantothenic acid (d-calcium pantothenate), biotin, PABA (para-aminobenzoic acid), folic acid, choline bitartrate, and inositol.

TWIN LABS, 150 Motor Parkway, Hauppauge, NY 11788; tel: 800-645-5626.

12 Ginsengs: Tablets. Blend of Korean, American, and Siberian ginsengs with other energy herbs.

AMERIFIT, 166 Highland Park Drive, Bloomfield, CT 06002; tel: 800-990- FIRM (3476) or 860-242-3476.

Colds and Flu

A cold is an acute infection—usually viral—of the upper respiratory tract characterized by sneezing, runny nose, head congestion, coughing, sore throat, and watery eyes. Inflammation of the mucosal lining of the nose (rhinitis) typically accompanies a cold. Influenza, or flu, is an acute viral respiratory infection, producing generalized muscle aches, fever, chills, and headache, often accompanied by a cold, cough, and sore throat.

Causes of Colds and Flu

The body is normally able to fight off the viruses that cause a cold or flu. It is when the immune system becomes weakened that a person contracts these ailments. Chronic nutritional deficiencies compromise immunity, as do overworked adrenal glands. Excess consumption or use of sugar, caffeine, alcohol, tobacco, and prescription or recreational drugs can over-stimulate and fatigue these glands, which help the body handle stress. Fatigued adrenals make a person more vulnerable to infection. The symptoms of colds, flu, asthma, and allergies often are greatly diminished when the adrenal glands are nutritionally supported.

See **Immune Support,**
in Part III,
pp. 462-483.

Nutrients and Herbs for Colds and Flu

For any respiratory condition, it is imperative to drink plenty of pure filtered water (six to eight 8-ounce glasses per day) and avoid smoke, exhaust, perfume, and chemical fumes.

■ **Vitamin C:** powerful antioxidant that assists in reducing the severity and duration of bacterial and viral infections, including the common cold.

■ **Zinc:** supplementation enhances immune function.

■ **Adrenal glandular products and adaptogenic herbal formulas:** adrenal glandular products support the adrenal glands and thereby raise the body's resistance to infection. We recommend using only organically-raised, chemical-free animal products. We also like Adrenal Glandular Plus, an adaptogenic glandular formula. Adaptogens are substances that support the body in handling stress. One of the best adaptogenic herbal products we have found is Adaptogem.

For Cough and Sore Throat

Loquat syrup, slippery elm, mullein flowers, and marshmallow root are useful to alleviate a chronic cough, especially in children. Combination formulas that include licorice root (soothing and expectorating herb), thyme (antibiotic and expectorant), and ephedra or lobelia (respiratory stimulant) are helpful for coughs with congestion. Lozenges or liquid throat formulas containing zinc, vitamin C, and slippery elm bark are effective for relieving the pain of a sore throat, as can a gargle made from tincture of goldenseal root or sage. Tea tree oil, an ingredient in some throat lozenges, is a powerful antiseptic and assists in fighting a broad range of infectious agents. Grapefruit seed extract, another good multipurpose antibiotic, can be used topically or internally for sore throats.

■ **Astragalus:** a Chinese herb for strengthening the body's resistance to disease; can reduce the length and frequency of occurrence of the common cold and other viral conditions.

■ **Echinacea:** has a broad spectrum of beneficial effects on the immune system and a history of use in the treatment of flu and the common cold, as well as other upper respiratory tract infections.

■ **Garlic:** helps combat numerous infectious agents, including bacteria, viruses, fungi, protozoa, and parasites.

■ **Goldenseal:** a potent antibiotic and an immune stimulator. Do not exceed a 4-week course of goldenseal unless under doctor's recommendation. Pregnant women should not take goldenseal.

■ **Grapefruit seed extract:** multipurpose antibiotic.

■ **Olive leaf extract:** antibacterial and antiviral; effective for colds, flu, bronchitis, and pneumonia, among other infections.[63]

Products for Colds and Flu

ACES Gold: Tablets. Antioxidant formula that contains coenzyme Q10, vitamins A, C, and E, and glutathione peroxidase support (selenium, glutathione, and N-acetyl-cysteine), superoxide dismutase support (zinc, copper, and manganese), alpha-lipoic acid, citrus bioflavonoids, quercetin bioflavonoid, and odorless garlic.

J.R. CARLSON LABS, INC., 15 College Drive, Arlington Heights, IL 60004-1985; tel: 800-323-4141 or 708-255-1600.

Adaptogem: Caplets. Combination of adaptogenic herbs traditionally recognized for their ability to help the body adapt to physical and emotional change; particularly recommended during periods of stress, overwork, and overconsumption of

---

sugar and caffeine in order to rebuild depleted body systems.
RAINBOW LIGHT, P.O. Box 600, Santa Cruz, CA 95061; tel: 800-635-1233 or 408-429-9089.

Adrenal Glandular Plus: Tablets. Combines bovine adrenal glandular extract and B vitamins involved in hormone production and regulation; nutritional support for adrenal function.
ETHICAL NUTRIENTS, 971 Calle Negocio, San Clemente, CA 92673; tel: 800-668-8743 or 949-366-0818.

Alkyrol: Capsules. Purified and standardized shark liver oil, which clinical studies have proven to be an immune stimulant; helps prevent colds and other infections, reduce symptoms of asthma and psoriasis, and lessen side effects of chemotherapy and radiation treatments.
SCANDINAVIAN NATURAL HEALTH & BEAUTY PRODUCTS, INC., 13 North 7th Street, Perkasie, PA 18944; tel: 800-688-2276.

Alpha CF: Tablets. Indicated for the cold and flu symptoms of sneezing, stuffy or runny nose, coughing, chills, fever, headache, and minor aches and pains; no side effects or contraindications such as drowsiness, excitability, or insomnia; contains no synthetic drugs, antihistamines, or vasoconstrictors.
BOERICKE & TAFEL, INC., 2381 Circadian Way, Santa Rosa, CA 95407; tel: 800-876-9505 or 707-571-8202.

Astragalus Deep Toning Formula: Liquid. Herbal tonic to nourish and strengthen the immune system, energy, and lungs; increases recovery and energy after colds, flu, and illness; lung tonic for people with a history of chronic respiratory problems.
ZAND HERBAL FORMULAS, 1722 14th Street #230, Boulder, CO 80302; tel: 800-800-0405 or 303-786-8558.

Belladonna: Homeopathic remedy. Helpful for sore throat, fever, headache, earache, toothache, and colic.
STANDARD HOMEOPATHIC CO., 201 West 131st, Los Angeles, CA 90061; tel: 800-624-9659 or 310-768-0700.

BHI Sinus: Homeopathic tablets. For temporary relief of sinusitis and rhinitis, headaches, congestion, sneezing, and runny nose.
HEEL/BHI, INC., 11600 Cochiti Road Southeast, Albuquerque, NM 87123-3376; tel: 800-621-7644 or 505-293-3843.

BioBoost: Capsules. Contains echinacea, goldenseal, and antioxidant vitamins and minerals to support your body's natural defenses.

BIODYNAMAX, 6525 Gunpark Drive #150-507, Boulder, CO 80301; tel: 800-926-7525 or 303-530-4665.

Buffered Vitamin C Powder or Beet Source "Buffered Vitamin C": Capsules or powder. Contains ascorbic acid, derived from a hypoallergenic, non-corn source, and buffered with the carbonates of potassium, calcium, and magnesium; some severely ill, allergic, or hypersensitive people are able to tolerate this formulation when unable to tolerate other vitamin C products.

ALLERGY RESEARCH GROUP/NUTRICOLOGY, P.O. Box 55907, Hayward, CA 94544; tel: 800-545-9960 or 510-487-8526.

Coldcalm: Homeopathic tablets. For temporary relief of one or more of these cold symptoms: sneezing, runny nose, nasal congestion, and minor sore throat.

BOIRON, 6 Campus Boulevard, Building A, Newtown Square, PA 19073; tel: 800-264-7661 or 610-325-7464.

ColdCare: Capsules. Relieves cold symptoms of the upper respiratory system without drowsiness; contains 100% of U.S. RDA per capsule, also a good source of vitamin C; no preservatives, sulfites, aspirin, or caffeine.

NATURE'S WAY PRODUCTS, INC., 10 Mountain Springs Parkway, Springville UT 84663; tel: 800-962-8873 or 801-489-1500.

Colds & Flu: Homeopathic liquid. Provides relief for symptoms of common cold and flu.

BIOENERGETICS, INC., P.O. Box 127, Sandy, OR 97055; tel: 800-334-4043 or 503-668-7478.

Cold & Flu: Capsules. Relieves nasal congestion and swelling of the nasal passages, shrinks swollen membranes, and restores free breathing through the nose; ingredients include Chinese ephedra herb, scute, pinella, cinnamon, ginseng, licorice, bupleurum, paeonia, jujube, and ginger.

RIDGECREST HERBALS, 1151 South Redwood Road #106, Salt Lake City, UT 84104-3729; tel: 800-242-4649 or 801-978-9633.

Cold & Flu by Jade: Tablets. Chinese herbal decongestant and pain-relieving formula. Relieves body aches and sluggishness, chills or fever, coughs and lung congestion, and runny nose or sinus congestion.

EAST EARTH HERB INC., P.O. Box 2802, Eugene, OR 97402; tel: 800-827-HERB (4372) or 541-687-0155.

Coldrin: Capsules. Relieves the most commonly described discomforts of the common cold, nasal congestion and discharge.

NATURE'S HERBS, 600 East Quality Drive, American Fork, UT 84003; tel: 800-437-2257 or 801-763-0700.

Cold Sentry: Capsules. Contains vitamin C, bioflavonoids, calcium, zinc, and the herbs garlic (odorless) and echinacea extract.

NATURE'S HERBS, 600 East Quality Drive, American Fork, UT 84003; tel: 800-437-2257 or 801-763-0700.

Cold Zinc Plus Vitamin C: Lozenges. Contains elemental zinc, an essential mineral that helps synthesize DNA and RNA; vitamin C, an important antioxidant for the health of teeth and gums, and for the structure of bones, muscles, and blood vessels; and slippery elm, an herb that soothes membrane discomfort.

IVC, 500 Halls Mill Road, Freehold, NJ 07728; tel: 800-666-8482 or 732-308-3000.

Colloidal Silver: Liquid. Combination of minute, electrically charged particles of silver and pure water that works as an antibiotic and immune system enhancer; use externally for cuts and abrasions; use internally for common colds and flu.

NUPRO, 735-L Park Street, Castle Rock, CO 80104; tel: 303-660-0562 or 800-704-8910.

Congestaway: Oil. Decongestant containing pure eucalyptus, dandelion and olive oils, and flower essences for relief of coughs due to colds, viruses, bronchitis, sinusitis, and lymphatic congestion; can be used as a vaporizer oil during colds and flu; also good for massaging and bathing feet, hands, and body.

OLYMPIC BOTANICALS, 231 Otto Street, Port Townsend, WA 98368; tel: 800-310-6924 or 360-385-9468.

Congest-Ease: Capsules. For relief of sinus congestion and sinus pressure without drowsiness.

NATURE'S HERBS, 600 East Quality Drive, American Fork, UT 84003; tel: 800-437-2257 or 801-763-0700.

Cough & Bronchial (B & T's): Homeopathic syrup. Soothes throat and bronchial irritation, relieves coughs caused by cold and flu viruses or air pollution (inhaled gases and dusts), loosens stubborn phlegm, thins bronchial secretions, and helps clear the lungs of mucus and drain the bronchial tubes; not habit-forming, no synthetic drugs or reported side effects.

BOERICKE & TAFEL, INC., 2381 Circadian Way, Santa Rosa, CA 95407; tel: 800-876-9505 or 707-571-8202.

Decongest Herbal Formula: Capsules. Herbal decongestant containing only four milligrams of ephedrine per capsule; helps relieve sinus congestion caused by colds, hay fever, and sinus infections; provides anti-inflammatory, astringent, and cooling properties to the mucous membranes while reducing the potentially stimulating effects of ephedra.

ZAND HERBAL FORMULAS, 1722 14th Street #230, Boulder, CO 80302; tel: 800-800-0405 or 303-786-8558.

Echinacea Ginger Wonder Syrup. Contains a combination of echinacea, ginger, and honey; helpful during the cold and flu season.

NEW CHAPTER, 22 High Street, Brattleboro, VT 05301; tel: 800-543-7279 or 802-257-9345.

Echinacea Glycerites: Liquid. Naturally sweet alternative to the traditional bitter-tasting echinacea liquid supplements.

PLANETARY FORMULAS, 23 Janis Way, Scotts Valley, CA 95066; tel: 800-606-6226.

Echinacea Goldenseal: Capsules or liquid. Provides resistance during cold and flu season.

FRONTIER COOPERATIVE HERBS, 3021 78th Street, Norway, IA 52318; tel: 800-669-3275 or 319-227-7996.

Echinacea • Goldenseal Compound: Liquid. Remedy for colds and flu accompanied by nasal congestion and other respiratory symptoms; can also be used as a strengthening, preventive tonic for those susceptible to colds and flu; ingredients include echinacea root, goldenseal rhizome and roots, osha root, spilanthes flowering herb and root, yerba santa leaf, horseradish root, elder flower, yarrow flower, watercress herb, and wild indigo root.

HERB PHARM, 20260 Williams Highway, Williams, OR 97544; tel: 800-348-4372 or 541-846-6262.

Echinacea & Goldenseal: Capsules. Immune-supporting herbs to help people through the cold and flu season.

NUTRITION NOW, 501 Southeast Columbia Shore Boulevard #350, Vancouver, WA 98661; tel: 800-929-0418 or 360-737-6800.

Echinacea & Goldenseal Herbal Blend: Capsules. Blend of concentrated organically grown echinacea (*E. angustifolia, E. purpurea,* and *E. pallida*) to boost immunity, goldenseal to help combat infections, and supporting herbs (red clover, garlic, stinging nettles, and ginger to help during the flu and common cold season.

CHAINATA CORP., 5965 205 A Street, Langley, British Columbia, Canada V3A8C4; tel: 800-406-7668 or 604-533-8883.

Echinacea PM: Syrup. Sedating, nighttime herbal syrup that stimulates the immune system to reduce the active symptoms of a cold or flu while promoting sleep; features antiviral and antibacterial herbs to reduce irritating symptoms and nervine herbs to relax the nervous system and facilitate recovery.

ZAND HERBAL FORMULAS, 1722 14th Street #230, Boulder, CO 80302; tel: 800-800-0405 or 303-786-8558.

Elder-Zinc Lozenges. For support during cold and flu season; contains herbs and vitamins, including elderberry extract.

NOW, 550 Mitchell Road, Glendale Heights, IL 60139; tel: 800-283-3500 or 630-545-9098.

E.N. Formula: Homeopathic lozenges. Eases congestion and discharge from the nose and sinuses, which can cause coughing; can be used for infants, children, and adults for an extended period of time.

SUPHERB LTD., P.O. Box 1135, Nahariya 22100, Israel; tel: 800-409-HERB (4372).

E-mergen-C: Powder. Replenishes electrolytes and muscle minerals and fights off free-radical damage; contains vitamin C mineral ascorbates, vitamins B1, B2, B6, and B12, potassium, magnesium, manganese, calcium, zinc, and chromium.

ALACER CORP., 19631 Pauling, Foothill Ranch, CA 92610; tel: 800-854-0249 or 949-454-3900.

Ester-C: Vegitabs. Ester-C, a special form of vitamin C, is bound to calcium to create a calcium ascorbate complex. Ester-C is non-acidic (pH neutral); contains vitamin C, calcium, naturally occuring metabolites of vitamin C, and active bioflavonoids.

COUNTRY LIFE, 101 Corporate Drive, Hauppauge, NY 11788; tel: 800-645-5768 or 516-231-1031.

Ester C Plus: Capsules. Contains a non-acidic form of vitamin C, which has antioxidant, antihistamine, anti-inflammatory, and immune-enhancing properties; strengthens blood vessels; and normalizes high cholesterol.

PHILLIPS NUTRITIONALS, 27071 Cabot Road #122, Laguna Hills, CA 92653; tel: 800-514-5115 or 702-898-8141.

Flu Formulae: Homeopathic liquid. Helps relieve chills, fever, aching joints, fatigue, headache, hoarseness, sore throat, cough, and other symptoms associated with the flu.

LIDDELL LABORATORIES, 1036 Country Club Drive, Moraga, CA 94556; tel: 800-460-7733 or 925-377-3000.

Flu-Tone: Phyto-homeopathic lozenges. Helps prevent the onset of flu or reduce the severity and duration of the illness; contains echinacea; does not interfere with any other medicine.

SUPHERB LTD., P.O. Box 1135, Nahariya 22100, Israel; tel: 800-409-HERB (4372).

Garlic, Echinacea, Goldenseal Plus: Tablets. Contains standardized echinacea extract and herbal blend, goldenseal, garlic, and other herbs.

FUTUREBIOTICS, 145 Ricefield Lane, Hauppauge, NY 11788; tel: 800-FOR-LIFE (367-5433) or 516-273-6300.

Garlic-Power: Tablets. Concentrated garlic extract from a Chinese formula of red and white garlic equivalent to 1,200 mg of fresh garlic; contains higher allicin potential (minimum 3 mg of total allicin potential calculated as allicin content and relative allinase enzyme activity per tablet) than any other garlic supplement; odor-controlled.

NATURE'S HERBS, 600 East Quality Drive, American Fork, UT 84003; tel: 800-437-2257 or 801-763-0700.

Han's Natural Honey Loquat Syrup. Chinese herbal beverage containing loquat, a sweet tasting fruit, in a base of honey; provides cool and soothing sensation for sore and irritated throats; alcohol-free.

PRINCE OF PEACE ENTERPRISES, INC., 3450 Third Street #3G, San Francisco, CA 94124; tel: 800-PEACE2U (732-2328).

HAS Fast-Acting Formula: Capsules. Provides temporary relief of nasal congestion in colds, sinusitis, hay fever, or allergies; active ingredients include plant extract of pseudoephedrine in an herbal base of Brigham tea, marshmallow root, burdock root, cayenne, goldenseal root, lobelia, parsley, cleavers, and rosemary.

NATURE'S WAY PRODUCTS, INC., 10 Mountain Springs Parkway, Springville, UT 84663; tel: 800-962-8873 or 801-489-1500.

Herbal Aloe Force: Juice or topical gel. Processed aloe vera juice containing vitamins, minerals, enzymes, amino acids, essential fatty acids, growth factors, glycoproteins, sterols, bioflavonoids, and polysaccharides (complex sugars), plus ionized colloidal silver and herbal extracts (cat's claw, chamomile, burdock root, hawthorn berry, *Astragalus membranaceus* root, sheep sorrell, pau d'arco bark, slippery elm bark, and rhubarb root).

HERBAL ANSWERS, INC., P.O. Box 1110, Saratoga Springs, NY 12866; tel: 888-256-3367 or 518-581-1968.

Herbal Cough Expectorant: Liquid. Helpful for coughs and sore throats; ingredients include clover honey, solid extract white pine, slippery elm (*Ulmus rubra*) bark, and oils of eucalyptus, camphor, and anise.

PHILLIPS NUTRITIONALS, 27071 Cabot Road #122, Laguna Hills, CA 92653; tel: 800-514-5115 or 702-898-8141.

HerbaLozenge. Available in three varieties: for winter time, Lemon Zinc HerbaLozenge contains zinc aspartate, lemon oil, and menthol in an herbal base; for optimal winter support, Orange C HerbaLozenge contains 125 mg of vitamin C; and to soothe coughs and minor throat irritation, Menthol HerbaLozenge contains 10 mg of menthol in an herbal base; contains no cane sugar, fructose, sorbitol, or artificial sweeteners.

ZAND HERBAL FORMULAS, 1722 14th Street #230, Boulder, CO 80302; tel: 800-800-0405 or 303-786-8558.

Herbal Resistance: Liquid. Contains osha root, lomatium, and echinacea, which were traditionally used by Native Americans for wellness and strengthening of respiratory functions during periods of health imbalance.

NOW, 550 Mitchell Road, Glendale Heights, IL 60139; tel: 800-283-3500 or 630-545-9098.

Hyland's Bronchial Cough: Tablets. For relief of cough due to colds; especially helps coughs with mucus production and a sensation of tickling in the throat.

P & S LABS, 210 West 131st Street, Los Angeles, CA 90061; tel: 800-624-9659 or 310-768-0700.

Hyland's Cough: Homeopathic liquid. For relief of symptoms of cough, especially when assistance in raising mucus is necessary.

P & S LABS, 210 West 131st Street, Los Angeles, CA 90061; tel: 800-624-9659 or 310-768-0700.

Hyland's Flu: Tablets. For relief of symptoms of flu, including common head cold with sore aching muscles.

P & S LABS, 210 West 131st Street, Los Angeles, CA 90061; tel: 800-624-9659 or 310-768-0700.

Hyland's Sore Throat: Homeopathic liquid. Relieves symptoms of dry, sore, irritated throat due to colds, smog, or dry weather.

P & S LABS, 210 West 131st Street, Los Angeles, CA 90061; tel: 800-624-9659 or 310-768-0700.

Katsu Herbal Garlic Complex: Tablets. Concentrated extract of garlic, coix, and rice bran with shark cartilage and vitamin C; garlic is well known for its ability to inhibit bacteria, fungi, yeast (including *Candida*) and parasites (protozoa and worms); promote immune functions; lower cholesterol; reduce platelet aggregation; and aid digestion.

KENSHIN TRADING, CORP., P.O. Box 7511, Torrance, CA 90504; tel: 800-766-1313 or 310-212-3199.

KYOLIC Formula 100: Capsules or tablets. Ingredients include Aged Garlic Extract (a Wakunaga product) plus whey to help normalize colon flora.

WAKUNAGA OF AMERICA, 23501 Madero, Mission Viejo, CA 92691; tel: 800-421-2998 or 949-855-2776.

Loquat Syrup: Liquid. Added to juice, warm water, or herbal tea, Loquat Syrup has a soothing effect on the throat; ingredients include honey, distilled water, loquat leaf, mullein leaf, stemona root, almond nut, ballon flower root, snakegourd seed, licorice root, fritillaria bulb, desert tea herb, and natural mint flavoring.

NATURE'S WAY PRODUCTS, INC., 10 Mountain Springs Parkway, Springville UT 84663; tel: 800-962-8873 or 801-489-1500.

Lymphomyosot: Homeopathic liquid or tablets. For temporary relief of edema (swelling of the tissues or glands) and symptoms of minor illnesses such as bronchitis, colds, and flu.

HEEL/BHI, INC., 11600 Cochiti Road Southeast, Albuquerque, NM 87123-3376; tel: 800-621-7644 or 505-293-3843.

NatureSoothe Sore Throat Syrup. Relieves irritations due to coughs, hoarseness, or dry throat; ingredients include slippery elm inner bark, loquat (a delicious yellow fruit) leaves, licorice, ginger, peppermint, fritillaria bulb (a bulbous lily plant), in a honey base; no alcohol, synthetic drugs, or artificial additives.

PRINCE OF PEACE ENTERPRISES, INC., 3450 Third Street #3G, San Francisco, CA 94124; tel: 800-PEACE2U (732-2328).

Nutussin: Liquid. Soothes, coats, and protects sore throats, and relieves singers' or smokers' dry throats, hoarseness, or loss of voice; contains slippery elm inner bark in a base of loquat, licorice, ginger, spearmint, fritillaria, and pure, raw honey; no alcohol, synthetic drugs, narcotic upset, preservatives, sucrose, or artificial colors.

NATURE'S HERBS, 600 East Quality Drive, American Fork, UT 84003; tel: 800-437-2257 or 801-763-0700.

Olive Leaf Extract: Capsules. Contains olive leaf extract guaranteed to contain a minimum of 17% (42.5 mg) of the active compound oleuropein.

SOLARAY, NUTRACEUTICAL CORP., P.O. Box 681869, Park City, UT 84068; tel: 800-669-8877.

Oregamax: Contains crushed wild oregano, rhus cariaria, garlic, and onion; wild oregano contains the active ingredients carvacrol (antimicrobial), bioflavonoids (antiseptic), and terpenes (anti-inflammatory).

PURITY PRODUCTS, 1804 Plaza Avenue, New Hyde Park, NY 11040; tel: 800-769-7873.

Oscillococcinum: Homeopathic tablets. Relieves flu symptoms such as fever, chills, and body aches and pains; all-natural ingredients, does not cause drowsiness, dizziness, addiction, or side effects.

BOIRON, 6 Campus Boulevard, Building A, Newtown Square, PA 19073; tel: 800-264-7661 or 610-325-7464.

OptiZinc: Tablets. Contains zinc combined with the essential amino acid methionine. Zinc is necessary for over 100 different enzyme systems, the health of the thymus gland and skin, wound-healing, and carbohydrate metabolism.

SOURCE NATURALS, THRESHOLD ENTERPRISES, 23 Janis Way, Scotts Valley, CA 95066; tel: 800-777-5677 or 831-438-1144.

Oxy-Caps by Earth's Bounty: Capsules. Releases molecular oxygen once it comes in contact with the stomach's hydrochloric acid; increased levels of oxygen can help the body work more efficiently and neutralize anaerobic bacteria.

MATRIX HEALTH PRODUCTS, 8400 Magnolia Avenue, Suite N, Santee, CA 92071; tel: 800-736-5609 or 619-448-7550.

PineBros: Liquid. Contains zinc, vitamin C, and slippery elm bark.

IVC, 500 Halls Mill Road, Freehold, NJ 07728; tel: 800-666-8482 or 732-308-3000.

Propolis Echinacea Herbal Throat Spray. Antiseptic, analgesic, and anti-inflammatory for inflamed and infected tissues of mouth, gums, throat, skin, and enlarged tonsils of tonsillitis; fights infection, relieves swelling, and soothes pain; contains echinacea seed, propolis resin, hyssop leaf and flower, sage leaf, St. John's wort flower and bud, and vegetable glycerine.

HERB PHARM, 20260 Williams Highway, Williams, OR 97544; tel: 800-348-4372 or 541-846-6262.

ProSeed Grapefruit Seed Extract: Liquid. Multi-purpose concentrate containing grapefruit seed extract; useful as a sore throat gargle, dental rinse, and for numerous skin and scalp conditions; also can be used as a broad-spectrum food cleanser.

IMHOTEP, INC., P.O. Box 183, Ruby, NJ 12475; tel: 800-677-8577 or 914-336-2070.

ProSeed Throat Relief: Spray. Contains concentrated extracts of *Echinacea purpurea*, calendula, aloe vera, and grapefruit seed extract in a base of pure vegetable glycerine to target dry, scratchy, and raw throats.

IMHOTEP, INC., P.O. Box 183, Ruby, NJ 12475; tel: 800-677-8577 or 914-336-2070.

Quietussin: Syrup. Expectorant and antitussive (anti-cough) to help reduce coughs and mucus congestion and soothe throat irritation; also aids wet and dry coughs in adults and children ages two and older;

contains the Chinese herbs fritillaria bulb and loquat with vitamin C and natural cherry flavor in honey-syrup base.

ZAND HERBAL FORMULAS, 1722 14th Street #230, Boulder, CO 80302; tel: 800-800-0405 or 303-786-8558.

Roxalia: Tablets. Helps relieve minor sore throat and hoarseness. BOIRON, 6 Campus Boulevard, Building A, Newtown Square, PA 19073; tel: 800-264-7661 or 610-325-7464.

Tea Tree Lozenges. Made with tea tree oil and honey to help fight sore throat and soothe coughs, colds, and congestion.

DESERT ESSENCE, 9700 Topanga Canyon Boulevard, Chatsworth, CA 91311; tel: 800-848-7331 or 818-734-1735.

Tea Tree Lozenges. Sore throat aid or breath freshener; contains the antiseptic qualities of tea tree oil with wild cherry, horehound, and lemon balm.

THURSDAY PLANTATION, INC., NATURE'S PLUS, 548 Broadhollow Road, Melville, NY 11747-3708; tel: 800-645-9500 or 516-293-0030.

Throat Soothe: Syrup. For dry, scratchy throats; ingredients include propolis, balm of Gilead, coltsfoot, echinacea, marshmallow, spearmint oil, organic alfalfa honey, and vegetable glycerin; inappropriate for children under one year of age due to the honey content.

NATURE'S APOTHECARY, P.O. Box 17970, Boulder, CO 80308; tel: 800-999-7422 or 303-664-1600.

Throat Soothe: Lozenges. Relieves sore throat pain and other minor mouth and throat irritations; ingredients include slippery elm, which is known for its demulcent (soothing) and emollient (softening) qualities, sorbitol, and natural flavors.

NATURE'S WAY PRODUCTS, INC., 10 Mountain Springs Parkway, Springville, UT 84663; tel: 800-962-8873 or 801-489-1500.

Vapor Balm Salve. Deep-breathing formula; ingredients include essential oils of camphor, peppermint, clove, wintergreen, lavender, and menthol.

NATURE'S APOTHECARY, P.O. Box 17970, Boulder, CO 80308; tel: 800-999-7422 or 303-664-1600.

Veggie Defense: Capsules. Provides dietary and nutritional support for a healthy immune system and for general well-being during cold and flu season; ingredients include vitamins, minerals, bioflavonoids, and herbs.

VegLife, Nutraceutical Corp., P.O. Box 681869, Park City, UT 84068; tel: 800-669-8877.

Warm Herbal Relief: Tea bags. Helps prevent colds and flu and speed recovery; contains echinacea, elderberry, willow bark, vitamin C, and zinc.

Nutrition Now, 501 Southest Columbia Shore Boulevard #350, Vancouver, WA 98661; tel: 800-929-0418 or 360-737-6800.

Wellness Formula: Tablets. Contains a mega-dose of vitamin C with antioxidants, herbs, and other vitamins to provide nutritional protection during the winter months and throughout the year.

Source Naturals, Threshold Enterprises, 23 Janis Way, Scotts Valley, CA 95066; tel: 800-777-5677 or 831-438-1144.

ZincEchinacea: Lozenges. Herbal cold defense that combines zinc with echinacea, propolis, slippery elm, and vitamins A and C.

Quantum, Inc., 754 Washington Street, Eugene, OR 97401; tel: 800-448-1448 or 541-345-5556.

Zinc Lozenges: Contains elemental zinc with the amino acid glycine; suitable for children.

AMNI, 2247 National Avenue, Hayward, CA 94540-5012; tel: 800-437-8888 or 510-783-6969.

Depression

Depression, as distinct from feelings of sadness in response to life events, is characterized by excessive grief, despair, anger, worry, and/or guilt, extreme fatigue, disturbance of normal sleep patterns and appetite, and withdrawal from normal activity. Physical manifestations such as back pain, headaches, and gastrointestinal disorders may also occur.

Causes of Depression

Depression can result from a variety of underlying factors, including mental/emotional conditions, biochemical imbalance, toxicity, thyroid problems, hypoglycemia (low blood sugar), food allergies, or nutritional deficiencies.[64]

Nutrients and Herbs for Depression

■ **Zinc:** deficiency is common in people suffering from depression.[65]

■ **Amino acid tyrosine:** helpful in cases of depression.[66]

■ **Stabilium:** contains *Garum armoricum* (a fish, salt, and herb preparation used for its high nutritive value). Stabilium is an adaptogen (assists the body in handling stress) that can also help balance mood, improve sleep, and increase energy and stamina.[67]

■ **St. John's wort:** has beneficial applications for depression, anxiety, and mood swings established by a large body of research. We have found that St. John's Wort Supreme (formerly Phyto-Proz Supreme) works well for mild to moderate depression as well as anxiety.

Do not attempt to replace your prescription anti-depressant drugs with antidepressant supplements and herbs without the guidance of a qualified physician. Stopping antidepressants abruptly can produce serious side effects.

Products for Depression

Beyond St. John's Wort: Tablets. Contains St. John's wort's active compound (hypericin), kava-kava, magnesium, royal jelly, calcium, vitamin B12, thiamine, and L-tyrosine; St. John's wort helps maintain a healthy central nervous system.

KAL, NUTRACEUTICAL CORP., P.O. Box 681869, Park City, UT 84068; tel: 800-669-8877.

For information on **testing for toxicity**, see Appendix: Great Smokies Diagnostic Laboratory Tests, pp. 484-485.

Depress-Ex Caps. Herbal combination formulated to help maintain peace and calm.

CRYSTAL STAR HERBAL NUTRITION, 4069 Wedgeway Court, Earth City, MO 63045; tel: 800-736-6015 or 314-739-7551.

Depression Release: Homeopathic liquid. For temporary relief of symptoms of depression including melancholy, sadness, despondency, and grief.

BIOENERGETICS, INC., P.O. Box 127, Sandy, OR 97055; tel: 800-334-4043 or 503-668-7478.

5HTP SeroTonic: Capsules. Scientists have discovered that conditions of depression, carbohydrate cravings (with resultant weight gain), anxiety, sleeplessness, obsessions, and compulsions are all connected to reduced levels of serotonin in the brain; if serotonin levels are restored, these conditions often disappear. The amino acid 5-HTP is a precursor of serotonin, and increases its production and availability; contains 5-HTP, St. John's wort and 5-pyridoxal phosphate plus cofactors magnesium hydroxide, inositol hexanicotinate, and calcium citrate.

LIFEENHANCEMENT PRODUCTS, INC., P.O. Box 751390, Petaluma, CA 94975-1390; tel: 800-543-3873 or 707-762-6144.

Mood Balance: Tablets. Helps deal with daily anxiety, stress, and irritability; contains standardized St. John's wort and valerian extracts; calming compounds such as lemon balm, kava-kava root extract, taurine, and GABA (gamma-aminobutyric acid); also contains amino acids that are used to synthesize neurotransmitters (chemical messengers) that support mental acuity and memory.

SOURCE NATURALS, THRESHOLD ENTERPRISES, 23 Janis Way, Scotts Valley, CA 95066; tel: 800-777-5677 or 831-438-1144.

Mood Swing Support: Capsules. Contains St. John's wort, which provides support for mild anxiety and depressed moods.

NUTRITION NOW, 501 Southeast Columbia Shore Boulevard #350, Vancouver, WA 98661; tel: 800-929-0418 or 360-737-6800.

Norival: Capsules. Contains a bioavailable form of the amino acid L-tyrosine, the precursor to the neurotransmitter norepenephrine, the rare vitamin biopterin, which serves as the co-factor to tyrosine hydroxylase and other enzymes involved in catecholamine biosynthesis; increasing levels of norepenphrine in the brain tissues has been used to treat depression. *Authors' note: We have found Norival to be very supportive in some cases of depression. Tyrosine, the amino acid used here, is also known to be helpful for people suffering from Parkinson's disease.*

ECOLOGICAL FORMULAS, 1061-B Shary Circle, Concord, CA 94518; tel: 800-888-4585 or 925-827-2636.

OptiZinc: Tablets. Contains zinc combined with the essential amino acid methionine. Zinc is necessary for over 100 different enzyme systems, the health of the thymus gland and skin, wound-healing, and carbohydrate metabolism.

SOURCE NATURALS, THRESHOLD ENTERPRISES, 23 Janis Way, Scotts Valley, CA 95066; tel: 800-777-5677 or 831-438-1144.

Stabilium (Garum armoricum): Softgels. *Garum armoricum*, a fish and salt preparation discovered by the ancient Celts, has been used since the time of the Roman Empire and traditionally used for its high nutritive value. An adaptogen and antidepressant, garum helps balance mood, correct sleep disturbances, and increase energy and stamina.

ALLERGY RESEARCH GROUP/NUTRICOLOGY, P.O. Box 55907, Hayward, CA 94544; tel: 800-545-9960 or 510-487-8526.

St. John's Positive Thoughts: Tablets. Contains St. John's wort, valerian, kava-kava, and lemon balm with key amino acids, vitamins, and minerals; designed to soothe and uplift one's mood.

SOURCE NATURALS, THRESHOLD ENTERPRISES, 23 Janis Way, Scotts Valley, CA 95066; tel: 800-777-5677 or 831-438-1144.

St. John's Special Formula: Capsules. Contains St. John's wort extract (hypericin), kava-kava, L-tyrosine, DL-phenylalanine, and ginkgo.

SOLARAY, NUTRACEUTICAL CORP., P.O. Box 681869, Park City, UT 84068; tel: 800-669-8877.

St. John's Wort: Capsules. Contains hypericin, the antidepressant compound of St. John's wort (research points to an extract containing 0.3% hypericin for treatment of depression).

BRONSON LABORATORIES, INC., 600 East Quality Drive, American Fork, UT 84003; tel: 800-235-3200 or 801-756-5670.

St. John's Wort Extract: Capsules. Standardized to 0.2% hypericin, the active ingredient in St. John's wort.

NATURE'S SOURCE, 15451 San Fernando Mission Boulevard, Mission Hills, CA 91345; tel: 800-423-2405 or 818-837-3633.

St. John's Wort Formula: Capsules. Contains St. John's wort and herbal energy tonics, adaptogens, and nervines to support the body's effort to overcome chronic fatigue, stress, and weak immunity; also contains tyrosine, magnesium, malic acid, and vitamin B6 to support neurotransmitter function and energy levels.

ZAND HERBAL FORMULAS, 1722 14th Street #230, Boulder, CO 80302; tel: 800-800-0405 or 303-786-8558.

St. John's Wort • Kava Compound: Liquid. Mild sedative, antispasmodic, and muscle relaxant; indicated in depression and despondency, and associated anxiety, nervous agitation, stress, restlessness, and sleeplessness; ingredients include St. John's wort flower and bud, kava-kava lateral root, skullcap flowering herb, and prickly ash bark.

HERB PHARM, 20260 Williams Highway, Williams, OR 97544; tel: 800-348-4372 or 541-846-6262.

St. John's Wort-Kava Compound: Tablets. Blend of Chinese and western herbs to promote mental well-being.

PLANETARY FORMULAS, 23 Janis Way, Scotts Valley, CA 95066; tel: 800-606-6226.

St. John's Wort • Melissa SuperComplex: Liquid. Herbal blend containing St. John's wort, lemon balm, and wild indigo.

RAINBOW LIGHT, P.O. Box 600, Santa Cruz, CA 95061; tel: 800-635-1233 or 408-429-9089.

St. John's Wort Supreme: Liquid. Herbal extracts with antidepressant properties that can be used in conjunction with other doctor-prescribed therapies in cases of mild depression or when being weaned off of antidepressant drugs; can also be used for symptoms related to chronic fatigue, recurrent viral infections (herpes, Epstein-Barr, and hepatitis C), compromised immune systems, or for cancer patients after chemotherapy; ingredients include kava-kava root, St. John's wort flower buds, passionflower, schisandra berry, wild oats, calamus root, Siberian ginseng, nettle seed, prickly ash bark, and gotu kola leaf and root.

GAIA HERBS, INC., 108 Island Ford Road, Brevard, NC 28712; tel: 800-831-7780 or 828-884-4242.

TranQaCalm: Tablets. Contains herbs for support of nervous system and a balance of minerals and digestive enzymes.

BIO NATIVUS, P.O. Box 3281, Ogden, UT 84401; tel: 888-628-4887 or 801-732-1294.

Valerian • Passionflower Compound: Liquid. Gentle, non-narcotic sedative, which is indicated in nervous excitement and hysteria, mental depression due to worry or imagined wrongs, nervous headache, insomnia, and in nervousness associated with menopause.

HERB PHARM, 20260 Williams Highway, Williams, OR 97544; tel: 800-348-4372 or 541-846-6262.

Viva-Lift: Tablets. Isolated, singular amino acid formula of L-tyrosine and pyridoxal-5-phosphate (the active form of vitamin B6); helps with moodiness due to stress or PMS.

THURSDAY PLANTATION, INC., NATURE'S PLUS, 548 Broadhollow Road, Melville, NY 11747-3708; tel: 800-645-9500.

Diabetes

Diabetes mellitus, commonly referred to as diabetes, is a chronic degenerative disease caused by a lack of, or resistance to, the hormone insulin, essential for the proper metabolism of blood sugar (glucose).

Types of Diabetes

Type I Diabetes Mellitus—Also called insulin-dependent diabetes, or juvenile-onset diabetes, Type I usually begins in childhood, but it may occur later in life if the pancreas is damaged by injury or disease. In Type I, the body manufactures little or no insulin. Symptoms include excessive thirst, hunger, and urination, hyperglycemia (high blood sugar), glycosuria (sugars in urine), dehydration, and, often, weight loss.

Type II Diabetes Mellitus—Known as non-insulin-dependent, or adult-onset diabetes, this form of diabetes typically occurs in people over 40 years of age. Here, the pancreas produces insulin, but the body is either resistant to insulin or cannot properly utilize it. Symptoms are the same as in Type I. Diet, nutritional supplementation, and exercise are often all that is needed to control Type II diabetes.

Causes of Diabetes

Although a genetic predisposition appears to govern susceptibility to both types of diabetes, other factors can determine whether or not a person develops the disease or not. Autoimmune processes, in which antibodies created to fight allergies or viral infections react against the body itself, may play a role in causing both types of diabetes.

Type II diabetes often occurs when a diabetes-prone person regularly eats a diet high in sugar and refined carbohydrates or a diet lacking sufficient nutrients. Over time, this type of diet can result in reduced pancreatic activity, which, in turn, causes the body to lose its ability to produce enough insulin. The result is excessive blood sugar levels and insufficiently metabolized carbohydrates that, instead of being burned off, accumulate and are eventually stored as fat. Obesity, a predisposing factor for diabetes, helps advance the onset of the disease.[68] Toxic overload, by impairing the function of the pancreas, can also contribute to the development of diabetes.

Nutrients and Herbs for Diabetes

A diet high in fiber and complex carbohydrates can help improve tolerance of sugar.[69] The following supplements and herbs are also useful for diabetes.

■ **Organic chromium or chromium-rich brewer's yeast:** glucose intolerance is a sign of chromium deficiency. Chromium is an essential component of glucose tolerance factor (GTF), which helps restore glucose tolerance. Supplementing with chromium has been shown to be beneficial in diabetes.[70]

■ **Copper, manganese, and zinc:** deficiencies are associated with glucose intolerance.[71]

■ **Vitamins B1, B6, and B12:** can help reduce diabetic neuropathy (numbness and tingling in the fingers and toes).[72]

■ **Vitamin C:** improves glucose tolerance in Type II diabetes.[73]

■ **Vitamin E:** can improve glucose utilization and insulin action.[74]

■ **Coenzyme Q10:** can help lower blood sugar[75] and is also beneficial for adult-onset diabetes because it plays a crucial role in cellular energy production, helps improve blood circulation, increases oxygenation of tissues, stimulates the immune system, and has various "anti-aging" properties.

■ **Enzymes:** can decrease pancreatic stress and improve the digestion of food, including sugars.

■ **Essential fatty acids (EFAs):** omega-3 EFAs have been shown to decrease insulin resistance and vascular risk factors in diabetics; omega-6 EFAs can reduce diabetic neuropathy.[76]

■ **Bilberry:** can aid in the reduction of retinopathy and small blood vessel disease in diabetes.[77]

■ **Bitter melon and fenugreek:** improve glucose tolerance.[78]

■ *Gymnema sylvestre:* has a general antidiabetic effect on Type II diabetes and has been shown to increase the pancreas' ability to produce insulin in Type I diabetics.[79]

Products for Diabetes

Broad Spectrum Enzymes: Chewable tablets or vegicaps. Enzyme replacement formula for people who eat cooked, processed food; when ingested with food, digestion can begin before the body's own enzymes go to work, reducing stress in the lower stomach and intestines and demand on the pancreas for digestive enzymes; contains protease, lipase, amylase, and cellulase.

Enzymes Inc., 8500 Northwest River Park Drive #223, Parkville, MO 64152; tel: 800-647-6377 or 816-746-6461.

Chromium Power-Herb: Capsules. Complete glycemic edge formula containing chromium and nutrients blended with *Gymnema sylvestre* extract.

Nature's Herbs, 600 East Quality Drive, American Fork, UT 84003; tel: 800-437-2257 or 801-763-0700.

Coenzyme Q-10 Rx (Q-Gel): Softgels. Cellular energizer that delivers up to four times more bio-availabile coenzyme Q10 than other delivery systems and is 100% dissolvable.

Phyto-Therapy, Inc., Optimum Health, 483 West Middle Turnpike, Manchester, CT 06040; tel: 800-228-1507 or 860-647-9729.

Diabetrol: Capsules. Contains GTF (glucose tolerance factor) chromium and vanadyl sulphate, which together help stabilize blood sugar; other ingredients include myo-inositol (a form of the B vitamin inositol), fenugreek, and rutin (a bioflavonoid).

Ecological Formulas, 1061-B Shary Circle, Concord, CA 94518; tel: 800-888-4585 or 925-827-2636.

GlucoBalance: Capsules. Contains micronutrients that help regulate blood glucose; ingredients include chromium (essential for glucose metabolism), niacin, niacinamide, vitamins B1, B6, B12, C, and E, biotin, copper, magnesium, manganese, carnitine, vanadium, zinc, and selenium.

Biotics Research, P.O. Box 36888, Houston, TX 77236; tel: 800-231-5777 or 281-344-0909.

GTF Chromium Complex: Tablets. Helps maintain healthy, balanced blood sugar levels; contains GTF chromium polynicotinate, a key mineral in the metabolism of sugars, and its essential co-factor L-glutathione, in a base of superfoods and herbs.

Rainbow Light, P.O. Box 600, Santa Cruz, CA 95061; tel: 800-635-1233 or 408-429-9089.

MSM (Methylsulfonylmethane): Capsules, eye and ear drops, lotion, or powder. Contains sulfur, which is a major component of the human body. MSM provides the body with building materials for healthy, flexible cells; sulfur is also a component of insulin.

Rich Distributing, P.O. Box 33830, Portland, OR 97292; tel: 877-245-5742 or 503-761-7450.

Regenex: Capsules. Diabetic support formula that helps maintain normal plasma glucose levels; ingredients include ginkgo, *Gymnema sylvestre*, and *Momordica charatia*, which have been shown in studies to be beneficial in maintaining normal blood glucose levels.
SCHIFF, WEIDER NUTRITION GROUP, 2002 South 5070 West, Salt Lake City, UT 84104; tel: 800-439-8042 or 801-975-5000.

Stevia: Liquid. Contains a concentration of stevia (*Stevia rebaudiana bertoni*) whole leaf and purified water. Stevia is a white-flowered herb native to Paraguay and has been used there by indigenous cultures as a natural sweetener; a powder form will soon be available. *Authors' note: Natural sweetener, sugar replacement.*
PLANETARY FORMULAS, 23 Janis Way, Scotts Valley, CA 95066; tel: 800-606-6226.

Stevita Stevia: Liquid. Stevia is a South American perennial shrub with sweet-tasting leaves; helps regulate blood sugar levels. *Authors' note: Natural sweetener, sugar replacement.*
STEVITA CO., INC., 7650 U.S. Highway 287 #100, Arlington, TX 76001; tel: 888-STE-VITA (783-8482) or 817-483-0044.

Ultra Antioxidant Plus: Softgels. Contains pycnogenol, coenzyme Q10, SOD (superoxide dismutase), glutathione, zinc, beta carotene, vitamins C and E, and selenium to neutralize free radical production.
PHILLIPS NUTRITIONALS, 27071 Cabot Road #122, Laguna Hills, CA 92653; tel: 800-514-5115 or 702-898-8141.

Ultra Oils: Capsules. Blend of oils supplying omega-3, -6, and -9 essential fatty acids, which have proven healing and balancing properties.
COUNTRY LIFE, 101 Corporate Drive, Hauppauge, NY 11788; tel: 800-645-5768 or 516-231-1031.

Vitamin B Complex. Tablets. Contains a combination of B vitamins plus catalytic-acting nervine herbs that support the body's nervous system, PABA (paraminobenzoic acid), choline inositol, thiamin (B1), riboflavin (B2), pyridoxine (B6), niacinamide, pantothenic acid (B5), folic acid, cobalamin (B12), and biotin, in a base of valerian root, hops, catnip, chamomile, barberry, and capsicum.
NATURAL ENERGY PRODUCTS, 21101 Welch Road, Snohomish, WA 98296; tel: 425-486-5956.

Ear Disorders

The ear, responsible for hearing and balance, is composed of an outer portion that collects sound waves and the middle and inner ear, which function in concert to convert vibrations into nerve impulses.

Types of Ear Disorders

Middle Ear Infection (Otitis Media)—Infection of the middle ear (otitis media) is often accompanied by an upper respiratory infection or allergy. Symptoms include earache, irritability, fever, chills, and a red, swollen eardrum. In chronic otitis media, fluid builds up in the middle ear due to blockage of the eustachian tube (connects the middle ear to the throat) caused by allergies or enlarged throat tissues. The result is increased pressure, inflammation, and dull, throbbing pain.

Excess Earwax—An accumulation of earwax (cerumen) can block the ear canal and cause itching, pain, and hearing loss.

Hearing Loss—Diminished hearing can be sudden or gradual in onset. Problems that develop over a short period of time usually signify a blockage in either the outer or inner ear. Outer-ear blockages are most often from wax buildup, while blockages of the inner ear are generally caused by fluid accumulation as a result of infection or allergy. Nutritional deficiencies or aging can contribute to gradual hearing loss. With age, the tympanic membrane (eardrum) tends to thicken and lose elasticity, leading to diminishment in hearing.

Tinnitus—Tinnitus is characterized by a continuous ringing or hissing in the ear, sometimes accompanied by pain. Causes include excess earwax, a blocked or impaired eustachian tube, dysfunction of the auditory nerve, decreased circulation in and around the ear (a problem in the elderly), sustained exposure to loud noise, and excessive drug use.

Ototoxicity—This condition is a reaction to drugs that are toxic to both hearing and balance. Symptoms include partial or total deafness, loss of balance, vertigo (dizziness), and difficulty walking (especially in the dark). Some antibiotics and diuretics, salicylates, and quinine and its synthetic counterparts can be toxic to the ear (or even produce permanent hearing loss). Salicylates (sodium salts for reducing pain and fever; the active ingredient in aspirin) can cause hearing loss and tinnitus (ringing in the ears), but these problems are usually reversible. Ototoxic antibiotics include streptomycin, neomycin, kanamycin, amikacin, vancomycin, viomycin, gentamicin, and tobramycin.[80]

Nutrients and Herbs for Ear Disorders

■ **For ear and upper respiratory infections related to food allergies:** vitamin C, *acidophilus* and other beneficial intestinal bacteria, N-acetyl-cysteine (which helps break down mucus), liquid chlorophyll, and echinacea.

■ **For general irritations of the ear, due to hay fever or other causes:** vitamin C, quercetin, and nettle.

■ **For tinnitus and hearing loss:** ginkgo improves blood flow to the inner ear and appears to help best in cases of tinnitus and general hearing loss if the root cause is noise damage or atherosclerosis (blockage of small blood vessels). Black cohosh can also relieve ringing in the ears.[81] Tea tree oil drops, diluted grapefruit seed extract drops, and the herbs goldenseal (*Hydrastis canadensis*) and echinacea are all

Ear problems can also be due to fungal infection. See **Fungal Infections,** pp. 190-197.

helpful for ringing in the ears, clogged ears, diminished hearing, ear pain or itching, or ear infections caused by yeast infections. Zinc and vitamin A are useful for tinnitus and hearing loss and we also recommend avoiding sugar in the diet and common food allergens.

■ **For excess earwax:** large accumulations of earwax are often caused by a deficiency of essential fatty acids.

■ **For age-related hearing loss:** we have found that MSM (methylsulfonylmethane, an organic form of sulfur) in liquid form used as eardrops can be beneficial for age-related hearing loss. Sulfur is essential to all cells in the body and a deficiency results in less permeable cells. MSM produces the effect of easier passage of fluids in and out of cells.[82] In the ears, this results in increased elasticity of the tympanic membrane, which, in turn, may improve hearing.

Products for Ear Disorders

Belladonna: Homeopathic remedy. Helpful for earache, fever, headache, toothache, sore throat, and colic.

STANDARD HOMEOPATHIC CO., 201 West 131st, Los Angeles, CA 90061; tel: 800-624-9659 or 310-768-0700.

Chamomilla: Homeopathic remedy. Helpful for earache, pain, fever, toothache, teething difficulties, colic, and temper.

STANDARD HOMEOPATHIC CO., 201 West 131st, Los Angeles, CA 90061; tel: 800-624-9659 or 310-768-0700.

Eardrops. Healing and soothing formula that contains 0.1% grapefruit extract in a base of tea tree oil and vegetable glycerine.

NUTRIBIOTIC, NUTRITION RESOURCES, INC., P.O. Box 238, Lakeport, CA 95453; tel: 800-225-4345 or 707-263-0411.

Ginkgo-Power: Capsules. Standardized extract of 24% flavonoid glycosides (bioflavonoids) of which 10% is quercetin, in a base of ginkgo leaf; helps increase blood circulation to the brain.

NATURE'S HERBS, 600 East Quality Drive, American Fork, UT 84003; tel: 800-437-2257 or 801-763-0700.

Ginkgo-Go!: Caplets. Daily formula containing 120 mg of ginkgo extract (50:1 extract) per caplet.

WAKUNAGA OF AMERICA, 23501 Madero, Mission Viejo, CA 92691; tel: 800-421-2998 or 949-855-2776.

MSM (Methylsulfonylmethane): Capsules, eye and ear drops, lotion, or powder. Contains sulfur, which is a major component of the human body. MSM provides the body with building materials for healthy, flexible cells.

RICH DISTRIBUTING, P.O. Box 33830, Portland, OR 97292; tel: 877-245-5742 or 503-761-7450.

Mullein/Garlic Compound: Liquid. Herbal ear drops that destroy bacteria or fungus in the ear canal, control inflammation and itching, relieve pain, and soften and disperse accumulated cerumen (earwax); can also help in certain cases of tinnitus (ringing in the ears) and vertigo; ingredients include calendula flower, St. John's wort flower and bud, mullein flower (no stalk), and garlic bulb.

HERB PHARM, 20260 Williams Highway, Williams, OR 97544; tel: 800-348-4372 or 541-846-6262.

ProSeed Ear Drops: Liquid. Contains grapefruit seed extract, mullein flower, and plantain extracts for both adults and children.

IMHOTEP, P.O. Box 183, Ruby, NJ 12475; tel: 800-677-8577 or 914-336-2070.

Eating Disorders

There are two major types of eating disorders: anorexia nervosa and bulimia nervosa.

Anorexia nervosa is clinically described as a self-imposed regimen of starvation, primarily affecting women (95% of all cases), mostly in their adolescence. Typically, there is a distorted body image (believing oneself to be fat when one is actually thin), a dissatisfaction with aspects of the physical body, an obsession with physical appearance, and an intense, even morbid, fear of gaining weight. Anorexics may refuse to eat and choose to exercise compulsively, induce vomiting, or abuse laxatives or diuretics. Other symptoms include a lack of menstrual bleeding, infertility, low blood pressure, fatigue, a diminishment of libido, cold intolerance, and constipation. An estimated 5% to 15% of anorexics die from the condition, 33% by suicide.

Bulimia nervosa, another food-related disorder which typically starts in adolesence or early adulthood, involves binge eating followed by feelings of guilt and shame and self-induced vomiting. The sufferer may also use laxatives, diuretics, or fasting to undo the effects of overeating. Medical risks include electrolyte imbalances and dehydration, leading to further physical complications. Of those afflicted, 90% are women; 2% of the adult female population in the United States meets the clinical definition of bulimia, while 5% to 15% are believed to manifest selected symptoms.

Nutrients and Herbs for Eating Disorders

■ **For anorexia:** zinc deficiency can be a major contributing factor in anorexia; zinc supplementation has proven successful in overcoming dietary deficiencies and in helping anorexics regain their appetite and weight.[83] Copper should always be taken in a balanced ratio with zinc. Recommended daily doses are 3 mg of copper and 50 mg of zinc.

Gentian root helps stimulate the appetite and has been useful in helping anorexics regain their appetite.[84]

■ **For bulimia:** liquid ionic multimineral complex and multivitamin complex supplements help overcome the extreme vitamin and mineral deficiencies associated with binge and purge eating and overuse of laxatives. We also recommend complex amino acids (protein building-blocks) to assist in balancing blood sugar levels, which helps reduce food cravings.

Products for Eating Disorders

AminoHealth: Capsules. Balanced complex of 18 isolated L-crystalline amino acids blended for maximum utilization during times of intense mental and physical stress.

NUTRI-SOURCE, 3290 Cessna Drive, Cameron Park, CA 95682; tel: 800-293-1683 or 530-676-8838.

Concentrated Mineral Drop Complex: Liquid. Contains complete, soluble, liquid ionic minerals and trace minerals in the proper balance needed for overall health and the functioning of the body's electrical system; dosage is a few drops daily.

BIO NATIVUS, P.O. Box 3281, Ogden, UT 84401; tel: 888-628-4887 or 801-732-1294.

Formula VM-2000: Tablets. Multi-nutrient system containing high levels of antioxidants, essential vitamins, and multi-chelated blend of minerals in their citrate, aspartate, amino acid, and picolinate forms; ingredients include B complex, buffered vitamin C, beta carotene, and nine essential amino acids.

SOLGAR VITAMIN & HERB CO, INC., 500 Willow Tree Road, Leonia, NJ 07605; tel: 800-645-2246 or 201-944-2311.

OptiZinc: Tablets. Contains zinc combined with the essential amino acid methionine. Zinc is necessary for over 100 different enzyme systems, the health of the thymus gland and skin, wound-healing, and carbohydrate metabolism.

SOURCE NATURALS, THRESHOLD ENTERPRISES, 23 Janis Way, Scotts Valley, CA 95066; tel: 800-777-5677 or 831-438-1144.

Zinc Status: Liquid. Simple screening method for zinc status; lack of taste or delayed taste perception after placing 10 ml of Zinc Status in the mouth suggests a possible zinc insufficiency.

ETHICAL NUTRIENTS, 971 Calle Negocio, San Clemente, CA 92673; tel: 800-668-8743 or 949-366-0818.

Our most dominant sense, vision, is facilitated by the eyes, two light-receptive organs located in the front of the face. The eye consists of three main sections: a protective layer (including the cornea); a middle layer dense in blood vessels (the choroid) to provide nutrients to the eye; and an inner layer of nerve endings (the retina).

Types of Eye Disorders

Cataracts—Commonly associated with aging, cataracts involve opacity (light blockage) of the lens and/or capsule of the eye, the progression of which increasingly impairs vision.

Diabetic Retinopathy—Long-term diabetes often affects the internal structures of the eye. Blood vessels of the retina may degenerate, burst, and bleed into the internal fluids of the eye, producing spots (known as floaters) and blurred vision.

Dry Eyes—Dryness of the mucous membranes of the eyes (conjunctivitis sicca), caused by reduced tear production, results in inflammation and the sensation of dry, gritty eyes.

Eye Fatigue—Eyestrain or fatigue results from prolonged periods of concentrated eye use (reading, writing, computer work, or driving).

Macular Degeneration—Another condition most commonly associated with aging, macular degeneration involves deterioration of the macula (area of the retina controlling fine vision), resulting in impairment of eyesight.

Night Blindness—Vitamin A is essential in the production of pigments in

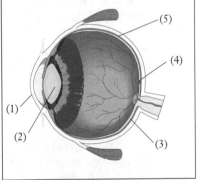

PARTS OF THE EYE. Light rays enter the eye through the cornea (1) to the lens (2) where light is focused as it travels to the retina (3). The retina, an extension of the brain, collects light through photo- or light-sensitive cells. The area of the retina with the highest concentration of photo-sensitive cells is the macula (4), responsible for central vision. Surrounding the retina is the choroid (5), which is filled with capillaries transporting nutrients to the eye.

the retina needed for night, day, and color vision. Vitamin A deficiency can cause night blindness, or impaired nighttime vision, by reducing the ability of the eyes to adapt to the dark.

Nutrients and Herbs for Eye Disorders

■ **For cataracts:** taking vitamins C and E and eating a diet rich in antioxidants (found in fresh fruits and vegetables) can lower the risk of developing cataracts.[85]

■ **For diabetic retinopathy:** magnesium levels are often low in diabetics, particularly those with retinopathy.[86] Ginkgo, which improves circulation and helps prevent free-radical damage, has been shown to aid in degenerative retinal conditions.[87] The incidence of floaters (bits of cellular debris in the eyes), which commonly occurs in degenerative eye conditions such as macular degeneration and diabetic retinopathy, can be reduced by using MSM (methylsulfonylmethane, an organic form of sulfur) eyedrops. Sulfur is essential to all cells in the body and a deficiency results in less permeable cells. MSM produces the effect of easier passage of fluids in and out of cells.[88] MSM eyedrops help soften eye membranes and remove floaters.

■ **For dry eyes:** evening primrose oil with vitamin A works well, since dry eyes can be the result of a vitamin A or essential fatty acid deficiency.

■ **For eye fatigue:** vision complex products, such as Ocudyne and OcuActin, can be effective for people whose work or hobbies produce eye fatigue. Vitamins A and B complex (especially B2) are also helpful for eyestrain.

■ **For macular degeneration:** zinc supplementation can reduce visual loss in macular degeneration patients.[89] Antioxidants (vitamins A, C, and E, pycnogenol, selenium, and carotenoids) can help prevent the free radical damage underlying macular degeneration. Free radicals are operative in all degenerative conditions and need to be inhibited if health is to be restored. Lutein (a carotenoid found in some green vegetables) is a dominant pigment in the macular region (area of the eye's retina). It also helps protect the macula from the harmful effects of sunlight. The herb ginkgo and the product MSM (an organic form of sulfur) may also be effective in degenerative conditions of the retina, which include macular degeneration.

■ **For night vision:** the herb bilberry has an extensive history of use in eye conditions. During World War II, pilots of night flights were given bilberry to nutritionally support night vision.

■ **For vision problems:** micellized or emulsified (both are processes to allow a fat-soluble vitamin to mix with water) vitamin A is the preferred product for vision problems. This nutrient is helpful for conditions of photophobia, the decreased ability of the eye to tolerate light.

■ **For lens protection:** the amino acids glutathione and NAC (N-acetyl-cysteine) show antioxidant properties in protecting the lens of the eye.

■ **For prevention of eye and vision degeneration:** avoid environmental pollutants and be sure to get sufficient minerals, proteins, vitamins A, C, and E, and other antioxidants in your diet. Food allergies and liver dysfunction can also contribute to eye degeneration, so if you have these conditions, it is advisable to alleviate them if possible.

Products for Eye Disorders

Advanced NutriVision: Capsules. Contains high potencies of beta carotene, vitamins C and E, zinc, and selenium, which studies suggest contribute to proper ocular nutrition; also contains the herbs bilberry (rich in anthocyanocide), eyebright, and ginkgo.

BRONSON LABORATORIES, INC., 600 East Quality Drive, American Fork, UT 84003; tel: 800-235-3200 or 801-756-5670.

Bilberry I Sight: Capsules. Helps protect against free-radical damage and UV light damage, nourish the lens of the eye, and maintain normal night vision; also helps the eye recover faster from glare .

NATURE'S LIFE, 7180 Lampson Avenue, Garden Grove, CA 92841-3914; tel: 800-854-6837 or 714-379-6500.

Carotene (Pro-Vitamin A): Capsules. One capsule supplies 25,000 IU of vitamin A activity from 15 mg of beta carotene.

TWIN LABS, 150 Motor Parkway, Hauppauge, NY 11788, tel: 800-645-5626.

Computer Eyes: Tablets. Antioxidants for eye stress and strain.

NUTRITION NOW, 501 Southeast Columbia Shore Boulevard #350, Vancouver, WA 98661; tel: 800-929-0418 or 360-737-6800.

Eye Care Kit: Drops, eyecup, and two filters. Contains herbal combination eye formula and packet of herbs (eyebright, fennel, goldenseal, red raspberry, and bayberry).

NATURE'S APOTHECARY, P.O. Box 17970, Boulder, CO 80308; tel: 800-999-7422 or 303-664-1600.

Eye-Power: Capsules. Vitamin, herb, and antioxidant formula for the eyes; ingredients include beta carotene, vitamins B2, C, and E, zinc, selenium, taurine, N-acetyl-choline, L-glutathione, chromium, quercetin, and extracts of bilberry and ginkgo.

NATURE'S HERBS, 600 East Quality Drive, American Fork, UT 84003; tel: 800-437-2257 or 801-763-0700.

Eye Support: Capsules. Helps maintain certain visual functions through the antioxidant nutrient lutein, a carotenoid (found in dark green leafy vegetables) and a dominant pigment in the macular region (area of the retina) of the eye.

NOW, 550 Mitchell Road, Glendale Heights, IL 60139; tel: 800-283-3500 or 630-545-9098.

Eye Support Formula with Bilberry Extract: Capsules. Bilberry contains the antioxidant compounds anthocyanosides, which help maintain capillary strength and microvascular integrity, especially capillaries in the retina; also contains barberry bark and the leaves of blueberry, eyebright, raspberry, and pulsatilla.

NATROL, INC., 21411 Prairie Street, Chatsworth, CA 91311; tel: 818-739-6000.

Hypericum: Homeopathic remedy. Helpful in eye, nerve, and tailbone injury, dental surgery, puncture wounds, splinters, bites, cuts, burns, and post-operative pain.

STANDARD HOMEOPATHIC CO., 201 West 131st Street, Los Angeles, CA 90061; tel: 800-624-9659 or 310-768-0700.

Lutein: Capsules. Lutein is a powerful antioxidant, which studies show can contribute to the protection of cells; benefits the eyes, particularly in regard to macular degeneration.

SOURCE NATURALS, THRESHOLD ENTERPRISES, 23 Janis Way, Scotts Valley, CA 95066; tel: 800-777-5677 or 831-438-1144.

Lutein I Care: Softgels. Antioxidant macular support with beta carotene, zinc, and copper; helps protect the lens, macula, and retina from damage by free radicals, blue-light, and UV light; also promotes SOD (superoxide dismutase) synthesis.

NATURE'S LIFE, 7180 Lampson Avenue, Garden Grove, CA 92841-3914; tel: 800-854-6837 or 714-379-6500.

MSM (Methylsulfonylmethane): Capsules, eye and ear drops, lotion, or powder. Contains sulfur, which is a major component of the human body. MSM provides the body with building materials for healthy, flexible cells.

RICH DISTRIBUTING, P.O. Box 33830, Portland, OR 97292; tel: 877-245-5742 or 503-761-7450.

OcuActin: Capsules. Supports ocular health, contains bilberry, zinc, and lutein.

NATURE'S PLUS, 548 Broadhollow Road, Melville, NY 11747-3708; tel: 800-645-9500 or 516-293-0030.

OcuDyne: Capsules. Contains vitamins, minerals, antioxidants, amino acids, and extracts of ginkgo and bilberry.

ALLERGY RESEARCH GROUP/NUTRICOLOGY, INC., P.O. Box 55907, Hayward, CA 94544; tel: 800-545-9960 or 510-487-8526.

OcuDyne II with Lutein and Added Minerals: Capsules. The original OcuDyne formula plus six mineral chelates and the bioflavonoid lutein; not a replacement for the original OcuDyne, but an additional formula for those who are taking OcuDyne as their only nutritional supplement.

ALLERGY RESEARCH GROUP/NUTRICOLOGY, INC., P.O. Box 55907, Hayward, CA 94544; tel: 800-545-9960 or 510-487-8526.

OcuGuard Plus with Lutein: Capsules. Vitamin and antioxidant supplement for the eyes.

TWIN LABS, 150 Motor Parkway, Hauppauge, NY 11788, tel: 800-645-5626.

OcuTone: Capsules. Combination of antioxidant nutrients that research has found to be important for maintaining normal eye function; also contains 10 key antioxidants including lutein, a carotene nutrient and major eye pigment in the retina.

AMNI, 2247 National Avenue, Hayward, CA 94540-5012; tel: 800-437-8888 or 510-783-6969.

Optique 1: Homeopathic drops. For relief of eye irritation symptoms, including redness, dryness, itching, burning, tired eyes, and sensitivity to light; no side effects, antihistamines, or decongestants.

BOIRON, 6 Campus Boulevard, Building A, Newtown Square, PA 19073; tel: 800-264-7661 or 610-325-7464.

Perfect Vision System: Vegicaps. Contains standardized bilberry extract, a broad spectrum of carotenes such as lutein, vegetable concentrates, and ginkgo extract for the overall health of the eyes.

RAINBOW LIGHT, P.O. Box 600, Santa Cruz, CA 95061; tel: 800-635-1233 or 408-429-9089.

Sightamins: Capsules. Fortifies the eyes, improve vision, and slows the progression of certain cataract conditions; ingredients include floraGLO lutein (a patented form of lutein), milk thistle, vitamin C, chelated (combined with an amino acid to improve assimilation) zinc, and ginger powder, and extracts of bilberry, grape seed, and cranberry.

PHILLIPS NUTRITIONALS, 27071 Cabot Road #122, Laguna Hills, CA 92653; tel: 800-514-5115 or 702-898-8141.

Strix: Tablets. Eye health formula that improves night vision, and relieves visual fatigue; can also be used in conjunction with conventional treatments for more serious eye conditions; contains extract of Swedish bilberries in a base of bilberry concentrate.

SCANDINAVIAN NATURAL HEALTH & BEAUTY PRODUCTS, INC., 13 North 7th Street, Perkasie, PA 18944; tel: 800-688-2276.

Vision Aid: Capsules. For failing eyesight, eyestrain, and blurred vision; clincial studies conducted in Japan by Dr. Shigenari Ogura (in 1957) and by Dr. Ken Fujihiri (in 1975) had an 80% success rate in treating senile cataracts in more than 700 patients with Pa-Wei-Ti-Huang-Wan (the Chinese formula comprising Vision Aid) for a 12-month period.

RIDGECREST HERBALS, 1151 South Redwood Road #106, Salt Lake City, UT 84104-3729; tel: 800-242-4649 or 801-978-9633.

VisualEyes: Tablets. Formula to support proper eye function; contains high potencies of vitamin A, bilberry, zinc, quercetin, N-acetyl-cysteine, ginkgo, copper sebacate (copper in its most bio-available form), and proanthocyanidins (an extract from grape seeds).

SOURCE NATURALS, THRESHOLD ENTERPRISES, 23 Janis Way, Scotts Valley, CA 95066; tel: 800-777-5677 or 831-438-1144.

Fatigue

A fast-paced, high-stress lifestyle leaves many people feeling exhausted. In these cases, we always consider supporting the adrenal glands and associated tissues with nutritional supplementation. The adrenal glands are responsible for helping the body adjust to stress and emotional changes. The adrenals produce adrenaline, the hormone active in the "fight or flight" response. Chronic stress requires constant production of adrenaline, which was meant to be released in crisis situations, not on an ongoing basis. Fatigued adrenal glands lead not only to overall exhaustion and lowered immunity, but to disturbances throughout the body, as adrenocortical hormones act in nearly all body systems. Degenerative diseases can result.

A diet high in sugar and refined carbohydrates (junk food), overuse of alcohol, excessive caffeine intake, and deficiencies in vitamins B and C can also cause adrenal stress and general fatigue.

See also **Chronic Fatigue Syndrome**, pp. 136-140, and **Stress**, pp. 369-384. For information on a **home test for nutritional status and toxicity,** see Appendix: Great Smokies Diagnostic Laboratory Tests, pp. 484-485.

Approximately 80% of our patients who are suffering from allergies have some degree of adrenal stress or adrenal exhaustion. Constant stress wears down the adrenal glands and immune system. When the immune system is overloaded, allergies often develop.[90] When we support the adrenal glands, the body is better able to handle stress, a burden is lifted from the immune system, and, in our clinical experience, allergies often subside or disappear entirely.

Another cause of fatigue, especially among women, is hormonal imbalance. Again, overworked adrenal glands may be contributing, since approximately one-third of the female hormones are produced by the adrenals.

Nutrients and Herbs for Fatigue

Antioxidant vitamins, especially vitamin C, play a role in easing fatigue. In one study, people with the lowest vitamin C intake had double the number of fatigue symptoms as those with the highest intake.[91]

There are many herbs which can alleviate tiredness. Cayenne, gotu kola, and ginseng are all stimulating, anti-fatigue herbs.[92] Caffeine-containing herbs, such as yerba maté, green tea, guarana, and kola nut, have been used worldwide for centuries to reduce fatigue. Prolonged use of

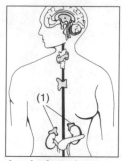

A major factor in cases of fatigue, the adrenal glands (1) are two triangular-shaped glands above the kidneys. They are the body's energy reserve tanks and control all hormone functioning.

any caffeinated products, however, puts stress on the adrenal glands.

The following are supplements and herbs for various categories of fatigue.

■ **For general fatigue:** vitamin B complex supports overall energy metabolism and is essential for red blood cell formation, a deficiency of B vitamins produces anemia (reduced red blood cells); the main symptom is fatigue. Deficiencies in magnesium (which is involved in energy metabolism and nerve function) and amino acids (especially glutamine, lysine, DLPA, carnitine, glutamine, and tyrosine) often cause fatigue and muscle weakness. Iodine is important for the production of thyroid hormones, involved in maintaining healthy energy levels. Kelp and other sea vegetables are good dietary sources of iodine. The herb astragalus is an energy tonic used to boost the immune system and relieve symptoms of tiredness. Ginkgo improves blood circulation and facilitates greater oxygen flow to the brain helping to lift mental fatigue.

Other supplements and herbs: *acidophilus*, American ginseng, antioxidants, ashwagandha, aspartic acid, bee pollen, beta carotene, brewer's yeast, bupleurum, calcium hydroxyapatite, chamomile, chromium picolinate, coenzyme Q10, copper, curcumin (turmeric), dandelion, DMG (dimethylglycine), ephedra, GABA (gamma-aminobutyric acid), germanium, glandular extracts (adrenal, thymus), ginger root, hawthorn, hops, iron (plant source), kava-kava, lecithin, lemon grass, maitake mushroom, manganese, milk thistle (silymarin), octacosanol (alcohol constituent in wheat germ), *Panax ginseng*, passionflower, peppermint, plant enzymes (systemic), potassium, psyllium or pectin fiber product, red clover, St. John's wort, schisandra, selenium, Siberian ginseng, suma (Brazilian ginseng), Stabilium, valerian root, vitamins D and E, wheat germ oil, wild oats, wild yam, yellowdock, and zinc.

■ **For adrenal stress and exhaustion:** Vitamin B5 (pantothenic acid) is vital for the synthesis of hormones and provides support for the adrenal glands. Licorice has beneficial effects on the endocrine system, adrenal glands, and liver; it is often prescribed for adrenal insufficiency. *Panax ginseng* in particular has a nutritive or tonic effect on the adrenal glands.

■ **For female adrenal stress:** DHEA (dehydroepiandrosterone), an adrenal hormone naturally produced by the human body, is a building block of estrogen and testosterone, an antioxidant, and hormone regulator. As we grow older, DHEA levels gradually decline. Supplementation is recommended if over 40 years of age and after salivary hormone test confirms a need for it.

Other supplements and herbs: alfalfa, bilberry, black cohosh (if not pregnant), black haw, blessed thistle, boron, chastetree berry (Vitex), corn silk, cramp bark, dong quai, essential fatty acids (black currant, flaxseed, or primrose oils), false unicorn root, fennel seed, feverfew, genistein, melatonin, motherwort, pau d'arco tea, red raspberry, rosemary, silica, squawvine, strawberry leaf, and vitamin A.

Products for Fatigue

Adaptogem: Caplets. Combination of adaptogenic herbs traditionally recognized for their ability to help the body adapt to physical and emotional change; particularly recommended after stress, overwork, and overconsumption of sugar and caffeine in order to help the body recover after depletion.

RAINBOW LIGHT, P.O. Box 600, Santa Cruz, CA 95061; tel: 800-635-1233 or 408-429-9089.

Adrenal Glandular Plus: Tablets. Nutritional support for adrenal function; combines bovine adrenal glandular extract and B vitamins involved in hormone production and regulation.

ETHICAL NUTRIENTS, 971 Calle Negocio, San Clemente, CA 92673; tel: 800-668-8743 or 949-366-0818.

Adrn-Active Caps. Herbal combination to increase energy, overcome exhaustion, and nourish the body.

CRYSTAL STAR HERBAL NUTRITION, 4069 Wedgeway Court, Earth City, MO 63045 tel. 800-736-6015 or 314-739-7551.

ADR-NL: Capsules. Dietary support for an active lifestyle; ingredients include mullein leaves, licorice root, gotu kola, cayenne, ginger root, Siberian ginseng root, and hawthorn berries.

NATURE'S WAY PRODUCTS, INC., 10 Mountain Springs Parkway, Springville, UT 84663; tel: 800-962-8873 or 801-489-1500.

AminoPlus: Capsules. Balanced complex of 14 isolated. L-crystalline amino acids to assist in maintaining energy.

NUTRI-SOURCE, 3290 Cessna Drive, Cameron Park, CA 95682; tel: 800-293-1683 or 530-676-8838.

Daily Fatigue: Capsules. Vitamin, mineral, and herbal fatigue formula.
NATURE'S HERBS, 600 East Quality Drive, American Fork, UT 84003; tel: 800-437-2257 or 801-763-0700.

Enada NADH: Tablets. NADH (coenzyme vitamin B3) is involved in production of cellular energy and is required for synthesis of neurotransmitters, which may explain its effects on maintaining healthy mood and mental functions; users report improved feelings of well-being and energy; in studies, exercising athletes have shown improvement in exercise performance (better use of oxygen) and improved reaction times (better brain function).
SCHIFF, WEIDER NUTRITION GROUP, 2002 South 5070 West, Salt Lake City, UT 84104; tel: 800-439-8042 or 801-975-5000.

Energy Green Caps. Green foods and herbs for energy and stamina.
CRYSTAL STAR HERBAL NUTRITION, 4069 Wedgeway Court, Earth City, MO 63045; tel. 800-736-6015 or 314-739-7551.

Energy Pak: Packets. Contains guarana, *Panax ginseng*, niacin, a blend of herbs, and a formula of complex carbohydrates, which together support intense athletic training and prolonged vigor.
UNIVERSAL, 3 Terminal Road, New Brunswick, NJ 08901; tel: 800-872-0101 or 732-545-3130.

Ener-Jet: Capsules. Contains ginseng, gotu-kola, *fo-ti*, damiana, licorice, and sarsaparilla, which help promote energy, endurance, and stamina.
HEALTH PLUS, 13837 Magnolia Avenue, Chino, CA 91710; tel: 800-822-6225 or 909-627-9393.

EnerMax: Liquid. Combination of vitamin B12, herbs, and metabolic activators that are intended to provide nutritive support for healthy energy levels in the body.
NATURAL MAX, NUTRACEUTICAL CORP., P.O. Box 681869, Park City, UT 84068; tel: 800-669-8877.

Exsativa: Caplets. Energizer for men and women containing green oats, nettles, and seat buckthorn, which clinical studies have proven to increase energy, vitality, muscle strength, and libido.

SCANDINAVIAN NATURAL HEALTH & BEAUTY PRODUCTS, INC., 13 North 7th Street, Perkasie, PA 18944; tel: 800-688-2276.

Formula B-Complex "50": Capsules. Contains high-potency, balanced B complex and the recognized B-complex factors.
SOLGAR VITAMIN & HERB COMPANY, INC., 500 Willow Tree Road, Leonia, NJ 07605; tel: 800-645-2246 or 201-944-2311.

Four Noble Gentlemen: Tablets. Contains ginseng, atractylodes, poria cocoas, and licorice to strengthen and revitalize.
PLANETARY FORMULAS, 23 Janis Way, Scotts Valley, CA 95066; tel: 800-606-6226.

Ginsana: Capsules. Herbal supplement to improve the way the body uses oxygen, which, in turn, enhances overall physical endurance and well-being. Contains G115, standardized ginseng extract; not an artificial stimulant and does not contain caffeine.
BOEHRINGER INGELHEIM PHARMACEUTICALS, INC., 900 Ridgebury Road, Ridgefield, CT 06877; tel: 800-243-0127 or 203-798-9988.

Ginseng-Gotu Kola Combination: Capsules. Helps supplement the body's nutritional needs during increased physical or mental activity; contains Siberian ginseng (*Eleutherococcus senticosus*), gotu kola, cayenne, and bee pollen
NATURE'S HERBS, 600 East Quality Drive, American Fork, UT 84003; tel: 800-437-2257 or 801-763-0700.

Ginseng Root-Siberian: Capsules. Siberian ginseng is milder than *Panax ginseng* and is often used to increase the body's resistance to environmental and physical stress.
NATURE'S SOURCE, 15451 San Fernando Mission Boulevard, Mission Hills, CA 91345; tel: 800-423-2405 or 818-837-3633.

Ginsenique: Homeopathic liquid. For relief of fatigue; increases energy and mental alertness; contains ginseng, alfalfa, echinacea, and *Avena sativa* (oats) as well as homeopathic dilutions of the plants menyanthese and cyclamen, for headaches due to fatigue, and the mineral kali phosporicum for mental and physical strain due to overwork.
BOIRON, 6 Campus Boulevard, Building A, Newtown Square, PA 19073; tel: 800-264-7661 or 610-325-7464.

Herbal Energy Liquid. Ingredients include Korean and Siberian ginseng root, ginger rhizome, oatstraw, milk, schisandra berry, milk thistle seed, hawthorn berry, licorice rhizome, and rose hips fruit, in a base of purified water, brown rice syrup, and natural honey.

NATURE'S APOTHECARY, P.O. Box 17970, Boulder, CO 80308; tel: 800-999-7422 or 303-664-1600.

High Performance Stress Relief: Tablets. Contains herbs and essential vitamins and minerals required to deal with stress.

BIO NATIVUS, P.O. Box 3281, Ogden, UT 84401; tel: 888-628-4887 or 801-732-1294.

Kijitsu: Tablets. Revitalizer derived from bitter orange, which according to traditional Chinese medicine is an energy regulator, yielding "cool" energy compared to *ma huang*'s "warm" energy.

SYNERGY PLUS, IVC, 500 Halls Mill Road, Freehold, NJ 07728; tel: 800-666-8482.

Korean Ginseng Power-Herb: Capsules. Nutritionally supports adaptogenic function.

NATURE'S HERBS, 600 East Quality Drive, American Fork, UT 84003; tel: 800-437-2257 or 801-763-0700.

Maca: Capsules. Native Peruvians have used Maca (*Lepidium meyenii*) for its nutritional and adaptogenic properties.

PERUVIAN RAINFOREST BOTANICALS, NUTRAMEDIX, 212 North U.S. Highway 1 #17, Tequesta, FL 33469; tel: 800-730-3130.

Maxi-Energizer: Caplets. For active people who need an energy boost; contains standardized extracts of *ma huang*, green tea, and kola nut, L-pyroglutamic acid (L-PCA), and Chinese herbal blend extract (epimedin, angelica, ginger, ginseng), in a base of *acidophilus*. Caution: Individuals with diabetes, hypertension, glaucoma, thyroid disease, or pregnant/lactating women should consult their health-care professional prior to using this product.

PHILLIPS NUTRITIONALS, 27071 Cabot Road #122, Laguna Hills, CA 92653; tel: 800-514-5115 or 702-898-8141.

MetaBoost: Capsules. Combines the thermogenic (heat-producing) and ergogenic (energy-producing) qualities of the botanical extracts of *Sida cortifolia* (a source of ephedrine), *Salix alba* (a source of aspirin), and kola nut (a source of caffeine).

NUTRIBIOTIC, NUTRITION RESOURCES, INC., P.O. Box 238, Lakeport, CA 95453; tel: 800-225-4345 or 707-263-0411.

Nine Ginsengs by Jade: Liquid or tablets. Chinese herbal tonic to help boost vitality, promote alertness and tranquillity, and help circulate and balance energy.
EAST EARTH HERB INC., P.O. Box 2802, Eugene, OR 97402; tel: 800-827-HERB (4372) or 541-687-0155.

OxyNutrients: Capsules. Supports molecular energy production (inadequate production contributes to fatigue); contains malic acid and magnesium, commonly used to treat chronic fatigue; coenzyme Q10, important in cellular energy production; TTFD (thiamine tetrahydro furfuryl disulfide), essential for the brain and nerves; L-carnitine, energy production; DMG (dimethylglycine), vital for synthesis of energy compounds and liver detoxification; and antioxidants.
ALLERGY RESEARCH GROUP/NUTRICOLOGY, P.O. Box 55907, Hayward, CA 94544; tel: 800-545-9960 or 510-487-8526.

Panax Ginseng: Liquid or tea bags. Made from six-year-old ginseng roots that have been preserved using steam and heat; ginseng is considered an adaptogen for replenishing vital energy.
PRINCE OF PEACE ENTERPRISES, INC., 3450 Third Street #3G, San Francisco, CA 94124; tel: 800-PEACE2U (732-2328).

Pfaffia Paniculata (Suma): Powder. Suma has been used to treat chronic diseases characterized by fatigue; provides relief from stress and helps enhance the immune system; it is a rich source of germanium, allantoin, vitamins, minerals, amino acids, and nutrients which help increase oxygen to the cells and coronary circulation.
SEDNA, P.O. Box 1453, Andrews, NC 28901; tel: 800-223-0858 or 828-321-2240.

PowerActin: Capsules. Supports the body's normal energy production; contains standardized Korean ginseng, Siberian ginseng, and *ashwagandha*, with coenzyme Q10 and vitamin B12.
NATURE'S PLUS, 548 Broadhollow Road, Melville, NY 11747-3708; tel: 800-645-9500 or 516-293-0030.

Premium North American Ginseng Pure Powdered Root: Capsules. Helps the body to maintain stable equilibrium when under stress.

CHAINATA CORP., 5965 205 A Street, Langley, British Columbia, Canada V3A8C4; tel: 800-406-7668 or 604-533-8883.

Raw Energy: Capsules. Energy product containing bee pollen, gotu kola, Siberian ginseng, royal jelly, and octacosanol.
PREMIER ONE, NUTRACEUTICAL CORP., P.O. Box 681869, Park City, UT 84068; tel: 800-669-8877.

Stabilium (Garum amoricum): Softgels. *Garum armoricum*, a fish and salt preparation discovered by the ancient Celts; An adaptogen and antidepressant; helps increase energy and stamina, balance mood, and correct sleep disturbances.
ALLERGY RESEARCH GROUP/NUTRICOLOGY, P.O. Box 55907, Hayward, CA 94544; tel: 800-545-9960 or 510-487-8526.

Stamina by Jade: Tablets. Chinese herbal endurance formula to help rebuild endurance, increase energy, nourish reproductive function, tonify the kidney and lung meridian, and support emotional balance.
EAST EARTH HERB INC., P.O. Box 2802, Eugene, OR 97402; tel: 800-827-HERB (4372) or 541-687-0155.

Stress Bee '60' Sustained Release: Tablets. Contains a high-potency B complex with vitamin C for energy, endurance, and replacement of water-soluble vitamins lost during stress.
NATURE'S PLUS, 548 Broadhollow Road, Melville, NY 11747-3708; tel: 800-645-9500 or 516-293-0030.

Stress-D: Capsules. Herbal formula to help calm the central nervous system and support the adrenal glands. Contains Siberian ginseng, American ginseng, magnesium, kava-kava root, passionflower, chamomile, vitamins B1, B2, B3, B5, B6, B12, and C.
BIODYNAMAX, 6525 Gunpark Drive #150-507, Boulder, CO 80301; tel: 800-926-7525 or 303-530-4665.

Stress Release: Capsules. Combination of vitamins and herbs to help replenish nutrients lost during illness, injury, physical overwork, dieting, or lack of sleep. Caution: May cause drowsiness.
NATURE'S HERBS, 600 East Quality Drive, American Fork, UT 84003; tel: 800-437-2257 or 801-763-0700.

T-Charge Plus: Capsules. Formula to help increase endurance and alertness; ingredients include ginseng, kola nut, ephedra (*ma huang*), guarana, *fo ti*, wood betony (*Stachys betonica*), gotu kola, cayenne, and garlic.

WGI, 35008 Emerald Coast Parkway, 5th Floor, Destin, FL 32541; tel: 800-854-8353 or 850-654-4744.

T/Lite Energy: Capsules. Energy-boosting blend of kola nut, ginger root, ginkgo, and gotu kola, which does not contain ephedrine or *ma huang*.

WGI, 35008 Emerald Coast Parkway, 5th Floor, Destin, FL 32541; tel: 800-854-8353 or 850-654-4744.

12 Ginsengs: Tablets. Contains a blend of Korean, American, and Siberian ginseng and other energy herbs.

AMERIFIT, 166 Highland Park Drive, Bloomfield, CT 06002; tel: 800-990- FIRM (3476) or 860-242-3476.

Veratrum Album: Homeopathic remedy. Helpful in heat exhaustion, sudden collapse, headache, nausea, and vomiting.

STANDARD HOMEOPATHIC CO., 201 West 131st Street, Los Angeles, CA 90061; tel: 800-624-9659 or 310-768-0700.

Vital K + Ginseng Extra: Liquid. Energy formula that contains Siberian, Korean, and American ginsengs, potassium, calcium, iron, and 16 invigorating herbal extracts.

FUTUREBIOTICS, 145 Ricefield Lane, Hauppauge, NY 11788; tel: 800-FOR-LIFE (367-5433) or 516-273-6300.

Zest-Aid: Capsules. Energy supplement containing vitamins and minerals combined with energizing herbs.

NATURE'S HERBS, 600 East Quality Drive, American Fork, UT 84003; tel: 800-437-2257 or 801-763-0700.

Fibromyalgia

Fibromyalgia, or myofascial pain syndrome, is a multiple-symptom syndrome primarily involving widespread muscle pain (myalgia) that can be debilitating in its severity. The pain seems to be caused by the tightening and thickening of the myofascia, the thin film or tissue which holds muscle together.

Typical tender sites in fibromyalgia include the neck, upper back, rib cage, hips, and knees. Other symptoms include general fatigue and stiffness, insomnia, anxiety, depression, mood swings, allergies, carpal tunnel syndrome, headaches, the sense of "hurting all over," tender skin, numbness, irritable bowel symptoms, dizziness, and exercise intolerance.

Post-traumatic fibromyalgia is believed to develop after a fall, whiplash, or back strain, whereas primary fibromyalgia has an uncertain origin. The majority of fibromyalgia sufferers are women between the ages of 34 and 56.

Nutrients for Fibromyalgia

■ **Vitamin B1:** supports proper oxygen metabolism; symptoms of a B1-deficiency are strikingly similar to those of fibromyalgia.

■ **Manganese:** supports normal body metabolism and, consequently, normal energy levels.

■ **Cetyl myristoleate:** oil derived from myristoleic acid (found in fish oils and cow's milk butter) with anti-inflammatory and lubricant properties, which can help alleviate the pain and swelling of joints, muscles, tendons, and other soft tissues in the body. Cetyl myristoleate also supports the immune system and seems able to stop the depletion of essential fatty acids which typically accompanies chronic inflammation.[93]

■ **Essential fatty acids:** decrease inflammation and pain in the body by supplying a source of lubrication for the tissues.

■ **Malic acid and magnesium:** helps to decrease fibromyalgia pain; low magnesium is what keeps the muscles in a state of spasm.[94]

See also **Arthritis**, pp. 84-96.

■ **Other supplements:** vitamins B2 and B6, amino acid complex and glycine, antioxidants (vitamins A, C, and E, beta carotene, and pycnogenol), and lecithin.

Products for Fibromyalgia

ACES: Softgels. Contains vitamins A, C, and E and the mineral selenium to help eliminate free radicals; beta carotene (pro-vitamin A) quenches single oxygen molecules, vitamin C protects tissues and blood components, vitamin E protects cell membranes, and selenium is a vital part of antioxidant enzymes.

 J.R. CARLSON LABS, INC., 15 College Drive, Arlington Heights, IL 60004-1985; tel: 800-323-4141 or 708-255-1600.

B-Complex-50: Capsules. Contains all of the B-complex vitamins, which are needed for numerous metabolic functions, including energy, detoxification, nerve transmission, blood formation, synthesis of proteins and fats, production of steroid hormones, maintenance of blood sugar levels, maintenance of the appetite, and toning of the muscles.

 HEALTH PRODUCTS DISTRIBUTORS, INC., 23847 Peaceful Ridge Road, Smithsburg, MD 21783; tel: 800-228-4265 or 301-416-0500.

Cetyl Myristoleate: Softgels. Concentrate from vegetable sources with anti-inflammatory and lubricant properties.

 FUTUREBIOTICS, 145 Ricefield Lane, Hauppauge, NY 11788; tel: 800-FOR-LIFE (367-5433) or 516-273-6300.

Elan Vital: Tablets. Multiple antioxidant that also supports structural integrity, energy generation, neurotransmitter production, and liver health; contains the antioxidants N-acetyl-cysteine, vitamins C and E, beta carotene, and selenium, plus niacin, biotin, chromium, coenzyme Q10, ginkgo, DMAE (an amino-acid complex originating from soybeans), silymarin, bilberry, N-acetyl-glucosamine, quercetin, N-acetyl L-tyrosine, and lipoic and succinic acids.

 SOURCE NATURALS, THRESHOLD ENTERPRISES, 23 Janis Way, Scotts Valley, CA 95066; tel: 800-777-5677 or 831-438-1144.

Flex: Tablets. For tissue structure and connective tissue support and formation; contains manganese and zinc (important for proper formation of connective tissue), pantothenic and folic acid (B vitamins that enable the body to deal with stress and lessen inflammation), NAG (N-acetyl-glucosamine) and glucosamine sulfate (which are the base of the tissue structure forming joints, ligaments, and tendons), vitamin C (which aids in body's utilization of NAG and glucosamine sulfate and helps form collagen, found in connective tissue), calcium, horsetail, magnesium, and potassium.

OPTIMAL NUTRIENTS, 1163 Chess Drive #F, Foster City, CA 94404; tel: 800-966-8874 or 415-525-0112.

Hemp Oil. Source of essential fatty acids for producing energy and maintaining cell structure, health, and longevity; contains a 3:1 balance of omega-6 to omega-3; also rich in active phospholipids and sterols, which promote cell membrane regeneration and improve immunity; does not contain active THC (tetrahydrocannabinol).

SPECTRUM NATURALS, 133 Copeland Street, Petaluma, CA 94952; tel: 800-995-2705 or 707-778-8900.

Magnesium Malate: Tablets. Contains magnesium (45% of the U.S. RDA) and malic acid (found in apples and also produced by the body); malic acid is involved in the manufacture of energy in the cells; it also crosses the blood-brain barrier and has been shown to bind to aluminum and flush it out of the body; by binding to aluminum, malic acid frees receptor sites for magnesium.

SOURCE NATURALS, THRESHOLD ENTERPRISES, 23 Janis Way, Scotts Valley, CA 95066; tel: 800-777-5677 or 831-438-1144.

Malic Magnesium: Tablets. For muscle function; contains magnesium (an essential co-factor for the production of energy in many cells of the body, including muscle cells) and malic acid (involved in the production of metabolites used by all cells to manufacture energy).

ETHICAL NUTRIENTS, 971 Calle Negocio, San Clemente, CA 92673; tel: 800-668-8743 or 949-366-0818.

Max Omega: Oil. Contains black currant seed oil, which is the most complete source of essential fatty acids (EFAs); contains linoleic acid (LA, an omega-6 essential fatty acid) and, unlike primrose or borage oil, alpha-linolenic acid (ALA, an omega-3 EFA). Also, unlike flaxseed, black currant seed oil contains 18% gamma-linolenic acid (GLA), twice the amount in primrose oil.

BIO-NUTRITIONAL FORMULAS, 106 East Jericho Turnpike, Mineola, NY 11501; tel: 800-950-8484.

Pycnogenol & Citrus Bioflavonoids: Capsules. Contains pycnogenol, from pine bark, a powerful antioxidant that crosses the blood-brain barrier helping to protect the body and the central nervous system from the damaging effects of free radicals; free radicals are unstable oxygen molecules with an extra electron that can damage cell walls, proteins, and genetic material.

AMERICAN HEALTH, 4320 Veterans Memorial Highway, Holbrook, NY 11741; tel: 800-445-7137.

Triple Action Antioxidant Plus: Capsules. Combination of proanthocyanidins, citrus bioflavonoids, and vitamin C to nourish the body, enhance joint flexibility, provide protection from free radicals, and promote healthy blood vessels and pliable, youthful skin.

NUPRO, 735-L Park Street, Castle Rock, CO 80104; tel: 800-704-8910 or 303-660-0562.

Ultra Antioxidants: Tablets. Contains 21 antioxidants, including selenium, zinc, grape seed extract, green tea, garlic, and others.

BIODYNAMAX, 6525 Gunpark Drive #150-507, Boulder, CO 80301; tel: 800-926-7525 or 303-530-4665.

Ultra Antioxidant Plus: Softgels. Contains pycnogenol, coenzyme Q10, SOD (superoxide dismutase), glutathione, zinc, beta carotene, vitamins C and E, and selenium to neutralize free radical production.

PHILLIPS NUTRITIONALS, 27071 Cabot Road #122, Laguna Hills, CA 92653; tel: 800-514-5115 or 702-898-8141.

Ultra Oils: Capsules. Supplies omega-3, -6, and -9 essential fatty acids, plant lignans, and GLA (gamma-linolenic acid)

COUNTRY LIFE, 101 Corporate Drive, Hauppauge, NY 11788; tel: 800-645-5768 or 516-231-1031.

Wheat Germ Oil: Softgels. Contain 73% wheat germ oil, which is an excellent source of vitamin E complex, and 27% flaxseed oil concentrate, which is a source of omega-3 essential fatty acids. Vitamin E is an antioxidant that stabilizes cell membranes and protects cells and tissues from damage.

SONNE'S ORGANIC FOODS, INC., P.O. Box 2160, Cottonwood, CA 96022; tel: 800-544-8147 or 530-347-5868.

Food Poisoning

Food poisoning is an acute illness resulting from eating contaminated or infected food.

Symptoms and Causes of Food Poisoning

Symptoms typically occur 12-48 hours after consuming the infected food, and include abdominal cramps, nausea, vomiting, diarrhea, headaches, chills, and fever. The severity of symptoms can range from mild to extreme and even fatal. Severe cases can cause dehydration, shock, and kidney failure. The easiest way to determine food poisoning is if other people who ate the same food also got sick. Many of these symptoms also occur in flu, gastrointestinal disorders, or severe allergic reactions.

Food poisoning may result from toxins produced by bacteria growing on the food, poisons in or on the food, or food-borne bacterial or viral infections. The most common forms are infective types such as salmonella found usually in farm animals or passed on by food handling. Other organisms such as *Staphylococcal* bacteria can be passed from food handlers, coughing, sneezing, or breathing onto the food itself. Botulism is associated with food preserved at home. Foods that remain at room temperature too long, such as large portions of meat, can encourage growth of *Clostridium*, often referred to as the "cafeteria" germ. Food poisoning can also be caused by eating poisonous mushrooms or contaminated shellfish.

If very severe vomiting and diarrhea occur, emergency medical intervention must be sought. Milder cases can be treated at home.

Nutrients for Food Poisoning

Food poisoning places great stress on the liver, as that organ bears the burden of processing toxins for elimination from the body. Products that support and cleanse the liver are therefore also important.

■ **Probiotics ("friendly" bacteria):** helps neutralize numerous pathogens (including *E. coli* and *Staphylococcus aureus*) in the intestines known to cause food poisoning.

■ **Lipoic acid:** unlike other antioxidants that are limited to attacking specific free radicals, lipoic acid is nonspecific and can perform the jobs of other antioxidants (such as vitamins C and E) when their supplies are low. Lipoic acid can also protect the liver from damaging free-radical attack caused by ingesting poisonous mushrooms.

Products for Food Poisoning

Inner Strength: Powder. Globulin concentrate from whey that nutritionally supports bowel defense and bowel changes for travelers; promotes and enhances the growth of beneficial intestinal bacteria; directly affects pathogenic intestinal organisms. *Authors' note: for food poisoning and traveler's diarrhea.*

ETHICAL NUTRIENTS, 971 Calle Negocio, San Clemente, CA 92673; tel: 800-668-8743 or 949-366-0818.

Lipoic Acid: Capsules. Lipoic acid, a powerful antioxidant, is one of two nutrients known to protect against mushroom poisoning and can protect other antioxidants (vitamins C and E, and glutathione);

HEALTH PRODUCTS DISTRIBUTORS, INC., 23847 Peaceful Ridge Road, Smithsburg, MD 21783; tel: 800-228-4265 or 301-416-0500.

Superdophilus: Powder. Contains nonfat milk, whey, *Lactobacillus acidophilus* (super strain DDS-1); produces hydrogen peroxide (H_2O_2) and other antimicrobial agents that can be used against the microorganisms *Staphylococcus aureus* (food poisoning and toxic shock syndrome), *Escherichia coli* (Montezuma's revenge and chronic kidney failure), *Candida albicans* (yeast overgrowth and thrush); used primarily for older children and adults; dairy-free formula also available.

For **products that support and cleanse the liver, see** Liver Disorders, pp. 257-262.

NATREN, 3105 Willow Lane, Westlake Village, CA 91361; tel: 800-992-3323 or 805-371-4737.

Fungal/Yeast Infections

Infections by fungal organisms (simple parasites including molds, mildew, and yeast) usually occur on the skin, but can also take place in organs and on a systemic level. Fungal infections may be more common and/or severe in people taking corticosteroids, oral contraceptives, or repeated courses of antibiotics. Such infections also occur more frequently in people with diabetes, leukemia, AIDS, or other immune-suppressing diseases.[95]

Symptoms and Types of Fungal Infections

Symptoms of localized fungal infection are listed below. Symptoms of systemic infection or infection of organs include loss of appetite, chills, fever, night sweats, weight loss, depression, and malaise.

Athlete's Foot—Infection between the toes, causing dry, itchy, scaly, cracked, bleeding, and tender skin.

Candidiasis—An overgrowth of *Candida albicans*, a yeast-like fungus normally found in the gastrointestinal and genitourinary tracts. If immunity is weakened or the beneficial bacterial populations that normally inhabit these tracts are depleted, the yeast is able to multiply rapidly, causing many far-reaching problems in the body. Systemic candidiasis (throughout the body) produces a wide variety of symptoms including intestinal problems, extreme fatigue, hypothyroidism (underactive thyroid gland), adrenal dysfunction, headaches, prostatitis, impotence, diabetes, and depression and other mood disorders, among many other conditions.[96]

Candidiasis is a reflection of serious imbalance in the body. Factors which can contribute to producing this imbalance include repeated courses of antibiotics (which kill the beneficial intestinal bacteria), a nutritionally poor diet, stress, fatigue, and the prolonged use of birth control pills or cortisone.

Fingernail and Toenail Infections—Thick, whitened, and crumbly nails; more common in toenails than fingernails and not usually affecting all ten nails.

Oral Thrush—An overgrowth of the yeast *Candida albicans* (see above) in the mouth, appearing as white sores.

Vaginal Yeast Infection—An overgrowth of *Candida albicans* (see above) in the vagina, producing itching, irritation, and inflammation of the vaginal tissues, accompanied by a foul odor, cottage cheese–like discharge, and pain with sexual intercourse; often passed back and forth between sexual partners.

Nutrients and Herbs for Fungal Infections

■ *Acidophilus*: these friendly intestinal bacteria (or probiotics) assist in reducing, or keeping in check, fungi in the gastrointestinal and genitourinary tracts and maintaining normal ratios of the bacterial populations.

■ **Colloidal silver:** an antimicrobial which can be used topically or internally. In addition to inhibiting fungal growth, this mineral compound also stimulates the immune system.

■ **Essential fatty acids:** contained in black currant, evening primrose, and salmon oils; can help maintain cellular integrity, protecting cells from fungal infection.

■ **Garlic:** can be effective against many strains of fungi, as can lavender, red thyme, and berberine-containing herbs (goldenseal, barberry, and Oregon grape root).

■ **Caprylic acid:** a fatty acid successfully used both on the skin and internally to control *Candida* overgrowth.[97]

■ **Grapefruit seed extract:** a multipurpose antibiotic, is also excellent for fungal (especially *Candida*) infections, and can be used topically or internally.

■ **Liquid stabilized oxygen:** provides electrolytes of stabilized oxygen, a form readily utilized by the body. It can be used to destroy fungi while preserving the important friendly intestinal bacteria. A product we have used with success is Oxy-Max.

■ **Oregano:** oil or capsules and products also containing pau d'arco are good antifungals.

■ **Tea tree oil:** has powerful antiseptic properties, assists in fighting a broad range of infectious agents, and is one of the best skin disinfectants for conditions of athlete's foot, infections of finger and toe nailbeds, vaginal area, and oral thrush. Nutrients, gargles, and mouthwashes containing tea tree oil, pau d'arco, or citrus seed extract can also be effective in treating oral thrush.

Products for Fungal Infections

Acidophilus Chewable: Wafers. Blend of the beneficial bacteria *B. bifidum* and *L. acidophilus* for intestinal health; for children or adults who prefer a chewable *acidophilus* product.

PHILLIPS NUTRITIONALS, 27071 Cabot Road #122, Laguna Hills, CA 92653; tel: 800-514-5115 or 702-898-8141.

All-Flora: Capsules or powder. Supplies billions of friendly flora, vitamins, and detoxifying and supportive enzymes to the digestive system.

NEW CHAPTER, 22 High Street, Brattleboro, VT 05301; tel: 800-543-7279 or 802-257-9345.

Anti-Fungal Foot Powder. Contains cassava-root base (does not contain talc or corn starch) with calcium undecylenate (derived from castor oil), grapefruit seed extract, and slippery elm.

IMHOTEP, P.O. Box 183, Ruby, NJ 12475; tel: 800-677-8577 or 914-336-2070.

Anti-Fungal Spray. Ingredients include black walnut, calendula, garlic, pau d'arco, glycerin, and essential oils of sage and tea tree.

NATURE'S APOTHECARY, P.O. Box 17970, Boulder, CO 80308; tel: 800-999-7422 or 303-664-1600.

Bee Kind Personal Feminine Care: Disposable douche. Soothes irritated vaginal tissue; also used as a cleansing aid after menstruation.

SEDNA, P.O. Box 1453, Andrews, NC 28901; tel: 800-223-0858 or 828-321-2240.

Begone: Drops. Herbal remedy for viral, yeast, fungal, and bacterial control; contains concentrated glycerine extract of echinacea, lovage root, and myrrh gum with herbal dilution and flower essences.

OLYMPIC BOTANICALS, 231 Otto Street, Port Townsend, WA 98368; tel: 800-310-6924 or 360-385-9468.

See **Biotonic** in Gastrointestinal Disorders product listing, p. 204.

Biocidin: Tablets. Herbal antimicrobial for intestinal dysbiosis (imbalance in the intestinal flora) in which fungal, bacterial, or parasitic pathogens have been identified. *In vitro* testing by Great Smokies Diagnostic Laboratory has shown that all strains of bacteria and yeast tested show high levels of sensitivity to this combination of medicinal plants. When used for an extended period of time, the cold nature of the herbs in Biocidin may weaken digestive energy, causing nausea or loss of appetite. In this case, appropriate tonic formulations can be chosen.

BIO-BOTANICAL RESEARCH, INC., 144 Pioneer Road, Corralitos, CA 95076; distributed by WELLNESS HEALTH PHARMACY, 2800 South 18th Street, Homewood, AL 35209; tel: 800-227-2627.

Candaid: Capsules. Helps maintain a proper yeast balance and relieves the symptoms of *Candida albicans*; ingredients include odorless garlic, pau d'arco, echinacea, black walnut leaves, and thymus substance.

RIDGECREST HERBALS, 1151 South Redwood Road #106, Salt Lake City, UT 84104-3729; tel: 800-242-4649 or 801-978-9633.

Candida-Pak: Capsules or tablets. Contains yeast-free vitamins, minerals, and fatty acids; replenishes helpful intestinal microorganisms.

AMNI, 2247 National Avenue, Hayward, CA 94540-5012; tel: 800-437-8888 or 510-783-6969.

Candida Yeast Formulae: Homeopathic liquid. Relieves vaginal yeast infections accompanied by burning or itching and thick, white discharge; should only be used after condition has been diagnosed by a physician; safe for children.

LIDDELL LABORATORIES, 1036 Country Club Drive, Moraga, CA 94556; tel: 800-460-7733 or 925-377-3000.

Caprylex: Tablets. Contains caprylic acid (a natural fatty acid), calcium, and magnesium; releases contents in lower gastrointestinal tract; helps to inhibit growth of *Candida albicans*; does not inhibit the growth of beneficial intestinal bacteria.

AMNI, 2247 National Avenue, Hayward, CA 94540-5012; tel: 800-437-8888 or 510-783-6969.

Eco-Harvest Tea Tree Oil: Liquid. Contains 100% pure, ecologically-harvested tea tree oil.

COUNTRY LIFE, 101 Corporate Drive, Hauppauge, NY 11788; tel: 800-645-5768 or 516-231-1031.

Flora Balance: Capsules or powder. Contains probiotic of the strain *Bacillus laterosporous*; unlike *acidophilus*, *B. laterosporous* is active in both intestines and feeds on *Candida albicans*.

BIO-NUTRITIONAL FORMULAS, 106 East Jericho Turnpike, Mineola, NY 11501; tel: 800-950-8484.

Flora Grow: Vegicaps. Restores the healthy intestinal bacteria (flora) normally depleted by the use of antibiotics and poor eating habits; beneficial bacteria are essential for a strong immune system, assimilation of vitamins, proteins, fats, carbohydrates, and the manufacture of B vitamins, vitamin K, and various amino acids.

ARISE AND SHINE, P.O. Box 1439, Mount Shasta, CA 96067; tel: 800-688-2444 or 530-926-0891.

Garlinase 4000: Tablets. Contains beneficial allicin (an active component of garlic).

ENZYMATIC THERAPY, 825 Challenger Drive, Green Bay, WI 54311-8328; tel: 800-558-7372 or 920-469-1313.

GSE Liquid Concentrate (Grapefruit Seed Extract): Capsules, liquid, or tablets. Use internally as a vaginal, dental, nasal, and ear rinse, and throat gargle or externally as a nail and scalp treatment, facial cleanser, skin rinse, and all-purpose cleaner.

NUTRIBIOTIC, NUTRITION RESOURCES, INC., P.O. Box 238, Lakeport, CA 95453; tel: 800-225-4345 or 707-263-0411.

Gy-Na•Tren: 14-day kit (capsules, vaginal inserts and applicator). Helps restore the healthy balance of vaginal and intestinal flora and inhibit recurring yeast infections.

NATREN, 3105 Willow Lane, Westlake Village, CA 91361; tel: 800-992-3323 or 805-371-4737.

Herbal Aloe Force: Juice or topical gel. Processed aloe vera juice containing vitamins, minerals, enzymes, amino acids, essential fatty acids, growth factors, glycoproteins, sterols, bioflavonoids, polysaccharides (complex sugars), ionized colloidal silver, and herbal extracts (cat's claw, chamomile, burdock root, hawthorn berry, astragalus root, sheep sorrel, pau d'arco bark, slippery elm bark, and rhubarb root).

HERBAL ANSWERS, INC., P.O. Box 1110, Saratoga Springs, NY 12866; tel: 888-256-3367 or 518-581-1968.

Hyland's Vaginitis: Sublingual tablets. For relief of symptoms of vaginal itching and burning from vaginal irritation or discharge; should be used after the condition is diagnosed by a physician.

P & S LABS, 210 West 131st Street, Los Angeles, CA 90061; tel: 800-624-9659 or 310-768-0700.

Immune-Neem by Farmacopia: Capsules or tea. Contains neem leaf (a mainstay of the Ayurvedic health system of India; laboratory studies have shown its antifungal, antibacterial, and antiviral activities), ginger, stevia, peppermint, lemon grass, cinnamon, licorice, and natural flavors.

BOTANICAL PRODUCTS INTERNATIONAL, P.O. Box 174, Hakalau, HI 96710; tel: 808-963-6771.

Katsu Herbal Garlic Complex: Tablets. Contains concentrated extracts of garlic, coix, and rice bran with shark cartilage and vitamin C. Garlic inhibits bacteria, fungi, yeast (including *Candida*), and parasites (protozoa and worms).

KENSHIN TRADING CORP., P.O. Box 7511, Torrance, CA 90504; tel: 800-766-1313 or 310-212-3199.

KYOLIC Formula 100: Capsules or tablets. Contains garlic extract plus whey to help normalize colon flora.

WAKUNAGA OF AMERICA, 23501 Madero, Mission Viejo, CA 92691; tel: 800 421-2998 or 949-855-2776.

Kyo-Dophilus: Capsules or tablets. Tablets contain one strain of the beneficial bacteria *L. acidophilus*; capsules contain three strains of beneficial bacteria *(L. acidophilus, B. bifidum,* and *B. longum)* prevalent in the intestines, helping to normalize the intestinal flora.

WAKUNAGA OF AMERICA, 23501 Madero, Mission Viejo, CA 92691; tel: 800-421-2998 or 949-855-2776.

Nail Rescue: Liquid. Contains the antifungal power of undecylenic acid (a castor oil derivative), grapefruit seed extract, and calendula, in a base of food-grade pure grain alcohol.

IMHOTEP, P.O. Box 183, Ruby, NJ 12475; tel: 800-677-8577 or 914-336-2070.

NH4 Redox: Capsules. Contains lactitol (a derivative of lactose), which is used after treatment of *Candida* overgrowth to normalize intestinal pH so that favorable bacteria can flourish.

ECOLOGICAL FORMULAS, 1061-B Shary Circle, Concord, CA 94518; tel: 800-888-4585 or 925-827-2636.

Oregamax: Capsules. Potent antifungal formula that can destroy yeasts and other fungi resulting from antibiotic treatment; contains crushed wild oregano, rhus cariaria, garlic (*Allium sativum*), and onion; wild oregano contains carvacrol (antimicrobial); flavonoids (antiseptic), and terpenes (anti-inflammatory).

PURITY PRODUCTS, 1804 Plaza Avenue, New Hyde Park, NY 11040; tel: 800-769-7873.

Oxy-Caps by Earth's Bounty: Capsules. Releases molecular oxygen once it comes in contact with the stomach's hydrochloric acid; increased levels of oxygen can help the body work more efficiently and neutralize anaerobic bacteria.

MATRIX HEALTH PRODUCTS, 8400 Magnolia Avenue, Suite N, Santee, CA 92071; tel: 800-736-5609 or 619-448-7550.

Oxy-Max by Earth's Bounty: Liquid. High potency, stabilized oxygen supplement that provides electrolytes of stabilized oxygen, a form readily utilized by the body. A shortage of oxygen in the body leaves it susceptible to bacterial, fungal, and viral infection, as well as a loss of mental acuity.

MATRIX HEALTH PRODUCTS, 8400 Magnolia Avenue, Suite N, Santee, CA 92071; tel: 800-736-5609 or 619-448-7550.

ProSeed Throat Relief: Spray. Uses concentrated extracts of echinacea, calendula, aloe vera, and grapefruit seed extract in a base of pure vegetable glycerine to relive sore throat and freshen breath.

IMHOTEP, P.O. Box 183, Ruby, NJ 12475; tel: 800-677-8577 or 914-336-2070.

Superdophilus: Powder. Contains nonfat milk, whey, *Lactobacillus acidophilus* (super strain DDS-1); produces hydrogen peroxide (H_2O_2) and other antimicrobial agents that can be used against the microorganisms *Candida albicans* (yeast overgrowth and thrush), *Staphylococcus aureus* (food poisoning and toxic shock syndrome), *Escherichia coli* (Montezuma's revenge and chronic kidney failure), and useful in the small intestines of older children and adults; dairy-free formula also available.

NATREN, 3105 Willow Lane, Westlake Village, CA 91361; tel: 800-992-3323 or 805-371-4737.

Tea Tree Antiseptic Cream. Herbal antiseptic for relief of minor skin irritations, sunburn, windburn, minor burns, and chafing.

THURSDAY PLANTATION INC., NATURE'S PLUS, 548 Broadhollow Road, Melville, NY 11747-3708; tel: 800-645-9500 or 516-293-0030.

Tea Tree Foot Powder and Foot Spray. Talc-free formula to keep feet dry with the odor-fighting properties of tea tree oil, the mildly astringent properties of zinc, and the cooling sensation of menthol and camphor.

THURSDAY PLANTATION INC., NATURE'S PLUS, 548 Broadhollow Road, Melville, NY 11747-3708; tel: 800-645-9500 or 516-293-0030.

Tea Tree Oil. Antiseptic, antibacterial, and antifungal that helps relieve infected nails, nasal blockage, mouth cankers, sore gums, athlete's foot, acne, pimples, ringworm, boils, muscle aches, sore joints, cuts, sunburn, bites, sprains, sinus congestion, sore throats, minor burns, thrush, stings, topical ulcers, rashes, coral cuts, and tick bites.

DESERT ESSENCE, 9700 Topanga Canyon Boulevard, Chatsworth, CA 91311; tel: 800-848-7331 or 818-734-1735.

Tea Tree Suppositories. Complements any internal cleansing program, allowing the natural defenses of the body to regain control when the system has become unbalanced.

THURSDAY PLANTATION INC., NATURE'S PLUS, 548 Broadhollow Road, Melville, NY 11747-3708; tel: 800-645-9500 or 516-293-0030.

Wild West Manuka Honey: Ointment. Has been found to be effective as a topical ointment when treating athlete's foot, scrapes, cuts, and boils.

WGI, 35008 Emerald Coast Parkway, 5th Floor, Destin, FL 32541; tel: 800-854-8353 or 850-654-4744.

Yeast Defense for Men: Capsules. Formula that can help a man's body fight against yeast; ingredients include caprylic acid, pau d'arco, deodorized garlic, grapefruit seed extract, chlorophyll concentrate, 100% natural cultures of *Lactobacillus acidophilus*, *Lactobacillus plantarum*, *Lactobacillus bulgaricus*, and *Lactobacillus casei*.

NUTRITION NOW, 501 Southeast Columbia Shore Boulevard #350, Vancouver, WA 98661; tel: 800-929-0418 or 360-737-6800.

Yeast Fighting Team: Liquid. For relief of vaginal itch, and discomfort caused by vaginal yeast infections.

NUTRITION NOW, 501 Southeast Columbia Shore Boulevard #350, Vancouver, WA 98661; tel: 800-929-0418 or 360-737-6800.

Gastrointestinal Disorders

The gastrointestinal or digestive system is made up of the organs and glands involved in ingestion and digestion, from the mouth to the anus, and including the stomach and large and small intestines. Digestion begins when food mixes with enzymes in saliva. The process is continued in the stomach by hydrochloric acid (HCl) and pepsin. Food is liquefied there then passes on to the small intestine, where it is further broken down by digestive enzymes into nutrients small enough to pass through the intestinal walls and be absorbed into the bloodstream.

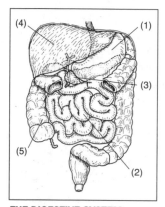

THE DIGESTIVE SYSTEM.
Digestion begins in the mouth, then food travels to the stomach (1), where it is further broken down by gastric juices. Next, the partially digested food goes to the small intestine (2) where enzymes from the pancreas (3) and bile produced by the liver (4) act upon the food to extract nutrients for absorption into blood and lymph cells. The unusable food materials are sent to the large intestine (5) for evacuation from the body.

Types of Gastrointestinal Disorders

Common gastrointestinal problems include constipation, diarrhea, colitis, Crohn's disease, gastritis, gastric ulcer, leaky gut syndrome, and malabsorption syndrome.

Constipation—Defined as infrequent or difficult evacuation of fecal material (stools), constipation is most often caused by lack of fiber and fluids in the diet. A low intestinal population of the beneficial bacteria *acidophilus*, magnesium deficiency, iron supplementation, and taking pain killers or antidepressants can also produce constipation. It is important to have at least one bowel movement per day. This avoids the formation and absorption of toxic by-products produced by poor digestion and assimilation.

Diarrhea—Abnormally frequent evacuation of watery stools, diarrhea is a common symptom of many disorders. Medical attention should be sought if it does not resolve in a few days, because prolonged diarrhea leads to dehydration from loss of fluids, and loss of electrolytes, which can result in death if they are not replaced. Common causes of diarrhea include lactose (milk sugar) intolerance; bacterial, viral, or parasitic infection; and gastrointestinal conditions such as colitis, Crohn's disease, and malabsorption syndrome (see below). Deficiencies of *acidophilus* or digestive enzymes, improper intestinal pH (SEE QUICK DEFINITION), stress, and emotional problems are also contributing factors.

Colitis and Crohn's Disease—Both of these disorders involve inflammation of the digestive tract. Colitis is confined to the colon, while Crohn's disease tends to affect the small intestine, but can also occur in the mouth, esophagus, and stomach. Symptoms of both include diarrhea, fever, weight loss, abdominal tenderness, and blood in the stool. Ulcerative colitis is characterized by open sores or lesions in the lining of the colon.

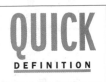

DEFINITION

The term **pH**, which means "potential hydrogen," represents a scale for the relative acidity or alkalinity of a solution. Acidity is measured as a pH of 0.1 to 6.9, alkalinity is 7.1 to 14, and neutral pH is 7.0. Normally, blood is slightly alkaline, at 7.35 to 7.45; urine pH can range from 4.8 to 8.0, but is usually somewhat acidic, with a normal reading between 5.0 and 6.0.

Gastritis and Gastric Ulcer—Gastritis is inflammation of the stomach and can be caused by viruses, bacteria, or chemical irritation from medications such as ibuprofen and aspirin. A gastric ulcer involves open sores or lesions in the lining of the stomach and shares the same causes as gastritis. Chronic stress and food allergies can also contribute.

Hemorrhoids—Hemorrhoids are veins in the lining of the anus that have become distended. They may be internal or protrude out of the anus. Symptoms include bleeding, pain, mucus discharge, and a feeling of incomplete evacuation of fecal material. Anal itching is not a symptom of hemorrhoids, but is a common side effect due to the difficulty of keeping the hemorrhoidal area clean.

Hemorrhoids are usually related to chronic constipation, pregnancy, improper diet, lack of exercise, prolonged sitting, heavy lifting, obesity, liver damage, and/or allergies. They can also be related to spinal misalignment in the lower back or sacrum (base of the spinal column). A chiropractor can rule out or identify this as a contributing factor.

Leaky Gut Syndrome—This intestinal disorder occurs when the intestinal mucosa is damaged (by disease, substance abuse, or medications, among other causes[98]) and large, incompletely digested food molecules

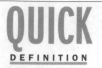

pass through the intestinal wall into the bloodstream and circulate throughout the body. The immune system regards these particles as antigens, or invaders, rather than as nutrients. It then mounts an antigen-antibody reaction, which is also known as a food allergy attack. When chronic, this condition places a heavy burden on the liver and the kidneys which must process these toxins in the bloodstream.

Malabsorption Syndrome—Involving impaired intestinal absorption of nutrients, malabsorption syndrome results in nutritional deficiencies and often anemia, usually due to iron, vitamin B12, or folic acid deficiencies.

Treatment of Gastrointestinal Disorders

To improve the digestive process and thereby promote gastrointestinal health, many people could begin by simply chewing their food more thoroughly (50% of digestion should take place in the mouth). Beyond this simple practice, there are four main criteria for optimal digestion and elimination: the correct type and amount of digestive enzymes (SEE QUICK DEFINITION); sufficient "friendly" intestinal bacteria (SEE QUICK DEFINITION); the correct pH in each area of the digestive tract; and an adequate amount of fiber in the diet.

Enzymes, found in plants and made by the pancreas, are crucial to the digestion of food, breaking it down so it can be absorbed by the body as nutrients. Fresh, raw foods contain the proper types and amount of enzymes needed for the body to digest that food. Unfortunately, the standard American diet contains little to no raw fruits and vegetables, consisting mainly of processed foods which have been depleted of enzymes. The pancreas is forced to provide the enzymes needed to digest this food.

Over time, such a diet exhausts the body's capacity for making pancreatic enzymes and digestion suffers. In addition, when the pancreas cannot keep up with the enzyme demand placed upon it, the digestive system recruits enzymes from the immune system's supply, leaving the body vulnerable to opportunistic infections and degenerative conditions. For optimal digestion and one's overall health, it is therefore important to get an adequate supply of enzymes either through consuming fresh, raw foods or taking plant enzyme supplements.

Lactobacillus acidophilus and other friendly intestinal bacteria, or probiotics, contribute to the efficiency of digestion and the synthesis of certain vitamins (vitamin B3, B6, folic acid, and biotin). Probiotics also produce antibacterial substances that can kill or deactivate disease-causing bacteria and other pathenogenic microorganisms such as yeast or fungus.

Use of antibiotics is one of the main causes of depleted beneficial bacteria, because antibiotics kill the good as well as the bad bacteria. Thus it is very important if you undergo antibiotic therapy, to reintroduce *acidophilus* and other probiotics while you are taking the antibiotics and especially after you finish the course of treatment. We have found in clinical practice that most people do well taking probiotic products on a regular basis to promote intestinal and digestive health.

To address another component of healthy digestion—pH balance in the digestive system which is typically too acidic—we suggest dietary changes involving reduced consumption of acid-forming foods and increased consumption of alkaline-forming foods. Sugar and red meat are the most acid-forming foods. Others are dairy products, eggs, animal proteins, fats and oils, flour-based products, fruit juices (especially citrus and cranberrry), and vinegar; coffee, alcohol, and colas are also acid-forming. The best alkaline-forming foods are vegetables and millet. Raw honey and molasses are sweeteners that alkalinize. Aloe vera juice and "green" foods (alfalfa, barley grass, chlorella, chlorophyll, wheat grass, and parsley) also promote alkalinity.

Finally, to ensure that you are getting enough fiber, eat high-fiber foods (such as whole grains and kidney beans) and, if necessary, take a fiber supplement. For most people, we recommend psyllium fiber products. To those with sensitive systems, we recommend vegetable or apple/pear pectin fiber.

See **Bacterial Infections**, pp. 105-112, **Fungal Infections**, pp. 190-197, and **Parasitic Infections**, pp. 298-302. For information on **colon cleansing**, see Detoxification in Part III, pp. 446-461.

Nutrients and Herbs for Gastrointestinal Disorders

■ **For constipation:** we recommend psyllium fiber products to most people. For people with sensitive bodies, however, we recommend vegetable or apple/pear pectin fiber. A good nutrient to loosen the stools is aloe vera juice. Strong herbal products such as cascara sagrada or senna work well as laxatives, but should not be used continuously for long periods of time because the body can become dependent on them.

■ **For diarrhea:** we often recommend a good *L. acidophilus/B. bifidum* supplement, plant-based digestive enzymes, and the product Inner Strength to assist in re-balancing intestinal flora.

■ **For gastritis and ulcers:** you must first rule out an infection by *Helicobacter bacteria*, parasites, or other microorganism; *Helicobacter* is often present in stomach ulcers and gastritis is frequently viral. Then digestion is worked on by using digestive enzymes, a product called Renewall, aloe vera, chlorophyll, and the herbs comfrey, ginger, marshmallow root, and slippery elm. Deglycyrrhizinated licorice (DGL) has proven effective in healing duodenal (small intestinal) and gastric ulcers and is safer than licorice root, which can raise blood pressure.[99]

■ **For hemorrhoids:** vitamins A, B complex, C, D, and E, beta carotene, calcium, coenzyme Q10, ionic liquid mineral complex, magnesium, potassium, aloe vera gel (topical), aloe vera juice, bilberry, buckthorn bark, butcher's broom, comfrey root (poultice), ginkgo, gotu kola, horse chestnut (topical), parsley, passionflower, and stone root.

■ **For intestinal cramps:** when the spasms are due to nervous tension, an allergic reaction to a food, indigestion, or to eating food that is spoiled, high in fat or sugar, or undercooked, we recommend the product MyoCalm.

■ **For inflammation and irritation associated with irritable gut, gastritis, and ulcerative colitis:** liquid chlorophyll reduces inflammation in the stomach and intestines, helps heal ulcers, and promotes colonization of beneficial flora and prevents the spread of yeast and fungi in the intestines.

■ **For pancreatitis:** liquid chlorophyll reduces inflammation in the stomach and intestines, soothes ulcers, promotes the growth of friendly bacteria, and prevents proliferation of yeast and fungi in the intestines.[100]

Products for Gastrointestinal Disorders

Acidophilus Chewable: Wafers. Blend of the beneficial bacteria *B. bifidum* and *L. acidophilus* for intestinal health; for children or adults who prefer a chewable *acidophilus* product.

PHILLIPS NUTRITIONALS, 27071 Cabot Road #122, Laguna Hills, CA 92653; tel: 800-514-5115 or 702-898-8141.

Acidophilus Liquid. Contains a blend of five strains of *Lactobacillus* bacteria with five billion viable organisms; available in natural yogurt and strawberry yogurt flavors.

AMERICAN HEALTH, 4320 Veterans Memorial Highway, Holbrook, NY 11741; tel: 800-445-7137.

Alkalizer: Powder. Concentrated source of organic potassium, sodium, calcium, phosphate, magnesium, and other alkaline electrolyte minerals for people with low alkaline reserves; not recommended for people who have sugar problems (hypoglycemia, diabetes, or candidiasis).

ARISE AND SHINE, P.O. Box 1439, Mount Shasta, CA 96067; tel: 800-688-2444 or 530-926-0891.

All-Flora: Capsules or powder. Supplies billions of friendly flora, vitamins, and detoxifying and supportive enzymes to the digestive system.

NEW CHAPTER, 22 High Street, Brattleboro, VT 05301; tel: 800-543-7279 or 802-257-9345.

Beans...Beans and More Rx: Softgels. Contains food enzymes that help stop gas, bloating and cramping; these enzymes are effective in digesting complex sugars found in gas-producing foods (beans, garlic, onions, Brussels sprouts, broccoli, cucumbers, cabbage, cauliflower, lentils, soy-based foods, and some fruits) into digestible sugars.

For **products recommended for acid Indigestion**, see Indigestion/ Heartburn, pp. 247-253.

PHYTO-THERAPY, INC., OPTIMUM HEALTH, 483 West Middle Turnpike, Manchester, CT 06040; tel: 800-228-1507 or 860-647-9729.

Bentonite Minerals: Liquid. Contains bentonite clay, zinc, copper, selenium, and chromium (50% of the U.S. RDA in each tablespoon); easily absorbable by the body and less likely to cause allergies.

WHITE ROCK MINERAL, P.O. Box 967, Springville, UT 84663-0967; tel: 888-328-2529 or 801-489-7138.

Biocidin: Tablets. Herbal antimicrobial for intestinal dysbiosis (imbalance in the intestinal flora) in which fungal, bacterial, or parasitic pathogens have been identified. *In vitro* testing by Great Smokies Diagnostic Laboratory has shown that all strains of bacteria and yeast tested show high levels of sensitivity to this combination of medicinal plants. According to Dr. Martin Lee, Ph.D., Great Smokies' laboratory director, "The herbal mixture Biocidin has been the most broadly acting and powerful natural or nonprescriptive substance evaluated. In separate experiments we have found that Biocidin was a potent inhibitor of growth for *Candida albicans*, as well as other *Candida* species." When used for an extended period of time, the cold nature of the herbs in Biocidin may weaken digestive energy, causing nausea or loss of appetite. In this case, appropriate tonic formulations can be chosen.

BIO-BOTANICAL RESEARCH, INC., 144 Pioneer Road, Corralitos, CA 95076; distributed by WELLNESS HEALTH PHARMACY, 2800 South 18th Street, Homewood, AL 35209; tel: 800-227-2627 or 205-879-6551.

Biotonic: Capsules. Based on Chinese herbal combinations that have been used to balance digestive function and energy metabolism; complements Biocidin by toning and supporting the gastrointestinal tract and liver; contains astragalus and Siberian ginseng for adaptogenic support, ginger for aiding digestion and stopping nausea, *Radix paeonia* and *Tuber curcuma* for supporting the liver and gallbladder, and artemesia for antifungal and antibacterial properties. Although specifically designed for use with Biocidin, Biotonic may be used whenever an adaptogenic combination is indicated.

BIO-BOTANICAL RESEARCH, INC., 144 Pioneer Road, Corralitos, CA 95076; distributed by WELLNESS HEALTH PHARMACY, 2800 South 18th Street, Homewood, AL 35209; tel: 800-227-2627 or 205-879-6551.

Body Balance: Capsules. Helps friendly bacteria normalize the colon pH, eliminate intestinal gas, evacuate wastes, improve immune function, form vitamins, produce lactase, and regulate cholesterol and hormonal levels; contains an enzymatic and bacterial mix including isolated soy protein, betaine, and seaweed.

NATURAL ENERGY PRODUCTS, 21101 Welch Road, Snohomish, WA 98296; tel: 425-486-5956.

Broad Spectrum Enzymes: Chewable tablets or vegicaps. Enzyme replacement formula for people who eat cooked, processed food; when ingested with food, digestion can begin before the body's own enzymes go to work, reducing stress in the lower stomach and intestines and demand on the pancreas for digestive enzymes; contains protease, lipase, amylase, and cellulase.

ENZYMES INC., 8500 Northwest River Park Drive #223, Parkville, MO 64152; tel: 800-647-6377 or 816-746-6461.

BWL Tone IBS Caps. Contains peppermint and slippery elm to soothe and tone the intestines.

CRYSTAL STAR HERBAL NUTRITION, 4069 Wedgeway Court, Earth City, MO 63045; tel: 800-736-6015 or 314-739-7551.

Celium: Powder. Daily supplement of soluble fiber to aid regularity and to help lower LDL (low-density lipoprotein) cholesterol levels; celium contains 98% pure psyllium husks for maximum bulking (contains 2% seed particles).

SIERRA HEALTH PRODUCTS, INC., 7949 Woodley Avenue, Van Nuys, CA 91406; tel: 818-375-5029.

Chewable Acidophilus With Bifidus: Wafers. Ingredients include *Lactobacillus acidophilus* and *B. bifidus*; available in natural banana, blueberry, and strawberry flavors sweetened with fructose.

AMERICAN HEALTH, 4320 Veterans Memorial Highway, Holbrook, NY 11741; tel: 800-445-7137.

Chloraid: Capsules. Source of premium chlorophyll, which reduces offensive body odors originating in the digestive and urinary tracts.

NATURE'S HERBS, 600 East Quality Drive, American Fork, UT 84003; tel: 800-437-2257 or 801-763-0700.

Chomper: Vegicaps. Herbal laxative that thoroughly cleanses the alimentary canal (passage from mouth to anus), liver, deep cell tissues, and other organs.

ARISE AND SHINE, P.O. Box 1439, Mount Shasta, CA 96067; tel: 800-688-2444 or 530-926-0891.

Cleaning Sweep 2: Capsules. Herbal laxative for occasional cleansing of the intestines; contains the pod of senna, a less irritating bowel stimulant, aged cascara, barberry, mullein, clove, and licorice.

NEW CHAPTER, 22 High Street, Brattleboro, VT 05301; tel: 800-543-7279 or 802-257-9345.

Cleansing Laxative Formula: Tablets. Herbal laxative for occasional constipation and colon-cleansing programs; contains the herb cascara sagrada, kaolin clay, and other ingredients to support bowel detoxification.

ZAND HERBAL FORMULAS, 1722 14th Street #230, Boulder, CO 80302; tel: 800-800-0405 or 303-786-8558.

Colon Balance: Tablets. Helps support the body's natural balance and a healthy elimination system.

VEDA HEALTH, INC., P.O. Box 1535, Soquel, CA 95073; tel: 888-856-8334 or 408-465-9084.

Colon Cleanse: Capsules. Contains psyllium husk (without seeds which may irritate the colon), an essential soluble fiber that expands and acts as a soft gentle brush inside the colon; lubricates the lining of the colon and helps in the removal of waste matter generated in the body.

HEALTH PLUS, 13837 Magnolia Avenue, Chino, CA 91710; tel: 800-822-6225 or 909-627-9393.

Colon-Fresh: Capsules. Gentle regulator that contains no harsh synthetics or mineral oils; ingredients include ginger root, fennel seed, bayberry, licorice, turkey rhubarb, red raspberry, slippery elm, and cascara sagrada.

WGI, 35008 Emerald Coast Parkway, 5th Floor, Destin, FL 32541; tel: 800-854-8353 or 850-654-4744.

Dairy Enzyme Formula: Capsules. Concentrated plant enzymes that aid in the digestion of dairy proteins, milk sugar, carbohydrates, and fat; many people have allergies to milk proteins and sugar (lactose) or their bodies don't produce enough lactase enzyme to digest lactose, causing abdominal pain, bloating, gas, and diarrhea.

PREVAIL CORP., 2204-8 Northwest Birdsdale, Gresham, OR 97030; tel: 800-248-0885 or 503-667-5527.

Dandelion Burdock: Capsules or liquid. Helps to enhance digestion and support the activity of the liver and gallbladder; includes dandelion and burdock roots, artichoke leaves, and milk thistle seed.

FRONTIER COOPERATIVE HERBS, 3021 78th Street, Norway, IA 52318; tel: 800-669-3275 or 319-227-7996.

Dandelion & Milk Thistle: Capsules. Herbal formula designed to help protect and detoxify the liver.

NUTRITION NOW, 501 Southeast Columbia Shore Boulevard #350, Vancouver, WA 98661; tel: 800-929-0418 or 360-737-6800.

Daytime/Nighttime Daily Cleanse: Tablets. Multiple herbs and fiber supplement program.

AMERICAN HEALTH, 4320 Veterans Memorial Highway, Holbrook, NY 11741; tel: 800-445-7137.

DetoxCleanse: Capsules. Herbal formula that assists in detoxifying the body and bloodstream through cleansing the liver, improving digestion, binding and excreting toxins within the gastrointestinal tract, and promoting regularity.

BIODYNAMAX, 6525 Gunpark Drive #150-507, Boulder, CO 80301; tel: 800-926-7525 or 303-530-4665.

Detox-Zyme: Vegicaps. Blend of enzymes necessary for the breakdown of proteins, fats, carbohydrates, and fiber, plus herbs traditionally used to support the cleansing and eliminating functions of the body.

RAINBOW LIGHT, P.O. Box 600, Santa Cruz, CA 95061; tel: 800-635-1233 or 408-429-9089.

Diar-Ease: Capsules. For relief of common diarrhea, gas pains, and abdominal cramps; contains pure kaolin, apple pectin, and activated charcoal in a base of agrimony, chamomile flowers, peppermint, and anise seed; no added sugar, starch, artificial colors, or excipients (inert substances used to give pills form).

NATURE'S HERBS, 600 East Quality Drive, American Fork, UT 84003; tel: 800-437-2257 or 801-763-0700.

Digest-Ease: Capsules. Relieves stomach and intestinal distress, bloating, distention, fullness, pressure, and cramps after eating; no animal-source ingredients.

NATURE'S HERBS, 600 East Quality Drive, American Fork, UT 84003; tel: 800-437-2257 or 801-763-0700.

Digest Eze Rx: Capsules. Multiple-enzyme digestive supplement formula; helps prevent gas, bloating, flatulence; effective when eating foods containing milk, beans, vegetables, soy-based foods, fruits, and lentils.

PHYTO-THERAPY, INC., OPTIMUM HEALTH, 483 West Middle Turnpike, Manchester, CT 06040; tel: 800-228-1507 or 860-647-9729.

Digestive Balance: Tablets. Helps support a healthy digestive system.

VEDA HEALTH, INC., P.O. Box 1535, Soquel, CA 95073; tel: 888-856-8334 or 408-465-9084.

Evacu Lax Rx: Caplets. Intestinal/colon probiotic and cleansing system that helps promote, cleanse, and reestablish a healthy colon.

PHYTO-THERAPY, INC., OPTIMUM HEALTH, 483 West Middle Turnpike, Manchester, CT 06040; tel: 800-228-1507 or 860-647-9729.

Everyday Fiber System: Powder. Fiber supplementation for maintaining daily regularity; contains a blend of three soluble fibers plus supporting herbs such as ginger, FOS (fructo-oligosaccharides), chlorophyll, and plant-source enzymes.

RAINBOW LIGHT, P.O. Box 600, Santa Cruz, CA 95061; tel: 800-635-1233 or 408-429-9089.

Fiber & Herbs Cleanse Caps. Balance of herbal nutrients for complete colon-cleansing.

CRYSTAL STAR HERBAL NUTRITION, 4069 Wedgeway Court, Earth City, MO 63045; tel: 800-736-6015 or 314-739-7551.

Fiber Support Barley Fiber with Beta Glucans: Capsules. Soluble dietary fibers such as beta glucans are important nutrients for maintaining healthy levels of cholesterol in the blood and boosting the immune system; also contains tocotrienols, an antioxidant related to vitamin E.

OPTIMAL NUTRIENTS, 1163 Chess Drive #F, Foster City, CA 94404; tel: 800-966-8874 or 650-525-0112.

Flora Grow: Vegicaps. Restores the healthy intestinal bacteria (flora) normally depleted by the use of antibiotics and from poor eating habits; beneficial bacteria are essential for a strong immune system, assimilation of vitamins, proteins, fats, carbohydrates, and the manufacture of B vitamins, vitamin K, and various amino acids.

ARISE AND SHINE, P.O. Box 1439, Mount Shasta, CA 96067; tel: 800-688-2444 or 530-926-0891.

Flora Therapy Rx: Softgels. Formula contains one billion beneficial microorganisms, which help reestablish and maintain intestinal health, in a base of alkyl-glycerols derived from shark liver oil.

PHYTO-THERAPY, INC., OPTIMUM HEALTH, 483 West Middle Turnpike, Manchester, CT 06040; tel: 800-228-1507 or 860-647-9729.

Fresh n' Free: Softgels. Contains chlorophyll complex, an anti-odor compound from plants, for the elimination of breath and body odors commonly found in people with fecal or urinary incontinence and odors associated with colostomies and ileostomies; prophylactic use may reduce the need for expensive sprays or deodorized protective briefs. PHILLIPS NUTRITIONALS, 27071 Cabot Road #122, Laguna Hills, CA 92653; tel: 800-514-5115 or 702-898-8141.

Gamma-Zyme Enzyme Formula: Capsules. Contains three enzymes to help digest fat, starches, and fiber plus other ingredients to soothe and restore damaged or irritated intestinal linings.
R GARDEN, 3881 Enzyme Lane, Kettle Falls, WA 99141; tel: 800-700-7767 or 425-271-0539.

Gasalia: Homeopathic tablets. For temporary relief of bloating, pressure, and pain associated with gas.
BOIRON, 6 Campus Boulevard, Building A, Newtown Square, PA 19073; tel: 800-264-7661 or 610-325-7464.

Gas Relief: Tablets. For relief of common bloating and flatulence; contains ginger root, peppermint leaves, and licorice root.
UNIVERSAL, 3 Terminal Road, New Brunswick, NJ 08901; tel: 800-872-0101 or 732-545-3130.

Gastone: Phyto-homeopathic lozenges. Contains homeopathic ingredients in a base of ginger, German chamomile, and caraway to diminish the accumulation of gases.
SUPHERB LTD., P.O. Box 1135, Nahariya 22100, Israel; tel: 800-409-HERB (4372).

Gastro Intestinal Support: Tablets. Combination of minerals, trace minerals, herbs, and enzymes that work to balance and increase the natural action of enzymes, which may result in permanent relief of heartburn, gas, indigestion, and ulcers.
BIO NATIVUS, P.O. Box 3281, Ogden, UT 84401; tel: 888-628-4887 or 801-732-1294.

Gentle-Cleanse: Capsules. Contains natural plant fiber (psyllium hydrophyllic mucilloid), which the body needs daily to help eliminate waste, and the extract casanthranol from aged cascara sagrada that gently promotes comfortable relief of occasional irregularity.
NATURE'S HERBS, 600 East Quality Drive, American Fork, UT 84003; tel: 800-437-2257 or 801-763-0700.

Ginger-Peppermint Combination: Capsules. For relief of stomach and intestinal distress, bloating, distention, fullness, pressure, and cramps (gas) after eating; contains ginger root, peppermint leaves, cramp bark, wild yam root, spearmint leaves, fennel seed, catnip herb, and papaya leaves.

NATURE'S HERBS, 600 East Quality Drive, American Fork, UT 84003; tel: 800-437-2257 or 801-763-0700.

Health Cleanse: Powder. Combination of highly soluble, sugar-free fibers and herbs that help cleanse and detoxify the colon and intestines.

BIODYNAMAX, 6525 Gunpark Drive #150-507, Boulder, CO 80301; tel: 800-926-7525 or 303-530-4665.

Herbal Aloe Force: Juice or topical gel. Processed aloe vera juice containing vitamins, minerals, enzymes, amino acids, essential fatty acids, growth factors, glycoproteins, sterols, bioflavonoids, and polysaccharides (complex sugars), plus ionized colloidal silver, and supportive herbal extracts (cat's claw, chamomile, burdock root, hawthorn berry astragalus root, sheep sorrell, pau d'arco bark, slippery elm bark, and rhubarb root).

HERBAL ANSWERS, INC., P.O. Box 1110, Saratoga Springs, NY 12866; tel: 888-256-3367 or 518-581-1968.

Herbal Nutrition: Vegicaps. Herbal nutritional formula that helps the body remove the mucoid plaque that lines the walls of the alimentary canal.

ARISE AND SHINE, P.O. Box 1439, Mount Shasta, CA 96067; tel: 800-688-2444 or 530-926-0891.

Herb Tablets (#9A). Herbal laxative containing *Aloe curacao* and cascara sagrada, which aid in the removal of consolidated, bacteria-laden waste matter that accumulates in the large intestine.

SONNE'S ORGANIC FOODS, INC., P.O. Box 2160, Cottonwood, CA 96022; tel: 800-544-8147 or 530-347-5868.

Hyland's Hemorrhoids: Sublingual tablets. For relief of itching and burning pains due to hemorrhoids; ingredients include *Aesculus hipp, Ratanhia, Nux vomica*, and *Calc fluorica*.

P & S LABS, 210 West 131st Street, Los Angeles, CA 90061; tel: 800-624-9659 or 310-768-0700.

Inner Strength: Powder. Contains patented globulin protein concentrate from whey that can help inhibit unfriendly microorganisms in the intestine. *Authors' note: Inner Strength is helpful for supporting bowel changes that occur while traveling.*

ETHICAL NUTRIENTS, 971 Calle Negocio, San Clemente, CA 92673; tel: 800-668-8743 or 949-366-0818.

Intestamine: Powder. Tissue-nourishing formula for general or intensive gastrointestinal support.

AMNI, 2247 National Avenue, Hayward, CA 94540-5012; tel: 800-437-8888 or 510-783-6969.

Intestinal Cleanser: Powder. Contains powdered psyllium seed and husk, which help remove old mucus, feces, and putrefying toxins that can accumulate in pockets of the large intestine.

SONNE'S ORGANIC FOODS, INC., P.O. Box 2160, Cottonwood, CA 96022; tel: 800-544-8147 or 530-347-5868.

Ipecac: Homeopathic remedy. Helpful in nausea and vomiting.

STANDARD HOMEOPATHIC CO., 201 West 131st, Los Angeles, CA 90061; tel: 800-624-9659 or 310-768-0700.

Kyo-Dophilus: Capsules or tablets. Capsules contain three strains of beneficial bacteria (*L. acidophilus, B. bifidum,* and *B. longum*) prevalent in the intestines helping to normalize the intestinal flora; tablets contain one strain of beneficial bacteria, *L. acidophilus.*

WAKUNAGA OF AMERICA, 23501 Madero, Mission Viejo, CA 92691; tel: 800-421-2998 or 949-855-2776.

KYOLIC Formula 102: Capsules or tablets. Contains Aged Garlic Extract (a Wakunaga product) and enzymes, which aid in breaking down and assimilating food.

WAKUNAGA OF AMERICA, 23501 Madero, Mission Viejo, CA 92691; tel: 800- 421-2998 or 949-855-2776.

Lactase Rx: Softgels. Dairy digestive aid containing lactase, which helps convert lactose (a milk sugar) found in dairy products into digestible sugars; helps prevent stomach cramps, gas, bloating, and diarrhea.

PHYTO-THERAPY, INC., OPTIMUM HEALTH, 483 West Middle Turnpike, Manchester, CT 06040; tel: 800-228-1507 or 860-647-9729.

Laxaco: Capsules. Herbal therapy for stomach distress and constipation; ingredients include cascara sagrada and senna leaves.

PHILLIPS NUTRITIONALS, 27071 Cabot Road #122, Laguna Hills, CA 92653; tel: 800-514-5115 or 702-898-8141.

LB Formula: Capsules or tablets. Vegetable laxative with cascara sagrada bark in a base of goldenseal root, barberry bark, ginger root, red raspberry leaves, rhubarb root, fennel seed, cayenne, and lobelia herb.

NATURE'S HERBS, 600 East Quality Drive, American Fork, UT 84003; tel: 800-437-2257 or 801-763-0700.

Lipex: Powder. Fiber supplement with lecithin, which contains dietary fibers, including carrageenan, guar gum, lecithin, and other nutrients that support metabolism of fat and cholesterol.

AMNI, 2247 National Avenue, Hayward, CA 94540-5012; tel: 800-437-8888 or 510-783-6969.

Liquid Bentonite. Bentonite clay has been used for centuries as an internal and external purification aid; absorbs metals, drugs, and toxins for release from the body.

ARISE AND SHINE, P.O. Box 1439, Mount Shasta, CA 96067; tel: 800-688-2444 or 530-926-0891.

LIV-WELL: Caplets or capsules. Contains the flavonoids silymarin, quercetin, cynarin, and capillarisin, which have been shown to improve liver metabolism and promote detoxification of the liver and body in general; aids in the elimination of excess water through the kidneys, and stimulates bile flow (through the gallbladder) and other digestive substances, which improves digestion; recommended for elimination of stored toxins or for those exposed to environmental pollutants or who consume alcohol.

EXTREME HEALTH, INC., 50 Oak Court, Suite 212, Danville, CA 94526; tel: 800-800-1285 or 925-855-1262.

Longest Living Acidophilus Plus: Capsules. Blend of the *Lactobacillus* strains *bacilli caucasicus, bulgarkus, foghurti,* and *bifktus.*

FUTUREBIOTICS, 145 Ricefield Lane, Hauppauge, NY 11788; tel: 800-FOR-LIFE (367-5433) or 516-273-6300.

LX-Elimination: Tablets. Helps digestion, assimilation, and elimination; contains aloe, buckthorn, bayberry, seaweed, white oak bark, myrrh, ginger, and cider vinegar.

NATURAL ENERGY PRODUCTS, 21101 Welch Road, Snohomish, WA 98296; tel: 425-486-5956.

MSM (Methylsulfonylmethane): Capsules, eye and ear drops, lotion, or powder. Contains sulfur, which is a major component of the human body.

MSM provides the body with building materials for healthy, flexible cells. RICH DISTRIBUTING, P.O. Box 33830, Portland, OR 97292; tel: 877-245-5742 or 503-761-7450.

Multi-Fiber Complex: Capsules. Daily fiber supplement to help maintain regularity or as part of a weight-loss program; contains fiber from five sources plus the herbs licorice root and slippery elm bark.
NATROL, INC., 21411 Prairie Street, Chatsworth, CA 91311; tel: 818-739-6000.

MyoCalm: Tablets. For relief of bowel spasm and muscle tension and spasm; also relieves anxiety by promoting relaxation and may facilitate sleep onset. Contains concentrates (four times the activity of unconcentrated herbs) of valerian, passiflora, and black cohosh, plus calcium, magnesium, vitamin B6, and niacinamide.
KARUNA CORP., 42 Digital Drive # 7, Novato, CA 94949; tel: 800-826-7225 or 415-382-0147.

Nature Cleanse: Tablets. Contains a blend of fiber and herbs with digestive enzymes to maximize the cleansing process.
NATURE'S PLUS, 548 Broadhollow Road, Melville, NY 11747-3708; tel: 800-645-9500 or 516-293-0030.

Oregamax: Capsules. Contains crushed wild oregano, *Rhus cariaria*, garlic, and onion; wild oregano contains carvacrol (antimicrobial), flavonoids (antiseptic properties), and terpenes (anti-inflammatory).
PURITY PRODUCTS, 1804 Plaza Avenue, New Hyde Park, NY 11040; tel: 800-769-7873.

Oxy-Cleanse by Earth's Bounty: Capsules. Oxygen colon conditioner that works without psyllium or herbs to break down debris into very small pieces that can be easily and gently eliminated.
MATRIX HEALTH PRODUCTS, 8400 Magnolia Avenue, Suite N, Santee, CA 92071; tel: 800-736-5609 or 619-448-7550.

PB 8 Lacto Safe: Capsules and chewable tablets. For people who are lactose intolerant; contains the enzymes lactase, protease, and lipase, plus *acidophilus* and FOS (fructo-oligosaccharides), to help digest dairy products.
NUTRITION NOW, 501 Southeast Columbia Shore Boulevard #350, Vancouver, WA 98661; tel: 800-929-0418 or 360-737-6800.

PB 8 Pro-Biotic Acidophilus: Capsules. Contains 14 billion viable "friendly" bacteria per capsule; also available as a vegetarian product called PB 8 Vegetarian.

NUTRITION NOW, 501 Southeast Columbia Shore Boulevard #350, Vancouver, WA 98661; tel: 800-929-0418.

pH Paper. pH Paper (to test acid/alkaline balance) is used for each of three pH tests to gauge the body's electrolyte levels during the cleansing program.

ARISE AND SHINE, P.O. Box 1439, Mount Shasta, CA 96067; tel: 800-688-2444 or 530-926-0891.

Plant Enzymes: Capsules. For gas, bloating, heartburn, maldigestion, food intolerance, and elimination of wastes; contains seven plant-source digestive enzymes, friendly bacteria, pantothenic acid, and papain (protein digestant) to help break down fat, protein, plant matter, sugars, and milk and encourage proper digestion of food.

NUPRO, 735-L Park Street, Castle Rock, CO 80104; tel: 800-704-8910 or 303-660-0562.

Primadophilus: Capsules. *Lactobacillus* supplement for adults containing *L. acidophilus* and *L. rhamnosus* at 10 billion microorganisms per gram (2.8 billion per capsule) at the time of manufacture.

NATURE'S WAY PRODUCTS, INC., 10 Mountain Springs Parkway, Springville, UT 84663; tel: 800-962-8873 or 801-489-1500.

Primadophilus Bifidus: Capsules. Senior adult formula containing selected strains of freeze-dried *Bifidobacterium* and *Lactobacillus* at 10 billion microorganisms per gram (3.4 billion per capsule) at the time of manufacture; primarily for people 50 years or older.

NATURE'S WAY PRODUCTS, INC., 10 Mountain Springs Parkway, Springville, UT 84663; tel: 800-962-8873 or 801-489-1500.

Proflora: Liquid. Nutritional and botanical support to optimize the climate and growth of beneficial flora in the intestinal tract, inhibit pathogenic or abnormal flora, and soothe irritated intestinal mucosa.

BIO-BOTANICAL RESEARCH, INC., 144 Pioneer Road, Corralitos, CA 95076; distributed by WELLNESS HEALTH PHARMACY, 2800 South 18th Street, Homewood, AL 35209; tel: 800-227-2627 or 205-879-6551

Pro-Gest: Tablets. Vegetarian digestive aid containing papain (protein digestant), papaya seed meal, Russian black radish, and betain

hydrochloride to help the body secrete digestive juices.
SONNE'S ORGANIC FOODS, INC., P.O. Box 2160, Cottonwood, CA 96022; tel: 800-544-8147 or 530-347-5868.

Propile: Phyto-homeopathic gel. Contains homeopathic ingredients in a base of butcher's broom and witch hazel to help soothe the pain, itching, and localized sensitivity of hemorrhoids and reduce minor swelling of the surrounding area.
SUPHERB LTD., P.O. Box 1135, Nahariya 22100, Israel; tel: 800-409-HERB (4372).

Psyllium Husk Powder. Fibrous bulking agent that gels and thickens when mixed with liquid and helps detoxify the alimentary canal.
ARISE AND SHINE, P.O. Box 1439, Mount Shasta, CA 96067; tel: 800-688-2444 or 530-926-0891.

Quintessence Clove-A-Day Garlic and Herbs: Capsules. Contains odor-free garlic, acerola cherry, rose hips, slippery elm, and marshmallow root for their ability to soothe the digestive tract.
PURE-GAR, 21411 Prairie Street, Chatsworth, CA 91311; tel: 800-537-7695 or 818-739-6046.

Quintessence Garlic Plus FOS: Capsules. Contains 100% pure odor-free garlic, combined with FOS (fructo-oligosaccharides), which selectively promote the growth of beneficial intestinal bacteria.
PURE-GAR, 21411 Prairie Street, Chatsworth, CA 91311; tel: 800-537-7695 or 818-739-6046.

Regucil: Capsules. For overnight relief of occasional irregularity. Combines the natural stimulant laxatives aloe vera and casanthranol (extract of cascara sagrada) in a base of fennel, ginger, raspberry leaves, goldenseal root, barberry bark, and cayenne.
NATURE'S HERBS, 600 East Quality Drive, American Fork, UT 84003; tel: 800-437-2257 or 801-763-0700.

Renewall: Capsules. Rebuilds the intestinal lining; contains quercetin, rutin, L-glutathione, L-cysteine-HCl, bioflavonoids, and L-selenium-methionine. For intestinal degenerative conditions such as colitis, diarrhea, giardiasis, candidiasis, and other toxic colon conditions from an improper diet or chronic constipation, and a history of antibiotic use.

ARISE AND SHINE, P.O. Box 1439, Mount Shasta, CA 96067; tel: 800-688-2444 or 530-926-0891.

Senna Extract (Cassia angustifolia): Capsules. For overnight relief of irregularity; suitable for cases of chronic constipation and for children.
NATURE'S HERBS, 600 East Quality Drive, American Fork, UT 84003; tel: 800-437-2257 or 801-763-0700.

Spectra Probiotic: Each capsule contains billions of bacteria in a base of FOS (fructo-oligosaccharides).
NF FORMULAS, INC., 9755 Southwest Commerce Circle C-5, Wilsonville, OR 97070; tel: 800-547-4891 or 503-682-9755.

Stomach Acid Balance: Tablets. Helps support the body's natural pH for health and well-being.
VEDA HEALTH, INC., P.O. Box 1535, Soquel, CA 95073; tel: 888-856-8334 or 408-465-9084.

Stomach Upset: Capsules. Contains the food enzymes amylase, lipase, cellulase, lactase, invertase, and glucoamylase; also contains botanicals and probiotics to support optimal digestive functions and maintain gastrointestinal integrity.
ALTERNATIVE THERAPY, INC., 1664 Fairlawn Avenue, San Jose, CA 95125; tel: 800-311-7922.

Stomach-Relief Rx: Softgels. Contains ginger (whole and extracts), parsley, peppermint, spearmint, ajowan, fennel, and anise, lemon oils, and enzymes with calcium carbonate to provide support and help the body neutralize excess acids and settle upset stomach.
PHYTO-THERAPY, INC., OPTIMUM HEALTH, 483 West Middle Turnpike, Manchester, CT 06040; tel: 800-228-1507 or 860-647-9729.

Super Colon Cleanse: Capsules or powder. Contains pure psyllium, herbs, and *acidophilus*; psyllium has lubricating properties; the herbs senna, fennel seed, celery seed, cascara sagrada, Oregon grape root, and buckthorn bark provide laxative action; digestive enzymes help digest food; and rose hips, peppermint, and Oregon grape root soothe an irritated colon.
HEALTH PLUS, 13837 Magnolia Avenue, Chino, CA 91710; tel: 800-822-6225 or 909-627-9393.

Superdophilus: Powder. Contains nonfat milk, whey, *Lactobacillus acidophilus* (super strain DDS-1); produces hydrogen peroxide (H_2O_2) and

GASTROINTESTINAL DISORDERS

other antimicrobial agents that can be used against the microorganisms *Staphylococcus aureus* (food poisoning and toxic shock syndrome), *Escherichia coli* (Montezuma's revenge and chronic kidney failure), and *Candida albicans* (yeast overgrowth and thrush); recommended for older children and adults; dairy-free formula also available.

NATREN, 3105 Willow Lane, Westlake Village, CA 91361; tel: 800-992-3323 or 805-371-4737.

Super Vegi-dophilus: Powder. Contains *Lactobacillus acidophilus* (DDS-1 super strain) developed from various vegetable sources that mimic the carbohydrate/protein ratio found in milk; defends the small intestine against harmful bacteria; milk-free.

NATREN, 3105 Willow Lane, Westlake Village, CA 91361; 800-992-3323 or 805-371-4737.

Tam—An Effective Natural Laxative: Tablets. Contains cascara sagrada, the "holy bark" that has been used as a laxative in folk medicine for centuries.

AMERICAN HEALTH, 4320 Veterans Memorial Highway, Holbrook, NY 11741; tel: 800- 445-7137.

Triphala: Tablets. Internal cleanser to invigorate, strengthen, and tone the gastrointestinal system; for long-term preventative maintenance or for a concentrated cleansing program; provides nutritional support for indigestion, carbohydrate intolerance, elevated cholesterol, diabetes, chronic lung disease, hypertension, anemia, yeast infections, eye disease, and skin disorders.

PLANETARY FORMULAS, 23 Janis Way, Scotts Valley, CA 95066; tel: 800-606-6226.

Vegetarian Enzyme Complex: Tablets. Contains seven enzymes derived from vegetarian sources to facilitate digestion of a wide variety of foods.

FUTUREBIOTICS, 145 Ricefield Lane, Hauppauge, NY 11788; tel: 800-FOR-LIFE (367-5433) or 516-273-6300.

Hair Problems

Hair on the human body goes through a natural cycle of gradual loss and replacement. The life span of hair ranges are from three to five months for eyebrow hair and two to five years for scalp hair.

Types of Hair Problems

Brittle Hair With Split Ends—Coarse, dry, brittle hair is one of the signs of an underactive thyroid gland (hypothyroidism), which is treatable by nutritionally supporting the thyroid with kelp products or thyroid glandular extracts.

Dandruff—Characterized by dry, white scales shed from the scalp, dandruff is associated with underlying nutritional deficiencies or health conditions such as seborrheica dermatitis.

Hair Loss (Alopecia)—The most common pattern of hair loss is called male pattern baldness or hereditary alopecia. Hair loss in women is usually less severe and typically occurs after the delivery of a child or after menopause (both associated with hormonal imbalance). Other causes of hair loss include stress, poor circulation, poor diet with excess salt and sugar, acute illness, surgery, chemotherapy or radiation, an underactive thyroid gland, skin disease, excessive tissue copper levels, sudden weight loss, diabetes, and mineral or vitamin deficiencies (particularly iron and biotin).

Nutrients and Herbs for Hair Problems

■ **For hair growth and maintenance:** Folic acid, biotin, vitamin B5, PABA (para-aminobenzoic acid), and silica help maintain the color and thickness of the hair. Kelp is a good source of the trace minerals needed for human metabolism and supports the maintenance of hair, nails, and skin. The amino acid cysteine supplies sulfur which is essential for strong, healthy hair and nails. Inositol and zinc regulate the oil content in hair and are necessary for hair growth.

■ **For dry hair:** Essential fatty acids are important for maintaining the oils of the hair.

■ **For dandruff:** minerals (particularly zinc), B vitamins, and beta carotene can alleviate dandruff.

■ **For maintaining the oxygen supply to the hair follicles and outer layers of the skin:** zinc, copper, and antioxidants such as vitamins A, C, and E are helpful.

Products for Hair Problems

Curetage: Shampoo. Blend of botanicals and antioxidant vitamins to cleanse hair follicles and remove toxins; also contains vasodilators that increase blood flow to the hair root.

AGE LESS PRODUCTS, INC., 24101 Highway 138, Albemarle, NC 28001; tel: 800-273-4246 (ext. 430) or 704-982-7551.

E • GEM Organic Shampoo. Contains vitamins E (d-alpha tocopherol acetate), A, and D, panthenol, and protein to bring out the natural highlights in hair; biodegradable.

J.R. CARLSON LABS, INC., 15 College Drive, Arlington Heights, IL 60004-1985; tel: 800-323-4141 or 708-255-1600.

Essential Oils Formula: Softgels. Contains flax seed, borage, and fish oils, which are sources of essential fatty acids; also contains vitamin E, an important antioxidant.

ATKINS NUTRITIONALS, INC., 185 Oser Avenue, Hauppauge, NY 11788; tel: 800-628-5467 or 516-951-7171; or CANADIAN AMERICAN RESOURCES, 327 West Fayette Street, Suite 211, Syracuse, NY 13202; tel: 315-476-4944.

Fundamental Sulfur: Tablets. Supplies biologically active sulfur, a mineral element that is indispensable as a structural component of hair, connective tissues, skin, nails, antibodies, and other body proteins.

AMNI, 2247 National Avenue, Hayward, CA 94540-5012; tel: 800-437-8888 or 510-783-6969.

Hair Clear 1-2-3: Spray. Contains essential oils of coconut, anise, and ylang-ylang.

QUANTUM, INC., 754 Washington Street, Eugene, OR 97401; tel: 800-448-1448 or 541-345-5556.

Hair Formula: Capsules. Combination of herbs and vitamins including horsetail extract, L-cysteine, vitamin C, biotin, and nettle leaf to help promote beautiful hair.

NATURE'S HERBS, 600 East Quality Drive, American Fork, UT 84003; tel: 800-437-2257 or 801-763-0700.

Hair It Is: Tablets. Contains vitamins and minerals required for healthy hair, including silica, to strengthen, nourish, and thicken hair.

PHILLIPS NUTRITIONALS, 27071 Cabot Road #122, Laguna Hills, CA 92653; tel: 800-514-5115 or 702-898-8141.

Hair & Nail Formula with Vegetal Silica: Capsules. Formula of horsetail, which contains silica to help fortify hair and nails, plus oatstraw and gotu kola.

NATROL, INC., 21411 Prairie Street, Chatsworth, CA 91311; tel: 818-701-6000.

Hair Rush: Liquid. Combines the stimulating herbs prickly ash and cayenne pepper with the nourishing botanicals nettle and horsetail to help promote vibrant and healthy hair.

NEW CHAPTER, 22 High Street, Brattleboro, VT 05301; tel: 800-543-7279 or 802-257-9345.

Hair Sensation: Tablets. For the maintenance of healthy hair, skin, and nails; contains antioxidant nutrients and herbs including horsetail, an herb containing silica (a mineral present in all of the connective tissues of the body).

RAINBOW LIGHT, P.O. Box 600, Santa Cruz, CA 95061; tel: 800-635-1233 or 408-429-9089.

Hair, Skin & Nails: Tablets. Contains 24 vitamins, minerals, herbs, and other nutrients to build and strengthen hair, nails, and skin.

FUTUREBIOTICS, 145 Ricefield Lane, Hauppauge, NY 11788; tel: 800-FOR-LIFE (367-5433) or 516-273-6300.

Hair, Skin & Nails: Tablets. Combination of vitamins A, B complex, and E, zinc, and calcium to help create healthy hair, skin, and nails; also contains the herbs butcher's broom (*Ruscus aculeatus*), bilberry, horsetail, and nettles, which provide nutritional support for hair, skin, and nails.

OPTIMAL NUTRIENTS, 1163 Chess Drive #F, Foster City, CA 94404; tel: 800-966-8874 or 650-525-0112.

Inner Beauty: Tablets. Ingredients include nourishing herbs with well-balanced vitamins to produce strong and healthy hair, skin, and nails.

BIO NATIVUS, P.O. Box 3281, Ogden, UT 84401; tel: 888-628-4887 or 801-732-1294.

Jojoba Oil Hydrating Hair Care: Shampoo. Contains jojoba oil and spirulina, which add body and shine to the hair; deeply cleanses the hair without stripping natural oils. Conditioners contain jojoba and kukui nut oils and aloe vera and comfrey extracts to help moisturize the scalp.

DESERT ESSENCE, 9700 Topanga Canyon Boulevard, Chatsworth, CA 91311; tel: 800-848-7331 or 818-734-1735.

Lustre: Tablets. Targets common deficiencies in American diets and the effects of pollution to provide nutrition for hair, skin, and nails; ingredients include silicon, vitamins A, B1, B2, B3, B5, B6, B12, and E, beta carotene, proline, manganese, copper, zinc, magnesium, folic acid, biotin, and inositol.

SOURCE NATURALS, THRESHOLD ENTERPRISES, 23 Janis Way, Scotts Valley, CA 95066; tel: 800-777-5677 or 831-438-1144.

MSM (Methylsulfonylmethane): Capsules, eye and ear drops, lotion, or powder. Contains sulfur, which is a major component of the human body. MSM provides the body with building materials for healthy, flexible cells.

RICH DISTRIBUTING, P.O. Box 33830, Portland, OR 97292; tel: 877-245-5742 or 503-761-7450.

Nutri~Hair: Tablets. Contains micronutrients (often lacking in our diets) necessary for biochemical support of healthy hair; ingredients include several B vitamin factors, lipotropics, minerals, trace minerals, copper, PABA (para-aminobenzoic acid), d-calcium pantothenate, and folic acid to maintain normal hair color and help fight premature graying.

AMERICAN HEALTH, 4320 Veterans Memorial Highway, Holbrook, NY 11741; tel: 800-445-7137.

Samson Hair Program: Liquid or tablets. Hair formula for balding men; increases blood flow to hair follicles and decreases the negative effects of testosterone on hair growth; contains silica and marine protein.

SCANDINAVIAN NATURAL HEALTH & BEAUTY PRODUCTS, INC., 13 North 7th Street, Perkasie, PA 18944; tel: 800-688-2276.

Shelly's Hair Care: Tablets. Contains vitamins, herbs, and amino acids, which can help give luster and body to hair.

HEALTH PLUS, 13837 Magnolia Avenue, Chino, CA 91710; tel: 800-822-6225 or 909-627-9393.

Skin and Hair Nutrients: Tablets. Combines vitamins, minerals, and concentrated herbal extracts for healthier-looking hair and skin.

NEW CHAPTER, 22 High Street, Brattleboro, VT 05301; tel: 800-543-7279 or 802-257-9345.

Tea Tree Oil Replenishment Hair Care System. Shampoo contains tea tree and lavender oil to cleanse and condition the hair and scalp; conditioner contains tea tree and jojoba oils to remove tangles and nourish hair shafts.

DESERT ESSENCE, 9700 Topanga Canyon Boulevard, Chatsworth, CA 91311; tel: 800-848-7331 or 818-734-1735.

Tea Tree Shampoo. Removes buildup in dull and lifeless hair.

THURSDAY PLANTATION INC., NATURE'S PLUS, 548 Broadhollow Road, Melville, NY 11747-3708; tel: 800-645-9500.

Headaches can have many causes, among them systemic infections, digestive disorders, allergies, stress, muscle tension, hormonal imbalance, caffeine withdrawal, oxygen deficiency, and problems in the ears, eyes, nose, throat, or teeth.

To permanently eliminate your headaches rather than simply treat the symptom of pain, it is necessary to identify the underlying causes. Once the relationship is established between the body's physiological state and the headache, proper treatment can begin.

Nutrients and Herbs for Headaches

■ **For all headaches:** we recommend essential fatty acid supplementation with evening primrose oil (EPO) which contains high levels of GLA (gamma-linolenic acid), known to work well for vascular headaches, hormonal, or allergy-related headaches. EPO improves circulation, helps regulate inflammation, and relieves pain.[101] White willow bark and feverfew, which have aspirin-like activity, can be an effective headache pain reliever.[102]

■ **For allergy headaches:** plant enzymes can both alleviate the current allergy-related headache and, by lowering the body's allergic load, reduce the incidence of future attacks. Quercetin, a bioflavonoid with anti-inflammatory properties, can reduce the mucus and sinus congestion contributing to headaches. Adaptogenic (assisting the body in coping with stress) herbs such as Siberian ginseng and *Panax ginseng* are useful to ease the adrenal stress which occurs with allergies and can produce headaches.

■ **For cluster headaches:** capsaicin, the active ingredient of cayenne pepper, has a long history of use in pain control. Applied topically, it can effectively relieve cluster headaches.

■ **For headaches related to digestive tract disorders:** digestive enzyme formulas can improve digestion, assimilation, and, with *acidophilus* (a beneficial intestinal bacteria), control harmful bacteria and toxins. By restoring digestive health, associated

CAUTION

If your headaches are accompanied by certain symptoms, they could be an indication of a more serious condition and you should consult your health-care practitioner immediately. These symptoms include: blurred vision, whole or partial loss of vision, or changes in color vision; extreme sensitivity to light; pressure behind the eyes, relieved by vomiting; excessive or continual throbbing of the head and/or temples (one or both sides); extreme pressure in the facial sinus area (behind the eyes and nose); and rapid heart beat and high blood pressure.

headaches can be eliminated.

■ **For hormonal headaches in women:** we first evaluate estrogen and progesterone levels and then treat any imbalance with natural progesterone topical creams and hormone-regulating herbs such as chastetree berry.

■ **For migraine headaches:** the herb feverfew has proven effective in decreasing both the frequency and intensity of migraine headache episodes.[103] Valerian root, a mild sedative and antispasmodic, will not cure migraine headaches, but can reduce the discomfort associated with them. The anti-inflammatory action of quercetin is sometimes beneficial for migraine headaches, as is niacin, due to its ability to dilate blood vessels. Ginger is an effective remedy for the nausea and vomiting which, in some people, accompany migraine headaches.

■ **For morning headaches:** low blood sugar (hypoglycemia) is another common cause of headaches, typically occurring upon waking in the morning when blood sugar is at its lowest. In these cases, free-form amino acids at bedtime can help maintain blood sugar levels through the night.

■ **For muscle tension headaches:** a deficiency of calcium and magnesium is a common cause of headaches, due to the increased muscle tension and constriction of blood vessels to the scalp and head produced by the deficiency. We often recommend Calcium Plus, which has the proper 2:1 ratio of magnesium to calcium, as a means of restoring these important minerals and thereby promoting muscle relaxation.

■ **For headaches caused by overconsumption of alcohol (hangover):** hangovers are partially the result of the dehydrating effects of alcohol, so drinking purified water is important to restore the body's liquids. As people who drink habitually or who abuse alcohol are typically deficient in vitamins B1, B2, B3, and B12, folic acid, calcium, magnesium, and zinc, these supplements are recommended.

■ **For headaches related to oxygen deficiency:** to promote better circulation and oxygenation of the blood, take coenzyme Q10, citrus bioflavonoids, pycnogenol (grape seed or pine bark extract), and ginkgo.

■ **For stress-related headaches:** we often recommend vitamin C, vitamin-B complex (especially B5, niacin, and niacinamide), calcium, and magnesium. The B vitamins

As feverfew is a uterine stimulant, it should not be used during pregnancy.

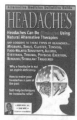

See *An Alternative Medicine Definitive Guide to Headaches* (Future Medicine Publishing, 1997; ISBN 1-887299-18-1); to order, call 800-333-HEAL.

For more on **natural progesterone**, see Premenstrual Syndrome, pp. 309-318; for **hormone-regulating herbs**, see Menopausal Symtoms, pp. 268-274. For information on a **home test for hormone levels**, see Appendix: Great Smokies Diagnostic Laboratory, pp. 484-485.

in general support proper function of the nervous system; niacin and niacinamide also improve circulation and B5, known as the anti-stress vitamin, is vital to production of adrenal hormones. Vitamin C is essential for adrenal gland function which is compromised by chronic stress. Calcium and magnesium are known to reduce muscle tension. Among herbs, wood betony can help relieve headaches due to nervous tension.

■ **For headaches related to toxicity:** as the liver is the body's main filter for toxins, cleansing and supporting this organ helps alleviate toxic overload, one symptom of which is headaches. Liver Guard or products containing blue-green algae, milk thistle (silymarin), and lipoic acid (sulfur-containing antioxidant involved in energy production; dietary sources are liver and yeast) provide nutritional and detoxification assistance to the liver.

Products for Headaches

Ache-Prin: Capsules. Provides relief of headaches and other body aches and pains; also effective in reducing fever; ingredients include magnesium salicylate, feverfew, white willow bark, and lupulin (hops).

RIDGECREST HERBALS, 1151 South Redwood Road #106, Salt Lake City, UT 84104-3729; tel: 800-242-4649 or 801-978-9633.

Aconitum Napellus: Homeopathic remedy. Helpful for headache, fright, injury, fear of dental treatment or surgery, earache, colic, and painful urination.

STANDARD HOMEOPATHIC CO., 201 West 131st, Los Angeles, CA 90061; tel: 800-624-9659 or 310-768-0700.

AspirActin: Capsules. Supports the body's normal adaptogenic functions; contains willow bark, kava-kava, ginkgo, and inositol hexanicotinate.

NATURE'S PLUS, 548 Broadhollow Road, Melville, NY 11747-3708; tel: 800-645-9500 or 516-293-0030.

Belladonna: Homeopathic remedy. Helpful for headache, fever, earache, toothache, sore throat, and colic.

STANDARD HOMEOPATHIC CO., 201 West 131st, Los Angeles, CA 90061; tel: 800-624-9659 or 310-768-0700.

Beyond Feverfew: Tablets. Contains feverfew for healthy blood vessels, purple willow, kava-kava, ginkgo, magnesium and DL-phenylalanine.

KAL, NUTRACEUTICAL CORP., P.O. Box 681869, Park City, UT 84068; tel: 800-669-8877.

BioE Headache: Homeopathic liquid. For temporary relief of headaches and migraines.

BIOENERGETICS, INC., P.O. Box 127, Sandy, OR 97055; tel: 800-334-4043 or 503-668-7478.

Calcium Plus: Tablets. Daily supplement of calcium, magnesium, essential minerals (which support the skeletal and muscular systems) co-nutrients, superfoods, and a blend of seven Chinese herbs considered supportive of skeletal health; for diets high in dairy products and low in magnesium-rich foods (grains and legumes).

RAINBOW LIGHT, P.O. Box 600, Santa Cruz, CA 95061; tel: 800-635-1233 or 408-429-9089.

Cayenne (Capsicum): Capsules. Cayenne, an internal disinfectant, provides effective support for migraine and cluster-type headaches; it is one of the highest sources of vitamins A and C, has the complete vitamin B complexes, and is rich in organic calcium and potassium.

ARISE AND SHINE, P.O. Box 1439, Mount Shasta, CA 96067; tel: 800-688-2444 or 530-926-0891.

Chamomilla: Homeopathic remedy. Helpful for pain, fever, earache, toothache, teething difficulties, colic, and temper.

STANDARD HOMEOPATHIC CO., 201 West 131st, Los Angeles, CA 90061; tel: 800-624-9659 or 310-768-0700.

Feverfew Scullcap: Capsules or liquid. Contains feverfew for reducing the body's production of prostaglandins (involved in inflammatory responses), plus skullcap, lavender, and rosemary for minor tension, and valerian for its relaxing effects on muscle tension.

FRONTIER COOPERATIVE HERBS, 3021 78th Street, Norway, IA 52318; tel: 800-669-3275 or 319-227-7996.

Gelsemium: Homeopathic remedy. Helpful for headache, stage fright, nervous dread of an ordeal, apprehension of dental work or surgery, dizziness, and flu.

STANDARD HOMEOPATHIC CO., 201 West 131st, Los Angeles, CA 90061; tel: 800-624-9659 or 310-768-0700.

The Hangover Formula: Tablets. Combination of antioxidants and herbs

that help prevent and relieve some of the symptoms of hangovers.
SOURCE NATURALS, THRESHOLD ENTERPRISES, 23 Janis Way, Scotts Valley, CA 95066; tel: 800-777-5677 or 831-438-1144.

Headache by Jade: Tablets. Chinese herbal pain-relief formula to relieve feelings of pressure, pent-up emotions, and tension.
EAST EARTH HERB INC., P.O. Box 2802, Eugene, OR 97402; tel: 800-827-HERB (4372) or 541-687-0155.

Hyland's Headache: Sublingual tablets. For relief of head pain due to stress, illness, or nerves.
P & S LABS, 210 West 131st Street, Los Angeles, CA 90061; tel: 800-624-9659 or 310-768-0700.

Hypericum: Homeopathic remedy. Helpful in eye, nerve, and tailbone injury, dental surgery, puncture wounds, splinters, bites, cuts, burns, and post-operative pain.
STANDARD HOMEOPATHIC CO., 201 West 131st Street, Los Angeles, CA 90061; tel: 800-624-9659 or 310-768-0700.

Liver Guard: Tablets. Provides nutrients and related substances identified in scientific studies as nourishing or protecting the liver; contains dandelion root and extract, turmeric, silymarin (from milk thistle seed extract), N-acetyl-cysteine, vitamins, minerals, and coenzyme Q10.
SOURCE NATURALS, THRESHOLD ENTERPRISES, 23 Janis Way, Scotts Valley, CA 95066; tel: 800-777-5677 or 831-438-1144.

MigraActin: Capsules. Contains feverfew, pantothenic acid, and ginkgo to support the body's normal adaptogenic function.
NATURE'S PLUS, 548 Broadhollow Road, Melville, NY 11747-3708; tel: 800-645-9500 or 516-293-0030.

Migracin: Capsules. Contains feverfew extract, white willow extract (concentrated and standardized for salicin), white willow bark, and DPLA (DL-phenylalanine, an important amino acid). Caution: Do not use if you are pregnant.
NATURE'S HERBS, 600 East Quality Drive, American Fork, UT 84003; tel: 800-437-2257 or 801-763-0700.

Migracin Plus: Softgels. Formula containing feverfew extract, magnesium, white willow and ginger root extracts, and vitamin E.

NATURE'S HERBS, 600 East Quality Drive, American Fork, UT 84003; tel: 800-437-2257 or 801-763-0700.

MigraGard: Capsules. Contains 0.7% parthenolide, the active ingredient in feverfew.

SOLARAY, NUTRACEUTICAL CORP., P.O. Box 681869, Park City, UT 84068; tel: 800-669-8877.

Migrahelp with Feverfew Extract: Capsules. Feverfew inhibits the body's production of prostaglandins (hormone-like, complex fatty acids involved in inflammation), suspected to play a role in migraines. Caution: Not to be used during pregnancy or lactation.

NATROL, INC., 21411 Prairie Street, Chatsworth, CA 91311; tel: 818-739-6000.

Migraine Formulae: Homeopathic liquid. Relieves the nausea, double vision, blind spots, chills, dizziness, throbbing severe headache, depression, and mood changes associated with migraine; safe for children.

LIDDELL LABORATORIES, 1036 Country Club Drive, Moraga, CA 94556; tel: 800-460-7733.

Pain Headaches Fever Relief Herbal Formula: Capsules. Ingredients include white willow (*Salix alba*) bark, a natural pain reliever, and meadowsweet herb.

PHILLIPS NUTRITIONALS, 27071 Cabot Road #122, Laguna Hills, CA 92653; tel: 800-514-5115 or 702-898-8141.

Pain Stop: Vegicaps. For relief of headaches, menstrual discomfort, joint pain, and other types of body pain; contains white willow bark extracts.

FLORA INC., 805 East Badger Road, Lynden, WA 98264; tel: 800-446-2110 or 360-354-2110.

Willow Bark: Capsules. Contains willow bark extract, standardized to 7%-9% salicin (the active ingredient in willow bark); like aspirin (derived from salicylic acid, an acid that is similar to salicin), willow bark is helpful for mild headaches and pain caused by inflammation, mild fevers associated with colds and infections (influenza), and acute and chronic rheumatic disorders, but does not have the side effects often associated with aspirin.

OPTIMAL NUTRIENTS, 1163 Chess Drive #F, Foster City, CA 94404; tel: 800-966-8874 or 650-525-0112.

Willowprin: Capsules. Contains white willow bark, extract, and concentrate; does not contain aspirin, caffeine, or synthetic drugs.

NATURE'S HERBS, 600 East Quality Drive, American Fork, UT 84003; tel: 800-437-2257 or 801-763-0700.

Vitamin B Complex: Tablets. Contains a combination of B vitamins plus catalytic-acting nervine herbs that support the body's nervous system, PABA (paraminobenzoic acid), choline inositol, thiamin (B1), riboflavin (B2), pyridoxine (B6), niacinamide, pantothenic acid (B5), folic acid, cobalamin (B12), and biotin in a base of valerian root, hops, catnip, chamomile, barberry, and capsicum.

NATURAL ENERGY PRODUCTS, 21101 Welch Road, Snohomish, WA 98296; tel: 425-486-5956.

Heart Disease

While heart disease is the leading cause of death in the United States,[104] it is also one of the most preventable degenerative diseases. Dietary changes, exercise, stress reduction, and nutritional supplementation are often sufficient to both prevent and reverse cardiovascular (pertaining to the heart and blood vessels) disorders.

Types of Heart Disease

Angina Pectoris–Characterized by discomfort, heaviness, pain, or pressure in the chest, angina results from a diminished supply of oxygen to the heart muscle. Angina is a warning sign of heart attack risk.

Arteriosclerosis–The most common form of arteriosclerosis (hardening of the arterial walls), atherosclerosis involves deposits of fatty substances on the walls of the arteries causing them to thicken. In advanced stages, blood flow is impeded.

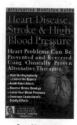

See *Alternative Medicine Guide to Heart Disease* (Future Medicine Publishing, 1998; ISBN 1-887299-10-6); to order, call 800-333-HEAL.

Heart Attack–A heart attack (myocardial infarction) occurs when blood supply and the oxygen it carries to the heart is cut off to the point that part of the heart literally dies. If blockage is extensive, death can result.

Congestive Heart Failure–Medically termed cardiomyopathy, this condition literally means failure of the heart muscle. When the heart has been weakened by a heart attack, for example, it is unable to pump fully, resulting in blood congestion in the heart. A typical sign of congestive heart failure is shortness of breath either with minimal exertion or when lying down at night.

For information about **lowering cholesterol levels**, see Cholesterol, Elevated, pp. 133-135.

High Blood Pressure–High blood pressure or hypertension is the most common cardiovascular disease in industrialized nations. It weakens and degenerates arteries and is a major cause of heart attack, stroke, and congestive heart failure. Lifestyle and dietary factors are the main causes of high blood pressure (SEE QUICK DEFINITION). Of these factors, a high-fat, high-salt diet and lack of exercise are particularly to blame.

Causes of Heart Disease

The standard American diet (refined, processed foods, saturated fats, and high levels of red meat and dairy products) and lifestyle are the main culprits in heart disease.

There is a significant body of evidence that homocysteine, a normal by-product of protein metabolism, may play a role in arteriosclerosis (hardening of the arteries). Homocysteine is normally converted into a harmless amino acid (cystathionine). But in some individuals, a genetic defect or nutritional deficiency (in folic acid and the B vitamins) prevents the normal conversion process of homocysteine from occurring. Excess homocysteine may generate free radicals which are capable of oxidizing cholesterol and damaging arterial walls.

The body actually needs cholesterol (SEE QUICK DEFINITION) for strong cell membranes, manufacturing hormones, and health of the immune system. Cholesterol presents a threat to the body when it has been oxidized by free radicals. Oxidized cholesterol initiates the formation of plaque on arterial walls, interfering with blood circulation, and leading to heart attacks and strokes.[105]

QUICK DEFINITION

The term **blood pressure** refers to the force of the blood against the walls of arteries, veins, and the chambers of the heart as it is pumped through the body. The additional force exerted by the blood against the arteries (when high blood pressure is present) begins to weaken the cellular walls and makes it easier for toxins and cholesterol to form deposits on the arterial walls. Blood pressure measurement involves systolic (when the heart contracts) and diastolic (when the heart rests and fills with more blood). The ratio of the two represents blood pressure. A healthy reading is 120/80. A typical reading indicative of early high blood pressure is 140/90.

Nutrients and Herbs for Heart Disease

A healthy diet emphasizing whole, unprocessed foods (including fruits, vegetables, and sources of essential fatty acids) can reduce the risk of developing heart disease. Specifically, essential fatty acids have demonstrated the ability to reduce hypertension.[106]

Possibly the most important nutritional fact to understand regarding the heart is the role of magnesium. All muscles in the body require this mineral for their ability to rest after contraction, but as the heart is a muscle that never stops working, it requires an estimated eight times the amount of magnesium needed by other muscles in the body.

Nutritional formulas designed for the cardiovascular system are an easy method of providing your heart with supplemental support for optimal functioning. A good formula will include most or all of the following: antioxidants such as coenzyme Q10 and pycnogenol, vitamins A, C, E, and B complex (B6, B12, and folic acid), selenium, and quercetin; the minerals magnesium, potassium, and calcium; bromelain (an enzyme derived from pineapple); and herbs such as hawthorn and garlic. Sufficient levels of B vitamins will prevent accumulation of toxic levels of homocysteine, while antioxidants will neutralize free radicals and prevent damage to the heart's arterial wall.

Coenzyme Q10 and vitamin E are particularly beneficial supplements for cardiovascular and coronary heart diseases, as evidenced by a large body of research. Co-Q10 helps increase exercise capacity, reduce arrhythmias (irregular heartbeat), improve oxygen delivery to the heart, and enhance healing and recovery in patients with heart and circulatory problems.[107] Vitamin E provides antioxidant protection, reduces platelet stickiness (a factor in atherosclerosis), and lowers cholesterol, all of which contribute to the prevention of cardiovascular disease.[108]

One of the most promising herbs for the treatment of heart disease is hawthorn, which has been found to improve circulation of blood to the heart by dilating the blood vessels and relieving spasms of the arterial walls.[109] Ginkgo is another herb with extensive research demonstrating its benefits for circulation and cardiovascular conditions.[110]

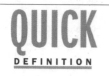

Products for Heart Disease

Basic Antiox: Capsules or tablets. Antioxidant nutrients to help support the heart and immune system.

AMNI, 2247 National Avenue, Hayward, CA 94540-5012; tel: 800-437-8888 or 510-783-6969.

Calcium Plus: Tablets. Contains calcium, magnesium, essential minerals (which support the skeletal and muscular systems) co-nutrients, superfoods, and a blend of seven Chinese herbs important for skeletal health; for diets high in dairy products and low in magnesium-rich foods (grains and legumes).

RAINBOW LIGHT, P.O. Box 600, Santa Cruz, CA 95061; tel: 800-635-1233 or 408-429-9089.

CardioHerb with Hawthorn Berry: Capsules. Contains hawthorn berry (which has promising attributes for heart function support), cayenne seed pod, ginger root, and motherwort leaf.

NATROL, INC., 21411 Prairie Street, Chatsworth, CA 91311; tel: 818-739-6000.

Cardio Protector Rx: Softgels. For optimum heart and vascular health.

PHYTO-THERAPY, INC., OPTIMUM HEALTH, 483 West Middle Turnpike, Manchester, CT 06040; tel: 800-228-1507 or 860-647-9729.

Cardi-Rite: Tablets. For normal function of the cardiovascular system; ingredients include the minerals (glycinate chelates), B complex vitamins, amino acids, coenzyme Q10, and the antioxidants beta carotene, buffered vitamin C, natural vitamin E, and organic selenium.

J.R. CARLSON LABS, INC., 15 College Drive, Arlington Heights, IL 60004-1985; tel: 800-323-4141 or 708-255-1600.

CholestaKit: Capsules. CholestaKit Formula I helps bind dietary fats and cholesterol and excrete them from the body; Formula II helps break down plaque in the arteries.

SIERRA HEALTH PRODUCTS, INC., 7949 Woodley Avenue, Van Nuys, CA 91406; tel: 818-375-5029.

Coenzyme Q-10 Rx (Q-Gel): Softgels. Cellular energizer; water-soluble coenzyme Q10 with enhanced bioavailability.

PHYTO-THERAPY, INC., OPTIMUM HEALTH, 483 West Middle Turnpike, Manchester, CT 06040; tel: 800-228-1507 or 860-647-9729.

CoQ10 (Coenzyme Q10): Capsules. Assists the antioxidant vitamins C and E; helps strengthen the heart muscle and provide oxygen to cells.

TWIN LABS, 150 Motor Parkway, Hauppauge, NY 11788; tel: 800-645-5626.

C.V. Support: Tablets. Designed to promote cardiovascular wellness.

HVL INC., 600 Boyce Road, Pittsburgh, PA 15205; tel: 800-245-4441.

Garlic-EDTA Chelator: Capsules. Chelation therapy can slow or reduce arteriosclerosis (hardening of the arterial walls) due to calcification. The chelating agents garlic and EDTA (ethylene diamine tetra-acetic acid) bind with heavy metals and minerals (lead, mercury, and calcium), which promote blood clotting and calcification of the arteries, and passes with them out of the body via the kidneys and the urine. Formulated by Gary Gordon, M.D., the founder of ACAM (the American College of Advancement in Medicine), Garlic-EDTA should be used as a general health measure not as a treatment of disease or pathology; use in conjunction with a complete multivitamin high in magnesium and zinc.

LIFEENHANCEMENT PRODUCTS INC., P.O. Box 751390, Petaluma, CA 94975-1390; tel: 800-543-3873 or 707-762-6144.

GarlioVascular: Capsules. Formula of garlic, hawthorn, bilberry, and butcher's broom to help support a healthy cardiovascular system.

SOLARAY, NUTRACEUTICAL CORP., P.O. Box 681869, Park City, UT 84068; tel: 800-669-8877.

Germanium: Capsules. Contains germanium Ge-132 (bis-carboxyethyl germanium sesquioxide); animal experiments suggest a role for organic germanium in hypertension and heart disease.

OPTIMAL NUTRIENTS, 1163 Chess Drive #F, Foster City, CA 94404; tel: 800-966-8874 or 650-525-0112.

Ginkgo Phytosome Plus Choline: Softgels. Helps increase blood circulation to the brain; contains herbal extracts, soybean phospholipids (lecithin), choline, and the antioxidant vitamin E.

NATURE'S HERBS, 600 East Quality Drive, American Fork, UT 84003; tel: 800-437-2257 or 801-763-0700.

Hawthorn Motherwort: Capsules or liquid. Contains hawthorn berry, Siberian ginseng, and the herbs valerian and motherwort. Caution: Do not use during pregnancy.

FRONTIER COOPERATIVE HERBS, 3021 78th Street, Norway, IA 52318; tel: 800-669-3275 or 319-227-7996.

Hawthorn Special Formula: Capsules. Contains standardized hawthorn extracts, coenzyme Q10, vitamin B6, magnesium, selenium, chromium, taurine, L-carnitine, and the herbs motherwort, rosemary, and ginger.

SOLARAY, NUTRACEUTICAL CORP., P.O. Box 681869, Park City, UT 84068; tel: 800-669-8877.

Heart Glandular Plus: Tablets. Contains raw bovine heart concentrate, magnesium, and hawthorn berry, which can help maintain healthy heart function and promote blood-vessel relaxation.

ETHICAL NUTRIENTS, 971 Calle Negocio, San Clemente, CA 92673; tel: 800-668-8743 or 949-366-0818.

Heart Science: Tablets. Helps protect the cardiovascular system, decrease homocysteine levels, fight cholesterol build up, supply energy, and regulate electrical rhythm.

SOURCE NATURALS, THRESHOLD ENTERPRISES, 23 Janis Way, Scotts Valley, CA 95066; tel: 800-777-5677 or 831-438-1144.

Hemp Oil. Source of essential fatty acids; contains a 3:1 balance of omega-6 to omega-3 and active phospholipids and sterols, which promote cell membrane regeneration and improve immunity; does not contain active THC (tetrahydrocannabinol).

SPECTRUM NATURALS, 133 Copeland Street, Petaluma, CA 94952; tel: 800-995-2705 or 707-778-8900.

Homocysteine Modifier Products: Tablets. Helps support healthy homocysteine levels; ingredients include folic acid, vitamin B6, vitamin B12, and trimethylglycine.

KAL, NUTRACEUTICAL CORP., P.O. Box 681869, Park City, UT 84068; tel: 800-669-8877.

Homocysteine Modulators: Vegicaps. Contains trimethylglycine (TMG), vitamins B6 and B12, and folic acid, which are important for maintaining proper levels of homocysteine.

SOLGAR VITAMIN & HERB COMPANY, INC., 500 Willow Tree Road, Leonia, NJ 07605; tel: 800-645-2246 or 201-944-2311.

KYOLIC Formula 106: Tablets. Contains Aged Garlic Extract (a Wakunaga product), natural vitamin E, hawthorn berry, and cayenne, which aid in the maintenance of a healthy heart and circulatory system.

WAKUNAGA OF AMERICA, 23501 Madero, Mission Viejo, CA 92691; tel: 800 421-2998 or 949-855-2776.

Max Omega: Oil. Source of essential fatty acids; contains black currant seed oil, linoleic acid, and alpha linolenic acid.

BIO-NUTRITIONAL FORMULAS, 106 East Jericho Turnpike, Mineola, NY 11501; tel: 800-950-8484.

#1 Garlic Plus Ester-C and FOS: Capsules. Contains garlic, an important herb for the cardiovascular and immune systems, ester-C (vitamin C), and FOS (fructo-oligosaccharides).

NUTRITION NOW, 501 Southeast Columbia Shore Boulevard, #350, Vancouver, WA 98661; tel: 800-929-0418 or 360-737-6800.

Ocean Nutrition of Canada Cardio Nutrition: Capsules. Helps maintain a healthy heart; contains omega-3, EPA (eicosapentaenoic acid), and DHA (docosahexaenoic acid).

OCEAN NUTRITION CANADA LTD., 757 Bedford Highway, Bedford, Nova Scotia, Canada B2A3Z7; tel: 888-980-8889 or 902-457-2399.

Oral Chelation and Age-Less Formulas: Liquid. Oral chelation, vitamin, mineral, and nutrient replenishment formula; Oral Chelation I Formula contains nutrients that can cross the blood-brain barrier to bind with and flush mercury and heavy metals out of the body; contains EDTA, alginate, garlic, attapulgite clay, chlorella, methionine, cysteine, lipoic acid, vitamin C, and other ingredients; Age-Less II Formula replenishes the nutrients that are removed by chelation and helps support and detoxify the liver; contains minerals, vitamins, phyto-nutrients, antioxidants, amino acids, and lipotropics; both formulas contain plant-based bromelain, lipase, and catalase enzymes for optimal digestion, assimilation, and utilization of nutrients.

EXTREME HEALTH, INC., 50 Oak Court, Suite 212, Danville, CA 94526; tel: 800-800-1285 or 925-855-1262.

PressuRest: Capsules. Strengthens the heart and circulatory organs; ingredients include Siberian ginseng, hawthorn berries, valerian root, yarrow flowers, garlic, rutin, and spirulina.

RIDGECREST HERBALS, 1151 South Redwood Road #106, Salt Lake City, UT 84104-3729; tel: 800-242-4649 or 801-978-9633.

Regenex: Capsules. Supports cardiovascular health; contains coenzyme Q10, pantetheine (a relative of vitamin B5), and carnitine (an amino acid).

SCHIFF, WEIDER NUTRITION GROUP, 2002 South 5070 West, Salt Lake City, UT 84104; tel: 800-439-8042 or 801-975-5000.

Resveratrol: Tablets. Contains antioxidants produced by grapevines and other plants in response to infection or environmental stress; can help prevent platelet aggregation.

SOURCE NATURALS, THRESHOLD ENTERPRISES, 23 Janis Way, Scotts Valley, CA 95066; tel: 800-777-5677 or 831-438-1144.

Thera Q Plus: Softgels. Combination of the cardio-supportive antioxidants coenzyme Q10, vitamin E, and alpha-lipoic acid.

NUTRIMEDIKA CORP., 101 Newport Street, Bayport, NY 11705-2224; tel: 800-688-7462 or 516-472-5761.

TMG Trimethylglycine: Tablets. Supports a healthy circulatory system; proper homocysteine levels can be maintained by trimethylglycine (a form of the amino acid glycine) and certain B vitamins.

SOURCE NATURALS, THRESHOLD ENTERPRISES, 23 Janis Way, Scotts Valley, CA 95066; tel: 800-777-5677 or 831-438-1144.

Trimethylglycine (TMG): Powder or tablets. Aids in the conversion of homocysteine to the amino acid methionine. TMG also benefits the liver and converts to a beneficial, energy-producing amino acid form (dimethylglycine or DMG).

KLABIN MARKETING, 2067 Broadway #700, New York, NY 10023; tel: 800-933-9440 or 212-877-3632.

Herpes

The herpes family of viruses include many different strains, among them Epstein-Barr, shingles, and herpes simplex I and II. The discussion here focuses on herpes simplex, also known as "herpes."

Types and Symptoms of Herpes

There are two forms of the herpes simplex virus: herpes simplex type 1 (HSV1), or oral herpes, and herpes simplex type 2 (HSV2), or genital herpes. Outbreaks of oral herpes consist of cold sores or fever blisters around the mouth. Outbreaks of genital herpes involve painful sores in the genital area.

Genital herpes is usually spread by sexual contact and is therefore classified as a sexually transmitted disease. The first signs of HSV2 infection can occur four to seven days after sexual activity with an infected partner. Tingling, burning, or a persistent itch usually herald an outbreak. A day or two later, small, pimple-like bumps appear over reddened skin and develop into painful blisters which eventually burst and then scab over. Symptoms typically subside in seven to ten days from the first sign of outbreak.

Once infected with herpes, a person carries the virus forever but it may remain dormant most of the time. Stress, nutritional deficiencies, and fever, among other factors, can precipitate an outbreak of either form of herpes simplex.

Nutrients and Herbs for Herpes

Research has demonstrated the antiviral effects of licorice root and its specific application to inactivating the growth of herpes simplex virus.[111] The flavonoid quercetin has also been shown to inhibit the herpes virus.[112] Herbal antimicrobials echinacea, goldenseal, and tea tree oil can also be helpful.

The amino acid lysine has proven effective in reducing the frequency of oral and genital herpes outbreaks.[113] Our clinical experience confirms these research results; lysine has worked well for most of our patients in both decreasing the episodes and lesion severity of herpes. Super Lysine Plus is a good product line, with both oral and topical applications. Topical zinc sulfate can also be effective in alleviating the symptoms of both oral and genital herpes outbreaks.[114]

Supplementing with essential fatty acids and B-complex vitamins, which support immune function and tissue healing, can be useful in both preventing and alleviating herpes outbreaks.

Products for Herpes

AminoMune: Capsules. Contains an arginine-free, balanced complex of 18 isolated L-crystalline amino acids and the amino acid L-lysine; for viral infections such as cold/lip sores, fever blisters, or underlying viral conditions.

NUTRI-SOURCE, 3290 Cessna Drive, Cameron Park, CA 95682; tel: 800-293-1683 or 530-676-8838.

BioPro Thymic Protein A: Sublingual powder. Contains thymic protein A, which increases the number of key white blood cells and allows the body to fight off infections (from flu to herpes).

KLABIN MARKETING, 2067 Broadway #700, New York, NY 10023; tel: 800-933-9440 or 212-877-3632.

Cold Sore Formula: Liquid. Relieves discomfort of fever blisters, dryness of lips and corners of mouth, eczema around mouth, and scaly or pustular eruptions with burning and itching.

LIDDELL LABORATORIES, 1036 Country Club Drive, Moraga, CA 94556; tel: 800-460-7733 or 925-377-3000.

Herpex: Phyto-homeopathic gel. Contains homeopathic ingredients in a base of melissa and Australian tea tree oil for relief of painful, itchy sores and to reduce local tension, soreness, and burning of herpes simplex type 1 and 2 eruptions on any part of the body.

SUPHERB LTD., P.O. Box 1135, Nahariya 22100, Israel; tel: 800-409-HERB (4372).

Hyland's Cold Sores & Fever Blisters: Ointment. For relief of symptoms of fever blisters and canker sores due to colds or stress.

P & S LABS, 210 West 131st Street, Los Angeles, CA 90061; tel: 800-624-9659 or 310-768-0700.

Lysine Herbal Formula: Capsules. Contains the amino acid L-lysine, additional nutrients, and traditional Chinese and Western herbs known for their cooling and relaxing properties.

ZAND HERBAL FORMULAS, 1722 14th Street #230, Boulder, CO 80302; tel: 800-800-0405 or 303-786-8558.

Super Lysine Plus:
   Cream. Contains L-lysine and 16 vitamins, herbs, and minerals.
   Coldstick. Moisturizes and relieves cracked lips, and heals, treats, and prevents sensitive skin problems; contains SPF-15 sunscreen, L-lysine, and 16 herbs and vitamins.
   Tablets. Contains L-lysine, echinacea, vitamin C, garlic, propolis, and goldenseal root; for best results use with cream.
   Liquid. Contains L-lysine, echinacea, gum benzoin, vitamin C, and licorice, propolis, and shiitake mushroom extracts.
   QUANTUM, INC., 754 Washington Street, Eugene, OR 97401; tel: 800-448-1448 or 541-345-5556.

Hypoglycemia

Hypoglycemia is an abnormally low level of blood sugar (glucose) or abnormal fluctuations in blood sugar levels.

Symptoms and Causes of Hypoglycemia

Symptoms include weakness, fatigue, extreme hunger, headache, irritability, dizziness, sweating, rapid heart rate, digestive disturbances, sugar cravings, and memory and concentration problems. Symptoms may vary in severity and frequency.

The root cause of hypoglycemia is oversecretion of insulin by the pancreas; insulin helps metabolize blood sugar. Common causes that can precipitate this dysfunction include stress, exhausted adrenal glands (which handle stress), excessive exercise, liver congestion or damage, underactive thyroid gland (hypothyroidism), irregular eating habits, nutritional deficiencies (such as vitamin B6, chromium, zinc, essential fatty acids, and the amino acid alanine), and excessive consumption of refined foods, caffeine, and sugar.

Blood sugar levels are ideally maintained by the breakdown of dietary proteins into amino acids, which can then be converted into glucose for use in the production of energy. This process is designed to keep a person's energy, stamina, and brain function steady for long periods of time. (People who are not able to adequately digest proteins often become hypoglycemic.)

By contrast, relying on sugar for energy wreaks havoc on blood sugar levels. Eating sugar to alleviate low blood sugar provides a sugar "rush," which then sends the body into a state of high blood sugar (hyperglycemia). After a short time (15-30 minutes), the body has used up the energy from the sugar and "crashes," or returns to a low-blood-sugar state. This roller-coaster effect is extremely hard on the body which operates best at a sustained blood sugar level.

Nutrients and Herbs for Hypoglycemia

Eat whole organic foods in small portions throughout the day. Avoid the following: skipping meals (especially breakfast), eating processed foods that are nutrient poor, or drinking excessive amounts of caffeinated beverages in the morning.

The following nutrients are also useful for hypoglycemia:

■ **Chromium picolinate and free-form amino acids:** these nutrients help normalize blood sugar; chromium is vital in glucose metabolism.

■ **Copper and zinc:** zinc is necessary for the proper production and utilization of insulin; copper and zinc levels must be maintained in relationship because an excess of one produces a deficiency of the other.

Products for Hypoglycemia

AminoPlus: Capsules. Balanced complex of 14 isolated L-crystalline amino acids to assist, along with a reduced-calorie diet and exercise program, in the reduction of body fat and aid in maintaining energy; helpful for people with blood sugar fluctuations, dieters with periodic sugar cravings, runners, swimmers, cyclists, boxers, aerobic enthusiasts and athletes, and circuit trainers.

NUTRI-SOURCE, 3290 Cessna Drive, Cameron Park, CA 95682; tel: 800-293-1683 or 530-676-8838.

Blood Sugar Balance: Capsules. Chinese herbal formula that controls blood sugar levels; ingredients include calcium sulfate, oryza seed, anamarrhena root, ginseng root, and licorice root.

RIDGECREST HERBALS, 1151 South Redwood Road #106, Salt Lake City, UT 84104-3729; tel: 800-242-4649 or 801-978-9633.

Chromium Picolinate: Capsules. Assists the body with the metabolism of sugar and protein utilization.

SPORTS ONE INC., 47 Capital Drive, Wallingford, CT 06492; tel: 800-624-8787 or 203-294-6370.

GlucoBalance: Capsules. For individuals with blood sugar disorder. Caution: If you are taking diabetes medication, do not use GlucoBalance without medical supervision.

PROBIOLOGIC, BIOTICS RESEARCH, 6801 Biotics Research Drive, Rosenberg, TX 77471; tel: 800-678-8218.

GTF Chromium Complex: Tablets. Helps maintain healthy, balanced blood sugar levels; contains GTF (glucose tolerance factor) chromium polynicotinate, a key mineral in the metabolism of sugars, and its essential co-factor L-glutathione in a base of superfoods and herbs.

RAINBOW LIGHT, P.O. Box 600, Santa Cruz, CA 95061; tel: 800-635-1233 or 408-429-9089.

Impotence

Impotence is a man's inability to achieve or maintain an erection.

Causes of Impotence

Among men over the age of 50 who are suffering from impotence, the main cause for almost half is arteriosclerosis (arterial hardening and narrowing which restricts blood flow) of the penile artery.[115]

Other physical factors contributing to impotence are diabetes, hypothyroidism, and the use of alcohol, antihypertensive medications, tranquilizers, or amphetamines.[116]

Nutrients and Herbs for Impotence

When atherosclerosis of the penile artery is the source of a man's impotence, we recommend a product called Oral Chelation. Chelation therapy (SEE QUICK DEFINITION) is a method used to "scrub" the arteries and get rid of arterial wall buildup, which can impede blood flow.

The following nutrients are also useful for impotence:

■ **Vitamins A, C, and E, and folic acid:** recommended for cases of low sex drive or impotence.

■ **Essential fatty acids and zinc:** important for sperm production and sexual energy.

■ **Ginkgo:** extract can improve blood flow in the penile artery.[117]

■ **Yohimbine:** extract of the bark of the yohimbe tree traditionally used as an aphrodisiac; has been shown to effectively restore erectile function, regardless of the cause of impotence.[118]

■ **Other Herbs:** Korean ginseng is a useful tonic for impotence,[119] as is suma (Brazilian ginseng), which is also used as an aphrodisiac. Muira puama (potency wood), a Brazilian herb, was traditionally used as a potent aphrodisiac and nerve stimulant and has demonstrating benefits in recent research.[120] Catuaba, guarana, and damiana leaf are sexual stimulants.

Yohimbine should be used with caution. In some cases, it can produce bronchospasm, increase blood pressure, or induce anxiety or mania in patients with bipolar depression. Do not use yohimbine if you have kidney disease or psychological disturbances.

Products for Impotence

Action Max for Men: Tablets. Herbal nutrient complex with yohimbe and *ashwagandha* to stimulate and improve sexual function and tonify the male reproductive organs and glands.

COUNTRY LIFE, 101 Corporate Drive, Hauppauge, NY 11788; tel: 800-645-5768 or 516-231-1031.

Arouse: Capsules. Combination of herbal extracts and amino acids that can help enhance the sexual experience; ingredients include L-arginine, yohimbe, *Avena sativa*, ginseng, saw palmetto, and *Ginkgo biloba*.

EMERALD LABORATORIES, 5933 Sea Lion Place #105, Carlsbad, CA 92008; tel: 800-775-1112 or 760-930-8091.

Herbal Male Complex: Vegicaps. Helps maintain male health and well-being; ingredients include the extracts of standardized saw palmetto, nettles, astragalus, Korean (*Panax*) and Siberian ginseng, soy isoflavone, and the raw powders of saw palmetto berry, astragalus root, Korean and Siberian ginseng, and nettle.

SOLGAR VITAMIN & HERB CO, INC., 500 Willow Tree Road, Leonia, NJ 07605; tel: 800-645-2246 or 201-944-2311.

In the Mood: Tablets. Helps support male functioning and enhance well-being, energy, and general health; ingredients include the herbs quebracho, pygeum bark, pumpkin seed oil, *Avena sativa*, damiana, nettle, and kava-kava, vitamins B and E, zinc, and the hormones DHEA and pregnenolone (derived from plant sources), which can be converted by the body into sex hormones.

SYNERGY PLUS, IVC, 500 Halls Mill Road, Freehold, NJ 07728; tel: 800-666-8482.

Love Male: Capsules. Contains damiana, guarana, suma, gotu kola, kava-kava, yohimbe, saw palmetto, Siberian ginseng, sarsparilla, muira puama, ginger root, wild yam, niacin, and zinc.

CRYSTAL STAR HERBAL NUTRITION, 4069 Wedgeway Court, Earth City, MO 63045; tel: 800-736-6015 or 314-739-7551.

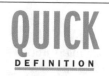

DEFINITION

Chelation therapy refers to a method of binding up ("chelating") toxins (e.g., heavy metals) and metabolic wastes and removing them from the body while at the same time increasing blood flow and removing arterial plaque. One type of chelation therapy involves the chelating agent disodium EDTA given as an intravenous infusion over a 3 1/2 hour period. Usually 20 to 30 treatments are administered at the rate of one to three sessions per week. Chelation therapy is especially beneficial for all forms of atherosclerotic cardiovascular disease including angina pectoris and coronary artery disease.

Male Drive: Capsules. Ingredients include yohimbe, vitamin E, green oats, zinc, Siberian ginseng, and I-histidine.

NUTRITION NOW, 501 Southeast Columbia Shore Boulevard #350, Vancouver, WA 98661; tel: 800-929-0418 or 360-737-6800.

Male Fuel: Capsules. Contains standardized yohimbe bark extract, L-arginine HCl, ginkgo extract, natural vitamin E, vitamins B5 and B6, zinc, L-tyrosine, choline bitartrate, saw palmetto, and phytosterol complex.

TWIN LABS, 150 Motor Parkway, Hauppauge, NY 11788; tel: 800-645-5626.

Male Plus: Liquid. Blend of herbs that support male sexual function; ingredients include muira puama, catuaba, sarsaparilla, and damiana.

RAINTREE GROUP, INC., 1601 West Koenig Lane, Austin, TX 78756; tel: 800-780-5902 or 512-467-6130.

Male Power: Tablets. Concentrated herbal/glandular formula that addresses nutritional deficiencies oftentimes causing fatigue and lackluster performance; ingredients include 15 herbal extracts, Chinese tonic herbs, high-energy foods, and nine male glandulars.

FUTUREBIOTICS, 145 Ricefield Lane, Hauppauge, NY 11788; tel: 800-FOR-LIFE (367-5433) or 516-273-6300.

Men's Formula APH: Capsules. Contains damiana leaves, sarsaparilla root, saw palmetto berries, *fo-ti* root, gotu kola, *Echinacea purpurea*, and Siberian ginseng root.

NATURE'S WAY PRODUCTS, INC., 10 Mountain Springs Parkway, Springville, UT 84663; tel: 800-962-8873 or 801-489-1500.

Men's Support: Tablets. For men concerned about sexual energy, hormonal balance, and vibrant health; contains zinc, vitamin E, selenium, and an herbal blend of saw palmetto, pumpkin seed, and ginseng.

RAINBOW LIGHT, P.O. Box 600, Santa Cruz, CA 95061; tel: 800-635-1233 or 408-429-9089.

Oral Chelation and Age-Less Formulas: Liquid. Oral Chelation I Formula contains nutrients that can cross the blood-brain barrier to bind with and flush mercury and heavy metals out of the body; ingredients include EDTA (an amino acid), alginate, garlic, activated attapulgite clay, chlorella, methionine, cysteine, lipoic acid, vitamin C, and lipotropics; Age-Less II Formula replenishes the nutrients that are removed by chelation and helps support and detoxify the liver; contains minerals, vitamins, phyto-nutrients, antioxidants, amino acids, and lipotropics; both formulas contain plant-based bromelain, lipase, and catalase enzymes for optimal digestion, assimilation, and utilization of nutrients.

EXTREME HEALTH, INC., 50 Oak Court, Suite 212, Danville, CA 94526; tel: 800-800-1285 or 925-855-1262.

Potent Potion: Capsules. Formula of five herbal extracts designed to act as an energizer, nervine tonic, and systemic cleanser; helps support men and women experiencing sexual inadequacy.

OPTIMAL NUTRIENTS, 1163 Chess Drive #F, Foster City, CA 94404; tel: 800-966-8874 or 650-525-0112.

Tribestan: Tablets. Non-hormonal preparation that helps stimulate sexual function in men and women.

SCHIFF, WEIDER NUTRITION GROUP, 2002 South 5070 West, Salt Lake City, UT 84104; tel: 800-439-8042 or 801-975-5000.

Vitality: Caplets. Combination of 13 herbs to help strengthen vitality and promote a healthy prostate and hormone levels.

NUPRO, 735-L Park Street, Castle Rock, CO 80104; tel: 303-660-0562 or 800-704-8910.

Yohimbe 1000: Capsules or liquid. Contains yohimbe bark, which has been shown to increase the body's testosterone levels.

SPORTS ONE, INC., 47 Capital Drive, Wallingford, CT 06492; tel: 800-624-8787 or 203-294-6370.

Indigestion/ Heartburn

Heartburn, a burning sensation below the sternum in the chest, is one of the symptoms of indigestion, or partial or improper digestion of food.

Symptoms and Causes of Indigestion and Heartburn

In addition to the uncomfortable and even painful burning sensation, symptoms of indigestion include a feeling of fullness, stomach pain, gas, belching, and regurgitation of acid from the stomach into the esophagus. The burning sensation of indigestion and heartburn is due to the return (reflux) of this stomach acid.

Indigestion is a common phenomenon after eating a large, rich, or spicy meal or certain foods that produce indigestion in the individual (citrus fruits, tomatoes, and legumes are common culprits). Consuming beverages and foods that irritate the stomach (such as alcohol, coffee, vinegar, and fatty, greasy foods) or taking medicine such as aspirin can also result in indigestion. Other causes include: enzyme deficiencies; food allergies or food intolerance, such as lactose intolerance; swallowing air as a result of eating too fast; not chewing food sufficiently (leads to poor digestion, as 50% of the breakdown of food should take place in the mouth); drinking large quantities of fluids with meals (which dilutes digestive enzymes and juices); ulcers or cancer of the stomach or small intestine; and excessive worry or anxiety.

We see many patients suffering from acid indigestion who are taking large amounts of antacids. Digestive enzymes and a basic review of how the stomach works and how antacids help create the problem are all most people need to end their indigestion. The stomach produces acid to break down proteins. Insufficient chewing and overconsumption of food, particularly proteins, can cause the stomach to compensate by producing extra acid. To counteract the acid, people often take antacids which makes the stomach alkaline. In order to restore the acid environment of the stomach, the body has to make more acid.

For more about promoting **healthy digestion**, see Gastrointestinal Disorders, pp. 198-217. For more about **enzymes**, see An A-Z Nutrient Guide in Part I, pp. 24-62.

In a related argument against antacids, taking them as a source of calcium is misguided. Calcium must be in an acidic environment in order to be properly assimilated. Antacids, as their name suggests, provide an alkaline environment that prevents the uptake of calcium.[121]

The cycle of poor digestion and the acid/alkaline roller coaster can be reduced or avoided by chewing food well, taking digestive enzymes with your meals, and limiting fluid intake while eating.

Nutrients and Herbs for Indigestion/Heartburn

■ **To improve digestion:** plant enzymes, taken as supplements before or an hour after meals, assist the body in proper digestion (breakdown) of foods; amylase breaks down carbohydrates, lactase breaks down milk sugars (found in dairy products), lipase for fats, and cellulase for fibers. Protease has deliberately been left off this list of the basic food enzymes because it can be irritating to an already upset stomach. Papain and bromelain are milder forms of proteolytic (protein-digesting) enzymes, which are not irritating and can help prevent inflammation.[122] Papain (enzymes found in unripe papaya), bromelain (enzyme compound from the pineapple plant), and the enzymes in papaya leaf facilitate healthy digestion by breaking down proteins and reducing inflammation.

Green tea, among many other healthful benefits, supports digestion and internal cleansing. Studies indicate a preventive effect on cancers of the gastrointestinal tract, including stomach, small intestine, pancreas and colon.[123] Aloe vera juice, taken internally, exerts tonic effects on the entire digestive tract and improves protein digestion and assimilation, reduces stomach acid, relieves and prevents constipation, and helps heal peptic ulcers.

Lactobacillus acidophilus, one of the main probiotics or "friendly" bacteria in the intestines, helps restore a healthy balance of intestinal flora. By improving the intestinal environment, *acidophilus* improves digestion, which in turn reduces heartburn and indigestion. Chlorophyll, a green plant pigment, brings beneficial effects to the entire digestive tract and digestion in general. It improves the digestive function of the liver and encourages the growth of healthy intestinal flora (such as *L. acidophilus* and *Bifidobacteria*),[124] neutralizes toxins, and aids in the elimination of fungal and yeast overgrowth in the digestive tract, and helps alleviate inflammation in the mouth, throat, stomach, and intestinal tract.

■ **To reduce inflammation and soothe the digestive tract:** slippery elm bark is high in mucilage (a plant substance similar to mucus), which soothes inflamed mucous membranes in the digestive tract; it has long been used for gastric and duodenal ulcer patients. Marshmallow root, like slippery elm bark, contains up to 35% mucilage and has a history of use for soothing digestive upsets, intestinal disorders, and inflammatory conditions. Known for its soothing and mildly stimulating effect on the stomach, ginger root is beneficial for a variety of stomach complaints including indigestion, stomachache, nausea, and ulcers. Gamma oryzanol, derived from rice bran oil, has shown benefits for gastrointestinal problems including chronic gastritis.[125]

■ **To reduce or eliminate excess gas:** mint has been used for thousands of years for the treatment of indigestion and intestinal colic (cramping). Specifically, peppermint and spearmint oils assist in the elimination of gas and the reduction of muscle spasms, as well as stimulate the flow of bile, which is an aid to digestion. Fennel oil, helpful in times of acid stomach, also assists in the elimination of gas, reduces muscle spasms in the intestinal tract, and relieves stomach and abdominal pains. Ajowan oil, pressed from wild celery seeds, has long been used in Ayurvedic medicine for indigestion and abdominal pains. It stimulates the digestive tract, reduces gas formation, and is antiparasitic.

Products for Indigestion/Heartburn

AbsorbAid: Capsules and powder. Contains stabilizing plant enzymes, which resist stomach acid and help digest every food group more effectively, preventing the symptoms of indigestion and heartburn.

NATURE'S SOURCE, 15451 San Fernando Mission Boulevard, Mission Hills, CA 91345; tel: 800-423-2405 or 818-837-3633.

Acid Arrest: Capsules. Relieves acid indigestion, calms the stomach, and reduces excess stomach acid normally associated with heartburn and upset stomach; ingredients include calcium carbonate, pepsin, pancreatin, bromelain, ox bile, papain, ginger, and peppermint. (Alternative to Maalox, Rolaids)

RIDGECREST HERBALS, 1151 South Redwood Road #106, Salt Lake City, UT 84104-3729; tel: 800-242-4649 or 801-978-9633.

Acid-Ease: Capsules. Soothing digestion formula for heartburn and acid indigestion; contains digestive enzymes that help break down and absorb foods; ingredients include pure plant enzymes, gamma oryzanol (found naturally in rice bran oil), slippery elm, and marshmallow root; suitable for sensitive digestive systems; does not contain antacid.

PREVAIL CORP., 2204-8 Northwest Birdsdale, Gresham, OR 97030; tel: 800-248-0885 or 503-667-5527.

Acidil: Homeopathic tablets. For temporary relief of occasional heartburn, acid indigestion, or sour stomach.

BOIRON, 6 Campus Boulevard, Building A, Newtown Square, PA 19073; tel: 800-264-7661.

Acidone: Phyto-homeopathic lozenges. Contains active homeopathic ingredients in a base of DGL (de-glycyrrhizinated licorice); especially suitable for dyspeptic (poor digestion) problems in the upper gastrointestinal tract, including peptic ulcers and reflux esophagitis; does not interfere with any other medicine.

SUPHERB LTD., P.O. Box 1135, Nahariya 22100, Israel; tel: 800-409-HERB.

Acidophilus Chewable: Wafers. Blend of the beneficial bacteria *B. bifidum* and *L. acidophilus* for intestinal health; for children or adults who prefer a chewable *acidophilus* product.

PHILLIPS NUTRITIONALS, 27071 Cabot Road #122, Laguna Hills, CA 92653; tel: 800-514-5115 or 702-898-8141.

Anti-Acid by Jade: Tablets. Chinese herbal digestive aid formula that neutralizes excess stomach acid, helps digestion, eases over-full sensation, and helps restore appetite.

EAST EARTH HERB INC., P.O. Box 2802, Eugene, OR 97402; tel: 800-827-HERB (4372) or 541-687-0155.

Beans...Beans and more Rx: Softgels. Helps stop gas, bloating, and cramping; contains food enzymes that are effective in digesting complex sugars found in gas-producing foods (beans, garlic, onions, Brussels sprouts, broccoli, cucumbers, cabbage, cauliflower, lentils, soy-based foods, and some fruits) into digestible sugars thereby preventing excess gas and discomfort.

PHYTO-THERAPY, INC., OPTIMUM HEALTH, 483 West Middle Turnpike, Manchester, CT 06040; tel: 800-228-1507 or 860-647-9729.

Broad Spectrum Enzymes: Chewable tablets or vegicaps. Enzyme replacement formula for people who eat cooked, processed food; when ingested with food, digestion can begin before the body's own enzymes go to work, reducing stress in the lower stomach and intestines and demand on the pancreas for digestive enzymes; contains protease, lipase, amylase, and cellulase.

ENZYMES INC., 8500 Northwest River Park Drive #223, Parkville, MO 64152; tel: 800-647-6377 or 816-746-6461.

Body Balance: Capsules. Helps friendly bacteria normalize colon pH, eliminate intestinal gas, evacuate wastes, improve immune function, form vitamins, produce lactase, and regulate cholesterol and hormonal levels; contains an enzymatic and bacterial mix including isolated soy protein, betaine, and seaweed (which provides trace minerals to support digestion).

NATURAL ENERGY PRODUCTS, 21101 Welch Road, Snohomish, WA 98296; tel: 425-486-5956.

Chamomile: Liquid. Standardized herbal extract; chamomile has been used for centuries as a gentle, soothing herb.

NATURE'S HERBS, 600 East Quality Drive, American Fork, UT 84003; tel: 800-437-2257 or 801-763-0700.

Digest-Ease: Capsules. Relieves stomach and intestinal distress, bloating, distention, fullness, pressure, and cramps after eating; no animal-source ingredients.

NATURE'S HERBS, 600 East Quality Drive, American Fork, UT 84003; tel: 800-437-2257 or 801-763-0700.

Digest Eze Rx: Capsules. Helps prevent gas, bloating, flatulence; effective when eating milk, beans, vegetables, and fruits.

R GARDEN, 3881 Enzyme Lane, Kettle Falls, WA 99141; tel: 800-700-7767 or 425-271-0539.

Gamma-Zyme Enzyme Formula: Capsules. Contains three enzymes to help digest fat, starches, and fiber, plus other ingredients to soothe and restore damaged or irritated intestinal linings.

R GARDEN, 3881 Enzyme Lane, Kettle Falls, WA 99141; tel: 800-700-7767 or 425-271-0539.

Gasalia: Homeopathic tablets. For temporary relief of bloating, pressure, and pain associated with gas.

BOIRON, 6 Campus Boulevard, Building A, Newtown Square, PA 19073; tel: 800-264-7661.

Gas Relief: Tablets. For relief of common bloating and flatulence; contains a blend of herbs and botanicals such as ginger root, peppermint leaves, and licorice root.

UNIVERSAL, 3 Terminal Road, New Brunswick, NJ 08901; tel: 800-872-0101 or 732-545-3130.

Gastone: Phyto-homeopathic lozenges. Contains homeopathic ingredients in a base of ginger, German chamomile, and caraway to diminish the accumulation of gases.

SUPHERB LTD., P.O. Box 1135, Nahariya 22100, Israel; tel: 800-409-HERB (4372).

Gastro Intestinal Support: Tablets. Contains minerals, trace minerals, herbs, and enzymes that work to balance and increase the natural action of enzymes; helps relieve heartburn, gas, indigestion, and ulcers.

BIO NATIVUS, P.O. Box 3281, Ogden, UT 84401; tel: 888-628-4887 or 801-732-1294.

Ginger-Peppermint Combination: Capsules. For relief of stomach and intestinal distress, bloating, and gas after eating; contains ginger root, peppermint leaves, cramp bark, wild yam root, spearmint leaves, fennel seed, catnip herb, and papaya leaves.

NATURE'S HERBS, 600 East Quality Drive, American Fork, UT 84003; tel: 800-437-2257 or 801-763-0700.

Lactase Rx: Softgels. Dairy digestive aid containing lactase, which helps convert lactose (a milk sugar in dairy products) into digestible sugars; helps prevent stomach cramps, gas, bloating, and diarrhea.

PHYTO-THERAPY, INC., OPTIMUM HEALTH, 483 West Middle Turnpike, Manchester, CT 06040; tel: 800-228-1507 or 860-647-9729.

Longest Living Acidophilus Plus: Capsules. Blend of the potent *Lactobacillus* strains *bacilli caucasicus, bulgarkus, foghurti* and *bifktus*; a diversity of bacterial strains can be important since each strain prospers under different conditions and in different parts of the intestines.

FUTUREBIOTICS, 145 Ricefield Lane, Hauppauge, NY 11788; tel: 800-FOR-LIFE (367-5433) or 516-273-6300.

Nighttime Heartburn Support: Capsules. Herbal digestive aid to ease the symptoms of nighttime heartburn; contains marshmallow root, slippery elm, licorice, *acidophilus*, and calcium.

NUTRITION NOW, 501 Southeast Columbia Shore Boulevard #350, Vancouver, WA 98661; tel: 800-929-0418 or 360-737-6800.

Plant Enzymes: Capsules. Contains seven plant-source digestive enzymes, friendly bacteria, pantothenic acid, and papain (protein digestant) to help break down fat, protein, plant matter, sugars, and milk and encourage proper digestion; helpful for gas, bloating, heartburn, maldigestion, food intolerance, and elimination of wastes.

NUPRO, 735-L Park Street, Castle Rock, CO 80104; tel: 303-660-0562 or 800-704-8910.

Primadophilus: Capsules. *Lactobacillus* supplement for adults containing *L. acidophilus* and *L. rhamnosus* at 10 billion microorganisms per gram (2.8 billion per capsule) at the time of manufacture.

NATURE'S WAY PRODUCTS, INC., 10 Mountain Springs Parkway, Springville, UT 84663; tel: 800-962-8873 or 801-489-1500.

Pro-Gest: Tablets. Vegetarian digestive aid containing papain (protein digestant), papaya seed meal, Russian black radish, and betain hydrochloride to help the body secrete digestive juices.

SONNE'S ORGANIC FOODS, INC., P.O. Box 2160, Cottonwood, CA 96022; tel: 800-544-8147 or 530-347-5868.

Spectra Probiotic: Capsules. Contains billions of bacteria from eight different strains in a base of FOS (fructo-oligosaccharides); each individual bacterium is coated with a protein matrix that protects the bacteria from harsh stomach acids for safe delivery to the upper intestinal tract; dairy-free and contains no yeast, soy, lactose or wheat.

NF FORMULAS, INC., 9755 Southwest Commerce Circle C-5, Wilsonville, OR 97070; tel: 800-547-4891 or 503-682-9755.

Stomach Acid Balance: Tablets. Helps support the body's natural pH balance for health and well-being.

VEDA HEALTH, INC., P.O. Box 1535, Soquel, CA 95073; tel: 888-856-8334 or 408-465-9084.

Stomach-Relief Rx: Softgels. Helps to neutralize excess acids and settle an upset stomach; contains ginger, parsley, peppermint, spearmint, ajowan, fennel, anise, lemon oil, enzymes, and calcium carbonate.

PHYTO-THERAPY, INC., OPTIMUM HEALTH, 483 West Middle Turnpike, Manchester, CT 06040; tel: 800-228-1507 or 860-647-9729.

Kidney Problems

The kidneys are two bean-shaped organs that filter the blood of water-soluble toxins and excess water, which are excreted from the body in the urine. Glucose and other substances that can be recycled are absorbed by the kidneys and reintorduced into the bloodstream. The kidneys also manage the body's strict water balance.

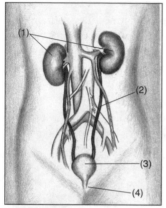

THE URINARY SYSTEM. The kidneys (1) filter water-soluble toxins and other wastes from the blood. These substances make up urine, which is sent through the ureter (2) to the bladder (3) for temporary storage until it can be expelled from the body through the urethra (4).

Types and Causes of Kidney Problems

Kidney Infection–Kidney infection produces chills and fever along with pain over the kidneys and is usually accompanied by frequent, urgent, and burning urination. The cause is typically a bacterial infection that has ascended from the urethra to the bladder and on to the kidneys. Women are particularly susceptible to kidney infections, having a higher incidence of urinary tract infections. Older men with prostate problems also have an increased rate of kidney infections.

Kidney Stones–Stones formed in the kidneys, ranging in size from a grain of sand to a walnut, can cause extreme pain when they pass through the urinary tract. Blockage can occur anywhere along the tract, from the ducts between the kidneys and bladder (ureters) to the urethra where the stones exit the body. Smaller stones may pass without symptoms, but when larger stones block the ureter, they cause sudden excruciating back pain which may be intermittent and often radiates from the back across the abdomen and into the genital area or inner thighs. The pain may be associated with nausea, vomiting, blood in urine, pain on urination, and chills and fever.

Kidney stone formation is linked to the following: insufficient water intake; a diet high in sugar, refined carbohydrates, acid-forming foods (especially meat proteins), and grains, with insufficient alkalinizing vegetables and fruits; and excessive consumption of coffee, sodas, and salt. Having once had a kidney stone episode, you are at high risk of having another. Changes in diet and nutrition are therefore strongly recommended.

Nutrients and Herbs for Kidney Problems

■ **Protease enzymes:** when taken on an empty stomach, enzymes can help treat numerous underlying causes of kidney stress, including infections, toxic exposure, lymphatic congestion, airborne and food allergies, and increased mucus production.

■ **Vitamins A and B6, the amino acid methionine, glutamic acid, lipoic acid, and magnesium:** we have found these as an effective combination for preventing stone formation in those who have had one or more kidney stones.

■ **Uva ursi and horsetail:** with diuretic (urine-increasing) and astringent properties, these herbs are helpful for urinary "gravel" and inflammation, bladder infections (cystitis), bladder cramps, and kidney stones. Horsetail is specifically indicated for bladder and kidney irritation involving "scalding" or burning urine.

■ **Dandelion root or extract:** helps the kidneys eliminate waste products.[126]

Products for Kidney Problems

KB Formula: Capsules. Ingredients include juniper berries, parsley herb, ginger root, uva ursi leaves, marshmallow root, cramp bark, and goldenseal root, which help to balance and support bodily functions.

NATURE'S WAY PRODUCTS, INC., 10 Mountain Springs Parkway, Springville, UT 84663; tel: 800-962-8873 or 801-489-1500.

KB-Kidney/Bladder: Tablets. Assists in eliminating toxic buildup in the kidneys and bladder, thereby supporting their healthy functioning; contains elecampane root, juniper, parsley, uva ursi, corn silk, cranberry, dandelion, and seaweed.

NATURAL ENERGY PRODUCTS, 21101 Welch Road, Snohomish, WA 98296; tel: 425-486-5956.

Kidney Aid: Capsules. Improves circulation to the kidneys, helping them eliminate accumulated debris; ingredients including cleavers, goldenrod tops, horsetail, hydrangea root, plantain leaf, and kidney glandular substance.

RIDGECREST HERBALS, 1151 South Redwood Road #106, Salt Lake City, UT 84104-3729; tel: 800-242-4649.

Kidney Glandular Plus: Tablets. Blend of nutrients and herbs designed to nutritionally support healthy kidney function and urination.

ETHICAL NUTRIENTS, 971 Calle Negocio, San Clemente, CA 92673; tel: 800-668-8743 or 949-366-0818.

Nephrochel: Capsules. Contains magnesium and potassium citrates with lipoic acid, glutamic acid, vitamin K, glycosaminoglycans, and the botanicals uva ursi and aloe vera.

ECOLOGICAL FORMULAS, 1061-B Shary Circle, Concord, CA 94518; tel: 800-888-4585 or 925-827-2636.

Stone Free: Tablets. Herbal support for the kidneys and gallbladder; softens and clears obstructions that result from the poor digestion of fats and mineral salts; also helps wash away sediment buildup that occurs as a result of inefficient fluid elimination.

PLANETARY FORMULAS, 23 Janis Way, Scotts Valley, CA 95066; tel: 800-606-6226.

Liver Disorders

The liver is the primary organ of detoxification, processing metabolic and environmental toxins for elimination and thereby protecting the body from their effects. In today's world, we are being bombarded with toxins and the liver is having to work overtime.

Many foods (especially processed and packaged foods) contain chemical ingredients, herbicide and pesticide residues, industrial pollutants, artificial (chemical) flavorings and colorings, hormones and hormone metabolites, antibiotics and antibiotic metabolites, preservatives, stabilizers, and synthetic or genetically altered ingredients.

In addition to dealing with the toxins commonly found in foods, if the body is further taxed by environmental toxins (as in air pollution) and chronic infection, the liver becomes exhausted and unable to keep up with the toxin-filtering demands. The result is a toxic liver, liver disorders, and, eventually, whole-body toxicity which can manifest in problems in any organ or system.

Types of Liver Disorders

Jaundice, or yellowing of the skin, eyes, and excretions, due to an excess of bile pigment in the blood and deposit of those pigments in body tissues, is a symptom of dysfunction in the liver or gallbladder (the storehouse of bile, manufactured by the liver). Hepatitis and cirrhosis are two common liver conditions. Hepatitis is inflammation of the liver produced by various strains of the hepatitis virus. Cirrhosis of the liver is a degenerative disease often caused by the toxic overload of chronic alcohol or drug abuse.

Nutrients and Herbs for Liver Disorders

Due to the load on the liver of agricultural pesticides and the chemicals used on dairy and beef cattle, we recommend eating only fruits, vegetables, meat, and dairy that have been organically produced. Vegetables having the highest amount of chemical residues are, in descending order, potatoes, spinach, green bell peppers, summer squash, and celery. Among fruit, raisins have the highest chemical concen-

See also
Detoxification in
Part III, pp. 446-461.

tration, followed by peaches, strawberries, apples, and pears.[127]

In addition to this dietary practice, the main nutrients we recommend to protect and detoxify the liver are lipoic acid (sulfur-containing antioxidant involved in energy production; dietary sources are liver and yeast), milk thistle (silymarin), artichoke extract, and dandelion root extract.

Products for Liver Disorders and Liver Detoxification

Biotonic: Capsules. Based on two Chinese herbal combinations that have been used to balance digestive function and energy metabolism and also complements the product Biocidin with tonifying support for the liver and gastrointestinal tract; contains astragalus and Siberian ginseng for adaptogenic support, ginger to aid digestion and stop nausea, *Radix paeonia* and *Tuber curcuma* for support of the liver and gallbladder; and artemesia for its antifungal and antibacterial properties; concentrated for maximum bio-availability, specifically designed for use with Biocidin but can be used whenever an adaptogenic combination is indicated.

For **Biocidin**, see the product listing in Gastrointestinal Disorders, p. 204.

BIO-BOTANICAL RESEARCH, INC., 144 Pioneer Road, Corralitos, CA 95076; distributed by WELLNESS HEALTH PHARMACY, 2800 South 18th Street, Homewood, AL 35209; tel: 800-227-2627 or 205-879-6551.

Bupleurum Calmative Compound (Xiao Yao Wan): Tablets. In traditional Chinese medicine, the liver is considered to be the organ primarily associated with emotional stability; works to cleanse and tonify the liver to restore a sense of peace and well-being to the entire body.

PLANETARY FORMULAS, 23 Janis Way, Scotts Valley, CA 95066; tel: 800-606-6226.

Dandelion Burdock: Capsules or liquid. Helps enhance digestion and support the activity of the liver and gallbladder; includes dandelion and burdock roots, artichoke leaves, and milk thistle (*Silybum marianum*) seed.

FRONTIER COOPERATIVE HERBS, 3021 78th Street, Norway, IA 52318; tel: 800-669-3275 or 319-227-7996.

Dandelion & Milk Thistle: Capsules. Herbal formula to help protect and detoxify the liver.

NUTRITION NOW, 501 Southeast Columbia Shore Boulevard #350, Vancouver, WA 98661; tel: 800-929-0418 or 360-737-6800.

Dandelion • Milk Thistle Compound: Liquid. Restorative and protective tonic for the liver and cleanser for the liver and gallbladder; helpful for sluggish bile and gallstones, hepatitis, and jaundice; can be used as an occasional maintenance tonic, after illness or abuse, as adjunct therapy in chronic constipation, or as post-surgical treatment of cholecystectomy (gallbladder removal); ingredients include dandelion root, leaf, and flower, Oregon grape root, mature seed of milk thistle, artichoke leaf, beet leaf, and fennel seed.

HERB PHARM, 20260 Williams Highway, Williams, OR 97544; tel: 800-348-4372 or 541-846-6262.

DetoxCleanse: Capsules. Herbal formula that helps detoxify the body and bloodstream through cleansing the liver, improving digestion, binding and excreting toxins within the gastrointestinal tract, and promoting regularity.

BIODYNAMAX, 6525 Gunpark Drive #150-507, Boulder, CO 80301; tel: 800-926-7525 or 303-530-4665.

Detox-Zyme: Vegicaps. Blend of enzymes necessary for the breakdown of proteins, fats, carbohydrates, and fiber, plus a combination of herbs traditionally used to support the cleansing and eliminative functions of the body.

RAINBOW LIGHT, P.O. Box 600, Santa Cruz, CA 95061; tel: 800-635-1233 or 408-429-9089.

Fundamental Sulfur: Tablets. Supplies biologically active sulfur (a mineral element missing from many diets) that supports connective tissues, immune function, and detoxification; the liver also depends on sulfur to detoxify food or airborne compounds that are foreign to the body.

AMNI, 2247 National Avenue, Hayward, CA 94540-5012; tel: 800-437-8888 or 510-783-6969.

Hepa Plus: Capsules. Nutritional support for liver function and detoxification; contains milk thistle extract (standardized to greater than 80% silymarin), dandelion root extract, alpha-lipoic acid, N-acetylcysteine (NAC), thiamin tetrahydrofurfuryl disulfide (TTFD), ornithine, alpha-ketoglutarate, glycine, taurine, and the minerals molybdenum and selenium.

HEALTH PRODUCTS DISTRIBUTORS, INC., 23847 Peaceful Ridge Road, Smithsburg, MD 21783; tel: 800-228-4265 or 301-416-0500.

Hepato-Pure: Tablets. Helps detoxify the system while directly supporting the liver.

PLANETARY FORMULAS, 23 Janis Way, Scotts Valley, CA 95066; tel: 800-606-6226.

Herbal Aloe Force: Juice or topical gel. Processed aloe vera juice containing vitamins, minerals, enzymes, amino acids, essential fatty acids, growth factors, glycoproteins, sterols, bioflavonoids, polysaccharides (complex sugars), ionized colloidal silver, and herbal extracts (cat's claw, chamomile, burdock root, hawthorn berry, astragalus root, sheep sorrell, pau d'arco bark, slippery elm bark, and rhubarb root).

HERBAL ANSWERS, INC., P.O. Box 1110, Saratoga Springs, NY 12866; tel: 888-256-3367 or 518-581-1968.

Herbal Liver Complex: Vegicaps. Formula for the support of normal healthy liver function.

SOLGAR VITAMIN & HERB CO, INC., 500 Willow Tree Road, Leonia, NJ 07605; tel: 800-645-2246 or 201-944-2311.

Lipoic Acid: Capsules. Lipoic acid is a powerful antioxidant that can protect other antioxidants (vitamins C and E and glutathione) in the body; it can also chelate (bind with) heavy metals, such as lead, cadmium, mercury, and free iron and copper, and eliminate them from the body.

HEALTH PRODUCTS DISTRIBUTORS, INC., 23847 Peaceful Ridge Road, Smithsburg, MD 21783; tel: 800-228-4265 or 301-416-0500.

LiverClean: Capsules. Nourishes, balances, and detoxifies the liver; ingredients include barberry root bark, blessed thistle, dandelion root, boldo leaves, black radish seed, wild yam root, fennel seed, and cloves.

RIDGECREST HERBALS, 1151 South Redwood Road #106, Salt Lake City, UT 84104-3729; tel: 800-242-4649 or 801-978-9633.

Liver Glandular Plus: Tablets. Formula that provides raw liver concentrate, methyl donors (which help carry oxygen, increase circulation, and metabolize fats), vitamin B6, and herbs designed to support liver function; the bovine glandular concentrate in this product is guaranteed raw (processed below 37° C).

ETHICAL NUTRIENTS, 971 Calle Negocio, San Clemente, CA 92673; tel: 800-668-8743 or 949-366-0818.

Liver Guard: Tablets. Provides 25 of the most important nutrients and related substances identified in scientific studies as either nourishment or protection for the liver.

SOURCE NATURALS, 23 Janis Way, Scotts Valley, CA 95066; tel: 800-777-5677 or 831-438-1144.

Liv-R-Actin: Vegicaps. Contains milk thistle extract and an herbal blend of dandelion, barberry, goldenseal, wild Oregon grape, and celery seed.

NATURE'S PLUS, 548 Broadhollow Road, Melville, NY 11747-3708; tel: 800-645-9500 or 516-293-0030.

Liver Support with Milk Thistle Extract: Capsules. Formula combines milk thistle extract (a powerful natural antioxidant, which helps maintain healthy liver functions while it deals with pollutants and other toxins, including alcohol) and dandelion root, ginger, burdock root, parsley root, and black radish root.

NATROL INC., 21411 Prairie Street, Chatsworth, CA 91311; tel: 818-739-6000.

LIV-WELL: Caplets or capsules. Contains the flavonoids silymarin, quercetin, cynarin, and capillarisin, which have been shown to improve liver metabolism and promote detoxification of the liver and the body in general; aids in the elimination of excess water through the kidneys and stimulates bile flow (through the gallbladder) and other digestive substances, which improves digestion; recommended for elimination of stored toxins or for those exposed to environmental pollutants or who consume alcohol.

EXTREME HEALTH, INC., 50 Oak Court, Suite 212, Danville, CA 94526; tel: 800-800-1285 or 925-855-1262.

Metabolic Liver Formula: Capsules. Combines plant enzymes with fat-processing lipotropic nutrients, herbs, and liver extract; ingredients include choline, methionine, inositol, milk thistle seed, Russian black radish, and beet leaf, all traditionally used for liver support.

PREVAIL CORP., 2204-8 Northwest Birdsdale, Gresham, OR 97030; tel: 800-248-0885 or 503-667-5527.

Milk Thistle: Tablets. Standardized to 80% silymarin, which has antioxidant properties and nutritionally supports healthy liver function and detoxification.

ETHICAL NUTRIENTS, 971 Calle Negocio, San Clemente, CA 92673; tel: 800-668-8743 or 949-366-0818.

Milk Thistle Extract: Capsules. Through its antioxidant properties, milk thistle seed extract helps maintain healthy liver function; used by people concerned about cigarette smoke, alcohol, or environmental toxins.

NATURE'S SOURCE, 15451 San Fernando Mission Boulevard, Mission Hills, CA 91345; tel: 800-423-2405 or 818-837-3633.

Milk-Thistle Power: Capsules. Concentrated, standardized extract of milk thistle combined with a base of artichoke and turmeric that supports healthy liver function.

NATURE'S HERBS, 600 East Quality Drive, American Fork, UT 84003; tel: 800-437-2257 or 801-763-0700.

Quick Cleanse Program Kit. One-week internal detoxification program that cleanses the colon and aids in the elimination of toxins from the liver and blood.

ZAND HERBAL FORMULAS, 1722 14th Street #230, Boulder, CO 80302; tel: 800-800-0405 or 303-786-8558.

Whole Beet Juice Tablets. Beets, which are high in iron, can help support liver function and detoxification, and also establish a favorable environment in the intestinal tract for support of healthy intestinal flora.

SONNE'S ORGANIC FOODS, INC., P.O. Box 2160, Cottonwood, CA 96022; tel: 800-544-8147 or 530-347-5868.

Lymphatic Disorders

The lymphatic system consists of lymph fluid and the structures (vessels, ducts, and nodes) involved in transporting it from tissues to the bloodstream. Lymph fluid occupies the space between the body's cells and contains plasma proteins, foreign particles, and cellular waste. Lymph nodes are clusters of immune tissue that work as filters or "inspection stations" for detecting and removing foreign and potentially harmful substances in the lymph fluid. While the body has hundreds of lymph nodes (more than 500), they are mostly clustered in the neck, armpits, chest, groin, and abdomen.

The lymphatic system is the body's master drain, collecting and filtering the lymph fluid and conveying it to the bloodstream, thereby clearing waste products and cellular debris from the tissues. The lymph system becomes particularly active during illness (such as the flu) when the nodes (particularly at the throat) visibly swell with collected waste products.

Causes of Lymphatic Disorders

Lymphatic disorders develop as a result of poor lymph circulation due to lack of exercise or chronic stress, which tightens muscles and impedes free circulation. Unlike the heart, the lymphatic system does not have a pump to move lymph; instead, its movement is dependent on muscle contraction, among other factors. A sedentary lifestyle can lead to lymph stagnation. Exposure to too many environmental chemicals or other toxins such as viruses or bacteria can also slow lymph circulation, as the system cannot keep up with the toxic filtering demands. A high intake of saturated fats, refined carbohydrates (junk food), and mucus-producing foods such as dairy products can also reduce lymphatic flow.

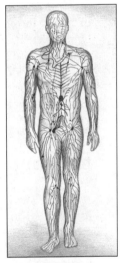

THE LYMPHATIC SYSTEM. A network of capillaries and nodes (primarily in the neck, groin, and armpits) and three organs (the tonsils, spleen, and thymus gland).

Poor lymphatic circulation or an overloaded lymph system results in lymphatic congestion. "Swollen glands" (lymph nodes) in the neck or throughout the body during colds and flu are a manifestation of lymph congestion, signaling that the body's immune and lymphatic systems are being challenged.

Typically bacteria (such as *Streptococcus*) cause congestion or inflammation as is the case in acute lymphangitis (inflammation of the lymphatic channels) and tonsillitis. A common childhood illness, tonsillitis (inflammation of the tonsils, small masses of lymphatic tissue located in the back of the throat) can also be caused by viral infections or food allergies. Common food allergens (substances that cause allergies) include dairy products, corn, wheat, certain spices, citrus, fruits, chocolate, and coffee.[128]

Treatment of Lymphatic Disorders—Deep breathing, mini-trampoline exercise (rebounding), and regular aerobic exercise can help stimulate the flow of lymph fluid. Brushing the skin with a dry, natural-bristle brush is also an aid to lymphatic health as it promotes the elimination of toxins through the skin and thereby relieves the burden on the lymph system. Avoiding exposure to heavy metals such as aluminum (found in food additives, antacids, certain deodorants, and cookware) and mercury (found in dental fillings) also alleviates some of the toxic load. Composite dental fillings which do not contain mercury can be used in lieu of the conventional "silver" fillings.

Nutrients and Herbs for Lymphatic Disorders

■ **For swollen lymph nodes, poor lymphatic flow, lymphatic congestion and toxicity, and lymph edema:** prickly ash bark can help activate sluggish circulation of the blood and lymphatic system. Two products we have used with success are Red Clover-Stillingia Compound and Collinsonia-Horse Chestnut Compound, both of which contain prickly ash bark and other beneficial herbs. Echinacea and goldenseal stimulate both the lymphatic and immune systems and are thus helpful for lymphatic disorders.[129] The homeopathic remedies *Arsenicum*, *Calendula*, and *Lycopodium* are indicated for swollen lymph nodes.

Protease enzyme formulas and pycnogenol (grape seed or pine bark extract) are useful supplements for edema. Taken on an empty stomach, protease enters the bloodstream and acts as a scavenger (much like white blood cells), breaking down proteins and clearing waste products present in swollen tissues.

Diuretic (urine-increasing) herbs can help the body eliminate excess water and ease edema. Such herbs include blue vervain, corn silk, dandelion, devil's claw, *dong quai*, echinacea, and ginkgo.

■ **For lymphatic system detoxification:** burdock root is helpful for lymph node enlargement and other conditions related to toxins in the lymphatic system and blood. Dandelion root stimulates the liver to detoxify the blood and lymph fluid. Poke root purifies blood and lymph.[130]

■ **For tonsillitis:** tea tree oil and colloidal silver have antiseptic properties and assist in fighting a broad range of infectious agents, such as viruses, and is recommended for many conditions, including sore throat and tonsillitis. The product Lymphomyosot is a homeopathic remedy that relieves swelling of the tonsils and other lymphatic tissues and organs. *Mercurius Vivus*, a homeopathic remedy, is specifically designed for tonsillitis.[131]

Products for Lymphatic Disorders

AquaActin: Capsules. Supports the body in maintaining a normal water balance; contains green tea, uva ursi, goldenseal, and vitamin B6.

NATURE'S PLUS, 548 Broadhollow Road, Melville, NY 11747-3708; tel: 800-645-9500 or 516-293-0030.

Catalyst Plus: Liquid. Oxygenator that helps to detoxify the body; helps make cell walls more permeable to oxygen; contains electrically charged minerals and trace elements.

OLYMPIC BOTANICALS, 231 Otto Street, Port Townsend, WA 98368; tel: 800-310-6924 or 360-385-9468.

Circu-Pressure: Vegitabs. Supports circulation and blood pressure function; contains hawthorn berry, dandelion root, grape skin extracts, and coleus.

COUNTRY LIFE, 101 Corporate Drive, Hauppauge, NY 11788; tel: 800-645-5768 or 516-231-1031.

Collinsonia • Horse Chestnut Compound: Liquid. Contains collinsonia, horse chestnut, butcher's broom, rosemary, and prickly ash. Improves tone of veins and reduces vascular fragility; reduces swelling (edema) by facilitating reabsorption of fluids back into the capillaries. For general edema, swollen lymph glands, and lymph blockage.

Herb Pharm, P.O. Box 116, Williams, OR 97544; tel: 800-348-4372 or 541-846-6262.

Colloidal Silver: Liquid. Antibiotic and immune system enhancer; combination of minute, electrically charged particles of silver and pure water; useful for colds and flu.

NUPRO, 735-L Park Street, Castle Rock, CO 80104; tel: 800-704-8910 or 303-660-0562.

Compounded Hoxsey/Red Clover: Liquid. Restores and replaces degenerated tissues with healthy, vital tissues; also has blood-purifying effects, which promote greater drainage and elimination through lymphatic glands; useful for the breakdown and removal of metabolic wastes from the body; contains red clover blossoms, buckthorn bark, fresh barberry root bark, fresh burdock root, fresh stillingia root, fresh poke root, cascara sagrada bark, licorice root, and prickly ash bark.

Herb Pharm, P.O. Box 116, Williams, OR 97544; tel: 800-348-4372 or 541-846-6262.

Congestaway: Oil. Contains pure eucalyptus, dandelion and olive oils, and flower essences for relief of lymphatic congestion, coughs due to bronchitis, sinusitis, colds, and viruses; can be used as a vaporizer oil during colds and flu; also good for massaging and bathing feet, hands, and body.

Olympic Botanicals, 231 Otto Street, Port Townsend, WA 98368; tel: 800-310-6924 or 360-385-9468.

Herbal Aloe Force: Juice or topical gel. Processed aloe vera juice containing vitamins, minerals, enzymes, amino acids, essential fatty acids, growth factors, glycoproteins, sterols, bioflavonoids, and polysaccharides (complex sugars), plus ionized colloidal silver and herbal extracts (cat's claw, chamomile, burdock root, hawthorn berry, astragalus root, sheep sorrel, pau d'arco bark, slippery elm (*Ulmus rubra*) bark, and rhubarb root).

Herbal Answers, Inc., P.O. Box 1110, Saratoga Springs, NY 12866; tel: 888-256-3367 or 518-581-1968.

KB Formula: Capsules. Contains juniper berries, parsley, ginger root, uva ursi leaves, marshmallow root, cramp bark, and goldenseal root; based on a classic Dr. John R. Christopher formula to balance and support bodily functions.

Nature's Way Products, Inc., 10 Mountain Springs Parkway, Springville, UT 84663; tel: 800-962-8873 or 801-489-1500.

Lymphomyosot: Homeopathic liquid or tablets. For temporary relief of edema (swelling of the tissues or glands) and symptoms of bronchitis, colds, and flu.

HEEL/BHI, INC., 11600 Cochiti Road Southeast, Albuquerque, NM 87123-3376; tel: 800-621-7644 or 505-293-3843.

Mercurius Vivus: Sublingual tablets. For relief of tonsillitis, sore throat, colds with profuse watery nasal discharge, foul or bad breath, certain types of earaches, or swollen gums.

STANDARD HOMEOPATHIC CO., 201 West 131st, Los Angeles, CA 90061; tel: 800-624-9659 or 310-768-0700.

Propolis • Echinacea: Liquid. Antiseptic, analgesic, and anti-inflammatory for inflamed and infected tissues of throat, mouth, gums, and skin; specifically indicated for tonsillitis and infected sore throat and can also be useful in the treatment of paryngitis and laryngitis and to heal sores and ulcerations of the mouth, gums and throat; ingredients include echinacea seed, propolis resin, hyssop leaf and flower, sage leaf, St. John's wort flower and bud, and vegetable glycerine.

HERB PHARM, 20260 Williams Highway, Williams, OR 97544; tel: 800-348-4372 or 541-846-6262.

Red Clover • Stillingia Compound (The Hoxsey Formula): Liquid. Blood-purifying formula, containing red clover blossom, stillingia root, licorice root, buckthorn bark, Oregon grape root, and prickly ash bark, among other herbs. Acts through the lymphatic, glandular, and mucous membrane systems and skin; indicated in disorders associated with a breakdown in elimination of metabolic wastes, especially chronic congestion and swelling in the lymphatic and glandular system. Caution: Do not use this product if you are pregnant or nursing.

HERB PHARM, P.O. Box 116, Williams, OR 97544; tel: 800-348-4372 or 541-846-6262.

Tonseals: Phyto-homeopathic lozenges. Relieves sore throats, difficulty when swallowing, and associated dryness and burning sensations caused by viral and bacterial infections; contains active homeopathic ingredients in a base including the herbal extracts of German chamomile flower, ribwort plantain, and echinacea root; does not interfere with any other medicine.

SUPHERB LTD., P.O. Box 1135, Nahariya 22100, Israel; tel: 800-409-HERB (4372).

Menopausal Symptoms

Menopause is marked by the cessation of menstruation, which can occur abruptly or gradually, with periods becoming less frequent over time. Symptoms commonly associated with menopause are hot flashes, insomnia, and irritability. For the majority of women, menstruation typically ends between the ages of 45 and 53,[132] but perimenopause (nearing menopause) with the same uncomfortable symptoms can begin ten to even 15 years before a woman's period actually stops. Caused by hormonal imbalance, these symptoms can be eased by proper hormonal and nutritional support. Contrary to popular belief, it is not always too little estrogen that creates menopausal and perimenopausal symptoms. In fact, some physicians point to an excess of estrogen in relation to declining progesterone levels (estrogen dominance) as the more frequent source of the symptoms.[133] In addition to hormonal influences, lifestyle factors such as stress, poor diet, and lack of exercise can worsen menopausal symptoms.

Other signs and symptoms of perimenopause and menopause are lack of sexual interest, calcium imbalance, mood swings, anxiety, depression, palpitations, and skin and vaginal dryness.

Nutrients and Herbs for Menopausal Symptoms

For information on a **home test for hormone levels**, see Appendix: Great Smokies Diagnostic Laboratory, pp. 484-485. See Osteoporosis, pp. 293-297, for more information about **preventing calcium imbalance and bone loss**.

■ **Genistein:** we have found genistein, derived from soy oil, to be an excellent nutrient for perimenopausal and menopausal women. Genistein is what is known as a phytoestrogen, that is, a substance found in plants that mimics estrogen in the body. By binding to estrogen receptor sites, genistein blocks the actual hormone from binding. The body, "fooled" into thinking it has all the estrogen it needs, dispatches the excess hormone to the liver to be processed out of the body. Since genistein performs only mild estrogenic actions itself, it thus aids in reversing estrogen dominance.

Genistein produces many of the beneficial results credited to estrogen, such as decreasing hot flashes and vaginal drying, osteoporosis, and cardiovascular disease and assisting in maintaining normal menstrual cycles—without the carcinogenic effects linked to synthetic estrogen. In fact, research shows that genistein can actually reduce the risk of breast cancer.[134]

■ **Phytoestrogenic herbs:** include *dong quai*, licorice root, and black cohosh. Yamcon sublingual (absorbed under the tongue) drops is one product containing phytoestrogens that women in our practice have successfully used to improve hormonal balance and decrease hot flashes. Chasteberry also helps balance hormones and alleviate menopausal symptoms, possibly through a progesterone-like constituent it is thought to contain.[135]

■ **DHEA (dehydroepiandrosterone):** a building block of estrogen, DHEA is another method of correcting imbalances in hormones. Produced in the adrenal glands, levels of DHEA gradually decline as people age. A person at age 80 is producing only a fraction of DHEA she did at age 20. But levels of DHEA vary significantly from person to person, and, for this reason, we recommend having your hormone levels tested before using DHEA or estrogen products.

From clinical experience, we have found that synthetic hormone products do not work as well as phytoestrogens and nutritional support in controlling menopausal symptoms and other problems of the female reproductive system.

In addition to the substances above, vitamins A, B complex, and E, calcium, magnesium, and zinc are helpful for premenopausal or menopausal symptoms of depression, fatigue, irritability, headaches, and hot flashes.

Products for Menopausal Symptoms

Beyond Vitex: Tablets. Contains vitex, black cohosh extract and powder, St. John's wort extract, wild yam, *dong quai*, licorice root, saw palmetto oil, *Pygeum africanum*, and soy.

KAL, NUTRACEUTICAL CORP., P.O. Box 681869, Park City, UT 84068; tel: 800-669-8877.

Change-O-Life Formula: Capsules. Ingredients include the roots of black cohosh, sarsaparilla, Siberian ginseng, licorice, and false unicorn and the herbs blessed thistle and squaw vine.

NATURE'S WAY PRODUCTS, INC., 10 Mountain Springs Parkway, Springville, UT 84663; tel: 800-962-8873 or 801-489-1500.

Chasteberry-Power: Capsules. Contains standardized extract of chasteberry in a base of wild countryside *dong quai* root and Siberian ginseng; chasteberry has been used since ancient times by women, especially in Europe.

NATURE'S HERBS, 600 East Quality Drive, American Fork, UT 84003; tel: 800-437-2257 or 801-763-0700.

Cimi-Fem: Tablets. Can help balance hormone activity.

SOURCE NATURALS, THRESHOLD ENTERPRISES, 23 Janis Way, Scotts Valley, CA 95066; tel: 800-777-5677 or 831-438-1144.

Climex: Phyto-homeopathic lozenges. Helpful for symptoms of menopause; contains active homeopathic ingredients in a base of *dong quai*; no side effects or hormones.

SUPHERB LTD., P.O. Box 1135, Nahariya 22100, Israel; tel: 800-409-HERB (4372).

DHEA- Power Women's Formula: Capsules. DHEA supplement combined with phytoestrogen herbs developed to help meet the nutritional needs of women over 40 years of age. Caution: Please review all warnings on label before using.

NATURE'S HERBS, 600 East Quality Drive, American Fork, UT 84003; tel: 800-437-2257 or 801-763-0700.

DHEA Sustained Release with Bioperine: Caplets. Eight-hour time-released DHEA supplement; also contains bioperine (a patented extract from black pepper), which assists the intestine in absorbing nutrients.

NUTRIMEDIKA CORP., 101 Newport Street, Bayport, NY 11705-2224; tel: 800-688-7462 or 516-472-5761.

Easy Change for Women Caps. Contains black cohosh, *dong quai*, cramp bark, and Ayurvedic herbs to encourage normality and balance in the female system.

CRYSTAL STAR HERBAL NUTRITION, 4069 Wedgeway Court, Earth City, MO 63045; tel: 800-736-6015 or 314-739-7551.

Emerald DHEA Plus Pregnenolone Women's Formula: Capsules. Research has shown that DHEA may improve mood, preserve muscle mass, and promote an overall feeling of well-being; pregnenolone can help improve brain function, mood, memory, and cognition.

EMERALD LABORATORIES, 5933 Sea Lion Place #105, Carlsbad, CA 92008; tel: 800-775-1112 or 760-930-8091.

Emotional Balance-Chaste Berry Extract: Liquid. Promotes hormonal balance.

PLANETARY FORMULAS, 23 Janis Way, Scotts Valley, CA 95066; tel: 800-606-6226.

Est-Aid Caps. Helpful for hormonal balance in menopausal women.

CRYSTAL STAR HERBAL NUTRITION, 4069 Wedgeway Court, Earth City, MO 63045 tel: 800-736-6015 or 314-739-7551.

EstroFem: Caplets. Supplies phytoestrogens and herbs for women during and after menopause; contains genisoy, a source for isoflavones, standardized for genistein content (recent studies suggest a link between isoflavones and tumor inhibition and between isoflavones and cholesterol reduction), chasteberry, evening primrose oil, southern blue and American ginseng, licorice, black cohosh, and *dong quai* plants with estrogenically active compounds.

IVC, 500 Halls Mill Road, Freehold, NJ 07728; tel: 800-666-8482 or 732-308-3000.

Estroven: Caplets. Helps ease the passage through menopause; contains natural plant estrogens from soy and black cohosh, calming herbal extract, calcium, and vitamins B6 and E.

AMERIFIT, 166 Highland Park Drive, Bloomfield, CT 06002; tel: 800-990- FIRM (3476) or 860-242-3476.

Every Woman II Menopause & Beyond: Tablets. Nutritional for women facing the changes that lead up to and accompany menopause.

NEW CHAPTER, 22 High Street, Brattleboro, VT 05301; tel: 800-543-7279 or 802-257-9345.

FemaMax: Capsules. Created for women over 40; ingredients include genistein, wild yam, black and blue cohosh, licorice, vitex, *dong quai*, and other support herbs.

NATURAL MAX, NUTRACEUTICAL CORP., P.O. Box 681869, Park City, UT 84068; tel: 800-669-8877.

FemChange: Capsules. Helps supplement the body's nutritional needs for women, commonly used during periods of stress such as menopause; contains the roots of false unicorn, blue and black cohosh, and cramp bark, ginger, and valerian, pennyroyal, red raspberry leaves, squaw vine, bayberry bark, uva ursi, and blessed thistle.

NATURE'S HERBS, 600 East Quality Drive, American Fork, UT 84003; tel: 800-437-2257 or 801-763-0700.

Fem-Gest: Cream. Transdermal progesterone cream for relief of PMS/menopausal symptoms, bone density, or hypothyroid.

BIO-NUTRITIONAL FORMULAS, 106 East Jericho Turnpike, Mineola, NY 11501; tel: 800-950-8484.

Golden Passage: Liquid or tablets. For symptoms of menopause.

FLORA INC., 805 East Badger Road, Lynden, WA 98264; tel: 800-446-2110 or 360-354-2110.

Hot Flash: Tablets. High potencies of phytoestrogens from soy and black cohosh to help balance hormonal surges that can cause extreme changes in skin temperature and subsequent hot flashes.

SOURCE NATURALS, THRESHOLD ENTERPRISES, 23 Janis Way, Scotts Valley, CA 95066; tel: 800-777-5677 or 831-438-1144.

MenoBalance Multiple: Tablets. Multivitamin and mineral for women over 40; contains phytoestrogens from soy and herbs, which function as hormone balancers.

SOURCE NATURALS, THRESHOLD ENTERPRISES, 23 Janis Way, Scotts Valley, CA 95066; tel: 800-777-5677 or 831-438-1144.

Meno-Fem: Capsules. Formula of herbs and nutrients for women during menopause; contains gamma oryzanol (from rice bran oil, which has been studied for its effects on menopausal women), vitamin E and magnesium (both essential for women going through menopause), and the herbs *dong quai* and wild yam (traditionally used to balance female hormones).

PREVAIL CORP., 2204-8 Northwest Birdsdale, Gresham, OR 97030; tel: 800-248-0885 or 503-667-5527.

Menopause Formulae: Homeopathic liquid. Relieves symptoms of hot flashes, palpitations, insomnia, nervous irritability, and emotional instability from the onset of menopause.

LIDDELL LABORATORIES, 1036 Country Club Drive, Moraga, CA 94556; tel: 800-460-7733 or 925-377-3000.

Menopause Nutritional Support: Tablets. Combination of herbs (some rich in estrogenic substances), minerals, trace minerals, and vitamins that help balance the entire system and maintain optimum health.

写

(real)

BIO NATIVUS, P.O. Box 3281, Ogden, UT 84401; tel: 888-628-4887 or 801-732-1294.

Meno-Select by Earth's Bounty: Tablets. Helps balance and harmonize the body during menopause; ingredients include black cohosh, sarsaparilla, eleuthero, Mexican wild yam, and chasteberry.
MATRIX HEALTH PRODUCTS, 8400 Magnolia Avenue, Suite N, Santee, CA 92071; tel: 800-736-5609 or 619-448-7550.

Phyto Estrogen-Power: Capsules. Contains soy germ isoflavone concentrate, kudzu root extracts, Mexican wild yam, and *dong quai*, Korean ginseng, boron, and natural vitamin E in a base of chasteberry powder and arrowroot.
NATURE'S HERBS, 600 East Quality Drive, American Fork, UT 84003; tel: 800-437-2257 or 801-763-0700.

PhytoGest: Cream. Natural progesterone cream helpful for menopause, PMS, and osteoporosis; natural progesterone is an estrogen antagonist and helps protect against breast and endometrial cancers, stimulates bone building, enhances energy and fat utilization, enhances thyroid hormone function, normalizes blood-sugar levels, restores libido, and acts as a natural antidepressant and diuretic; contains wild yam, aloe vera, and AHA (alpha-hydroxy acid).
KARUNA CORP., 42 Digital Drive # 7, Novato, CA 94949; tel: 800-826-7225 or 415-382-0147.

PhytoGyn: Liquid. Phytoestrogen (plant-derived) nutritional support for women with hormone-related complaints including the symptoms of menopause, dysmenorrhea, amenorrhea, and PMS. Contains concentrated extracts of chasteberry, *dong quai*, black cohosh, and licorice in a fluid for improved absorption.
KARUNA CORP., 42 Digital Drive # 7, Novato, CA 94949; tel: 800-826-7225 or 415-382-0147.

Pregnenolone: Capsules. Pregnenolone is a hormone precursor, which the body normally manufactures using cholesterol, for other hormones, including DHEA, estrogen, testosterone, and progesterone; many physicians and scientists believe that replacement of pregnenolone to youthful levels is an important step in dealing with the symptoms of aging, and many people report a sense of enhanced well-being and increased energy after taking it.

LIFE ENHANCEMENT PRODUCTS, INC., P.O. Box 751390, Petaluma, CA 94975-1390; tel: 800-543-3873 or 707-762-6144.

Rejuvenal: Capsules. Pregnenolone, a natural hormone secreted by the body, plays a role in menopause, PMS, arthritis, memory, mood, energy, and stress reduction.

PHILLIPS NUTRITIONALS, 27071 Cabot Road #122, Laguna Hills, CA 92653; tel: 800-514-5115 or 702-898-8141.

Remifemin: Tablets. Nutritional support containing black cohosh root for women experiencing menopause.

ENZYMATIC THERAPY, 825 Challenger Drive, Green Bay, WI 54311-8328; tel: 800-558-7372 or 920-469-1313.

Valerian • Passionflower Compound: Liquid. Gentle, non-narcotic sedative indicated in nervousness associated with menopause, nervous excitement and hysteria, mental depression due to worry or imagined wrongs, nervous headache, and insomnia.

HERB PHARM, 20260 Williams Highway, Williams, OR 97544; tel: 800-348-4372 or 541-846-6262.

Women's Care Menopausal Formula: Capsules. Daily multivitamin, mineral, and herbal supplement for the nutritional needs associated with menopause.

NATURE'S HERBS, 600 East Quality Drive, American Fork, UT 84003; tel: 800-437-2257 or 801-763-0700.

Women's Change: Tablets. Provides nutrients to support health and well-being during menopause.

ETHICAL NUTRIENTS, 971 Calle Negocio, San Clemente, CA 92673; tel: 800-668-8743 or 949-366-0818.

Yamcon: Sublingual drops. Contains yam extract, natural orange oil, and water.

PHILLIPS NUTRITIONALS, 27071 Cabot Road #122, Laguna Hills, CA 92653; tel: 800-514-5115 or 702-898-8141.

Menstrual Problems

Menstruation is ruled by the rise and fall of estrogen, progesterone, and other hormones which produce cyclic changes in the endometrium (lining of the uterus where a fertilized egg implants). The popular belief that a normal menstrual cycle is 28 days is erroneous and does a disservice to women whose cycles depart from that standard. Menstrual cycles actually vary widely and 24-day to 37-day cycles are still within the normal range.

Types and Causes of Menstrual Problems

Hormonal imbalance is a primary cause of menstrual disorders, which include amenorrhea, menorrhagia, and dysmenorrhea. Possible imbalances may include deficient levels of progesterone and/or dominant levels of estrogen. Diet, stress, and lack of exercise are also common influencing factors.

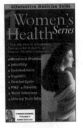

See **Menstrual Problems** in *Alternative Medicine Guide to Women's Health 1* (Future Medicine Publishing, 1998); ISBN 1-887299-12-2); to order, call 800-333-HEAL.

Amenorrhea—This disorder is the absence of the menstrual period for at least three months, not due to pregnancy, lactation, or menopause; common causes include extreme thinness and excessive exercise (as in marathon training) as well as the causes mentioned above.

Menorrhagia—Excessive bleeding during menstruation, or menorrhagia, means that your period is too heavy, flows too fast, or the bleeding persists for too long. Endometriosis, deficiencies in iron and vitamin A, hypothyroidism, or intrauterine devices are additional causes.

See also **Premenstrual Syndrome**, pp. 309-318. For information on a **home test for hormone levels**, see Appendix: Great Smokies Diagnostic Laboratory, pp. 484-485.

Dysmenorrhea—Erroneously considered normal by many women, dysmenorrhea is pain (spasmodic in the lower abdomen, back, and/or thighs) and cramping during menstruation. Dysmenorrhea is an indicator of hidden imbalances, such as hormones, food allergies, vaginal yeast infections, endometriosis (functioning endometrial tissue outside the uterus), or pelvic inflammatory disease.

Nutrients and Herbs
for Menstrual Problems

Supplementing with natural progesterone can help restore the body's normal hormonal equilibrium and reduce symptoms related to menstrual problems. Natural, plant-based progesterone is normally derived from wild yam *(Dioscorea)* roots and is available in topical creams. Two products that we recommend are PhytoGest and Fem-Gest. Although there have been no significant side effects reported from the use of natural progesterone, we encourage consultation with a qualified health-care provider to measure hormonal levels and monitor use of natural progesterone.

■ **For nutritional support during menstruation:** calcium and magnesium (taken together as the function of one depends upon the other), B vitamins, and vitamin E are particularly important nutrients for menstrual health.

■ **For amenorrhea:** research has shown that black haw bark can be effective in restoring menstruation.[136]

■ **For dysmenorrhea:** the plant enzymes bromelain and papain, and the herbs bilberry, black haw bark, *dong quai*, and feverfew are beneficial for this condition.[137] We also recommend magnesium glycinate (more easily assimilated than other forms of magnesium).

■ **For heavy menstrual cramps:** avoid sugar in the diet and supplementing with calcium and magnesium (in a 1:2 ratio). The product Calcium Plus provides the correct ratio of these minerals in combination with helpful herbs. Taking this formula along with Fema-Gen, an overall tonic for the female system, has produced good results for our patients. Passionflower, a mild sedative and nervine (supports the nervous system), helps reduce muscle tension and menstrual cramps. Kava-kava, cramp bark, red raspberry, wild yam root, and *dong quai* can also diminish menstrual cramping.

■ **For menorrhagia:** the antioxidant vitamins A, C, and E, chlorophyll, pycnogenol, essential fatty acids, and botanical "female" formulas that contain blue cohosh and/or shepherd's purse are useful for women whose menstrual flow is excessive.

■ **For menstrual cycles that are consistently too long or too short:** we often recommend an herbal formula called Fema-Gen. Black cohosh can also help restore healthy menstrual cycles.[138]

■ **For prevention of iron deficiencies:** women's need for iron is high due to iron being lost in the menstrual blood flow, especially in cases of menorrhagia. We have had good success with the products

Floradix and Gentle Iron, both of which contain an easily assimilable form of iron.

■ **For spotting (slight bleeding) between periods:** pycnogenol or organic adrenal glandular extracts are helpful.

Products for Menstrual Problems

Aqua-Trim. Gentle diuretic with potassium for relief of the bloating, puffiness, and fatigue associated with menstrual periods; ingredients include uva ursi, natural caffeine, potassium, and the extracts of buchu leaf, juniper berry, and horse chestnut seed.

NATURE'S HERBS, 600 East Quality Drive, American Fork, UT 84003; tel: 800-437-2257 or 801-763-0700.

Beyond Vitex: Tablets. Contains vitex (chasteberry), black cohosh extract and powder, St. John's wort extract, wild yam, *dong quai*, licorice root, saw palmetto oil, *Pygeum africanum*, and soy.

KAL, NUTRACEUTICAL CORP., P.O. Box 681869, Park City, UT 84068; tel: 800-669-8877.

Blessed Thistle Combination: Capsules. For use during menstrual cycle or other stressful times; contains blessed thistle herb, goldenseal root, red raspberry leaves, squaw vine, ginger root, cramp bark, uva ursi leaves, marshmallow root, cayenne, and false unicorn (*Chamaelirium luteum*) root.

NATURE'S HERBS, 600 East Quality Drive, American Fork, UT 84003; tel: 800-437-2257 or 801-763-0700.

Blood-Booster: Capsules. Easily assimilated iron supplement combined with herbs rich in trace minerals; contains odorless garlic, wheat grass, alfalfa juice extract, pau d'arco extract, yellowdock, parsley, red clover, and iron.

NATURE'S HERBS, 600 East Quality Drive, American Fork, UT 84003; tel: 800-437-2257 or 801-763-0700.

Chasteberry-Power: Capsules. Contains standardized extract of chasteberry in a base of wild countryside *dong quai* root and Siberian ginseng; chasteberry has been used since ancient times by women, especially in Europe.

NATURE'S HERBS, 600 East Quality Drive, American Fork, UT 84003; tel: 800-437-2257 or 801-763-0700.

Cramp-Prin: Capsules. Relieves cramp pains, premenstrual tension, irritability, headache, and backache associated with the menstrual cycle; ingredients include magnesium salicylate, white willow, *dong quai*, peppermint, cnidium, pleurisy root, and uva ursi.

RIDGECREST HERBALS, 1151 South Redwood Road #106, Salt Lake City, UT 84104-3729; tel: 800-242-4649 or 801-978-9633.

CrampRelax for Women by Farmacopia: Capsules or tea bags. Capsules contain kava-kava; tea bags contain kava-kava, peppermint, spearmint, lemongrass, and natural flavors.

BOTANICAL PRODUCTS INTERNATIONAL, P.O. Box 174, Hakalau, HI 96710; tel: 808-963-6771.

Emotional Balance-Chaste Berry Extract: Liquid. For promoting hormonal balance.

PLANETARY FORMULAS, 23 Janis Way, Scotts Valley, CA 95066; tel: 800-606-6226.

FEM: Capsules. Monthly supplement for women; contains goldenseal root, blessed thistle herb, cayenne, uva ursi leaves, cramp bark, red raspberry leaves, squaw vine, ginger root, and false unicorn root.

NATURE'S WAY PRODUCTS, INC., 10 Mountain Springs Parkway, Springville, UT 84663; tel: 800-962-8873 or 801-489-1500.

Fema-Gen: Caplets or liquid. Blend of herbs traditionally used for women needing balancing support, especially as it applies to the female cycle.

RAINBOW LIGHT, P.O. Box 600, Santa Cruz, CA 95061; tel: 800-635-1233 or 408-429-9089.

Female Balance: Capsules. Combination of herbal extracts and borage oil (rich in essential fatty acids) for general hormone support.

NOW, 550 Mitchell Road, Glendale Heights, IL 60139; tel: 800-283-3500 or 630-545-9098.

Female Balance: Tablets. Helps support a woman's natural balance for a healthy monthly cycle by utilizing herbal combinations created by Ayurvedic physicians. These formulas are in harmony with the science of Ayurveda, which incorporates a holistic view of health by balancing the body's mechanisms and organs.

VEDA HEALTH, INC., P.O. Box 1535, Soquel, CA 95073; tel: 888-856-8334 or 408-465-9084.

Female Formula: Tablets. Herbal/glandular formula; supports the endocrine system and the female hormones for hormonal and glandular balance; contains the raw glandulars DHEA, heart, kidney, pancreas, thymus, adrenal, ovarian, RNA powder, whole pituitary, and spleen in a base of blue cohosh, catnip, chamomile, seaweed, and hawthorn berry.

NATURAL ENERGY PRODUCTS, 21101 Welch Road, Snohomish, WA 98296; tel: 425-486-5956.

Female Harmony Caps: Capsules. PMS monthly balancer and female system toner.

CRYSTAL STAR HERBAL NUTRITION, 4069 Wedgeway Court, Earth City, MO 63045; tel: 800-736-6015 or 314-739-7551.

Fem-Gest: Cream. Natural progesterone cream (900 mg of progesterone per two-ounce jar) used topically to relieve PMS and menopausal symptoms, improve bone density, and help restore balance in hypothyroidism (an underactive thyroid gland); comes with a free educational booklet outlining proper cycling and transdermal application.

BIO-NUTRITIONAL FORMULAS, 106 East Jericho Turnpike, Mineola, NY 11501; tel: 800-950-8484.

Feminique: Capsules. Combination of seven nurturing herbs that help strengthen, revitalize, and support the distinctive needs of the female body; also helps promote healthy hormone levels.

NUPRO, 735-L Park Street, Castle Rock, CO 80104; tel: 800-704-8910 or 303-660-0562.

Floradix Iron Plus Herbs: Liquid. Contains organic iron, extracts of herbs, fruits, vitamins, cultured yeast, ocean kelp, extracts of wheat germ, and rose hips; easily and completely absorbed, does not cause constipation. Also available without yeast or added sugar or honey as the product Floravital Iron Plus Herbs.

FLORA INC., 805 East Badger Road, Lynden, WA 98264; tel: 800-446-2110 or 360-354-2110.

Gentle Iron (Iron Bisglycinate): Vegicaps. Contains a chelated (combined with an amino acid to improve assimilation) form of iron that is nonconstipating, nonirritating, and easily absorbed.

SOLGAR VITAMIN & HERB COMPANY, INC., 500 Willow Tree Road, Leonia, NJ 07605; tel: 800-645-2246 or 201-944-2311.

Herbal Female Complex: Vegicaps. For maintaining the health and well-being of women; contains extracts of chasteberry, *dong quai*, isoflavone, milk thistle, black cohosh, and motherwort as well as powders of the raw roots of astragalus, Korean ginseng, and *dong quai*.

SOLGAR VITAMIN & HERB COMPANY, INC., 500 Willow Tree Road, Leonia, NJ 07605; tel: 800-645-2246 or 201-944-2311.

Hyland's Menstrual Cramps: Sublingual tablets. For relief of cramps associated with the menstrual period, especially those that radiate and are made better from pressure and heat.

P & S LABS, 210 West 131st Street, Los Angeles, CA 90061; tel: 800-624-9659 or 310-768-0700.

Mega Primrose: Softgels. Contains gamma-linolenic acid (GLA), a precursor to prostaglandin E1, a compound that may help reduce the discomforts of breast tenderness and irritability that accompany fluctuating estrogen levels.

SOURCE NATURALS, 23 Janis Way, Scotts Valley, CA 95066; tel: 800-777-5677 or 831-438-1144.

Menstrual-Ease: Capsules. Helps supplement the nutritional needs of women during the menstrual cycle; contains vitamin B6, DLPA (DL-phenylalanine), *dong quai*, white willow, valerian, juniper berry, and uva ursi extracts and leaves, licorice, valerian root, black cohosh, cramp bark, and ginger; contains no caffeine, aspirin, or artificial chemicals.

NATURE'S HERBS, 600 East Quality Drive, American Fork, UT 84003; tel: 800-437-2257 or 801-763-0700.

PhytoGest: Cream. Natural progesterone cream for PMS, menopause, and osteoporosis; natural progesterone is an estrogen antagonist, helps restore libido, protects against breast and endometrial cancers, stimulates bone building, enhances energy and fat utilization, acts as a natural diuretic, enhances thyroid hormone function, normalizes blood-sugar levels, and acts as a natural antidepressant; contains wild yam, aloe vera, and AHA (alpha-hydroxy acid).

KARUNA CORP., 42 Digital Drive # 7, Novato, CA 94949; tel: 800-826-7225 or 415-382-0147.

PhytoGyn: Liquid. Phytoestrogen (plant-derived estrogens) nutritional support for women with hormone-related complaints including dysmenorrhea, amenorrhea, PMS, and the symptoms of menopause. Contains concentrated extracts of chasteberry (*Vitex agnus-castus*), *dong quai*, black cohosh, and licorice in a fluid form for improved absorption.

KARUNA CORP., 42 Digital Drive # 7, Novato, CA 94949; tel: 800-826-7225 or 415-382-0147.

Positive Menstrual Support: Tablets. Blend of nutrients, superfoods, and herbs for the problems often accompanying the female cycle; contains B vitamins, calcium, potassium, and the herbal extracts of chasteberry and *dong quai* traditionally used as hormonal balancers.

RAINBOW LIGHT, P.O. Box 600, Santa Cruz, CA 95061; tel: 800-635-1233 or 408-429-9089.

Premium North American Ginseng Women's Formula: Capsules. Builds stamina, assists in balancing the body cycles, tonifies, and regulates; contains a blend of damiana, cranberry, North American ginseng (*Panax quinquefolius*), chasteberry, and other natural ingredients.

CHAINATA CORP., 5965 205 A Street, Langley, British Columbia, Canada V3A8C4; tel: 800-406-7668 or 604-533-8883.

Vitex Black Cohosh: Capsules or liquid. Female monthly balance blend containing the herb chasteberry, motherwort (*Leonurus cardiaca*), partridge berry, and black cohosh to help balance the reproductive system, cramp bark to relax pelvic muscles and release cyclic tension, licorice to help soothe and support the reproductive system, nettle for general nourishment, and ginger for its warming properties. Caution: Do not use during pregnancy.

FRONTIER COOPERATIVE HERBS, 3021 78th Street, Norway, IA 52318; tel: 800-669-3275 or 319-227-7996.

Woman's Select by Earth's Bounty: Tablets. Herbal formula used for over ten years by naturopathic doctors; contains herbs selected for their traditional ability to safely balance and harmonize a woman's body; ingredients include holy thistle, *dong quai*, red raspberry, squaw vine, false unicorn, echinacea, cramp bark, bearberry, black cohosh, Oregon grape, ginger, sarsaparilla, and licorice.

MATRIX HEALTH PRODUCTS, 8400 Magnolia Avenue, Suite N, Santee, CA 92071; tel: 800-736-5609 or 619-448-7550.

Women's Best Friend: Capsules. Herbal balancing formula for women.

CRYSTAL STAR HERBAL NUTRITION, 4069 Wedgeway Court, Earth City, MO 63045; tel: 800-736-6015 or 314-739-7551.

Women's Comfort: Tablets. Combines herbs that help balance and ease women through premenstrual and menstrual cycles, including *dong quai* extract, European chasteberry, and cramp bark.

PLANETARY FORMULAS, 23 Janis Way, Scotts Valley, CA 95066; tel: 800-606-6226.

Women's Essence by Jade: Tablets. Helps regulate the menstrual cycle and nourish the blood, liver, and heart.

EAST EARTH HERB, INC., P.O. Box 2802, Eugene, OR 97402; tel: 800-827-HERB (4372) or 541-687-0155.

Women's Ginseng Formula: Capsules or liquid. For the energy needs of women, supports the adrenals, builds depleted blood after menstruation, and balances the hormonal system; contains American and Siberian ginseng, *dong quai*, and chasteberry; for women of all ages for one to three weeks a month (do not use during menstruation).

ZAND HERBAL FORMULAS, 1722 14th Street #230, Boulder, CO 80302; tel: 800-800-0405 or 303-786-8558.

Women's Nutritional System: Tablets. Multiple for women of all ages, especially those who are active or concerned with supporting the delicate balance of the female system; contains amino acids, enzymes, and extracts of herbs supportive of the female system (including the balancing herb chasteberry) in a base of superfoods and herbs.

RAINBOW LIGHT, P.O. Box 600, Santa Cruz, CA 95061; tel: 800-635-1233 or 408-429-9089.

Women's Treasure: Tablets. Modified version of a classical Chinese herbal formula (Dong Quai Four) to tonify and normalize the female cycle; contains the Chinese herbs *dong quai*, lingusticum, rehmannia, and peony along with Native American "female" herbs (cramp bark, false unicorn, and blue cohosh).

PLANETARY FORMULAS, 23 Janis Way, Scotts Valley, CA 95066; tel: 800-606-6226.

Mouth and Dental Conditions

Good oral hygiene and proper nutrition are the basis for maintaining the health of the mouth, gums, and teeth. Bad hygienic habits, poor diet, lifestyle practices such as smoking, and underlying diseases can create a variety of mouth and dental disorders.

Types of Mouth and Dental Conditions

Bad Breath–Medically known as halitosis, bad breath is an unpleasant odor emanating from the mouth. The foul smell of the breath may be accompanied by a bad taste in the mouth. Bad breath is usually caused by a health problem in the mouth, teeth, gums, throat, or digestive system. Conditions such as diabetes, respiratory infections, or liver problems can also produce bad breath. The mouth is a window into the body. As such, if there is a bad odor, it is a sign that there is some underlying cause and imbalance which needs to be treated.

For information on **oral herpes**, see Herpes, pp. 238-240.

Dry Mouth–Xerostomia, or dry mouth, is caused by underfunctioning of the salivary glands associated with aging, but may also be triggered by smoking, snoring, alcohol consumption, long periods of talking, or exposure to dust, paints, or irritants. Dry mouth is also associated with depression, nervousness, asthma, allergies, diabetes, Sjögren's syndrome, and rheumatoid arthritis, among other conditions. Medical treatments such as chemotherapy, radiation, and beta-blocker administration can affect the production of saliva.

Gingivitis–Inflammation of the gums, or gingivitis, is characterized by bleeding, swelling, and redness in the tissues around the teeth. The most common cause is poor dental hygiene, which allows for a buildup of plaque (sticky mass of microorganisms) on the teeth at the gum line. As the plaque hardens, gums become inflamed, bleed, and recede from the teeth. Chronic gingivitis often leads to periodontal disease. Regular brushing and flossing is the best prevention against plaque buildup and gingivitis.

Periodontal Disease–The inflammation or degeneration of the tissues surrounding and supporting the teeth, including the gums, bone, ligaments, and the connective tissue at the root tip, is called periodontal disease. It manifests as painful and bleeding gums, deepening pockets in the gums, bone loss, and loosening or loss of teeth. It can also produce bad breath (halitosis) and lead to abscesses in the jaw. Causes of periodontal disease include poor diet (high sugar and junk food intake), nutritional deficiencies (especially vitamins A, C, or D, calcium, folic acid, or niacin), improper hygiene (brushing and flossing), excessive use of alcohol, tobacco, or drugs, and chronic disorders such as diabetes, glandular problems, and diseases of the blood.

Demineralized or "Soft Teeth"—In our clinical practice, we have seen a correlation between mineral-deficient patients and general health problems in the mouth, including softening of the enamel of the teeth.

Nutrients and Herbs for Mouth and Dental Conditions

■ **For overall oral hygiene:** vitamin C with bioflavonoids is the primary nutrient for the maintenance of tissues in the mouth; deficiencies cause bleeding gums and loosening of the teeth. Toothpaste or other oral hygienic products that contain vitamin C, tea tree oil, citrus seed extract, or baking soda promote the health of the mouth, gums, and teeth.

■ **For bad breath:** digestive enzymes and *acidophilus* can prevent and reverse halitosis by improving digestion. Fiber (psyllium or pectin fiber) helps remove toxins from the colon and thereby decreases bad breath. Chlorophyll products (wheat grass juice, chlorella, barley juice) act as a blood purifier and can be effective in reducing and preventing bad breath, taken both with food and on an empty stomach. For stubborn cases of bad breath, we recommend a short course of the antibiotic herbs goldenseal and odorless garlic to help eliminate bacteria contributing to the bad breath.

■ **For demineralized teeth:** a liquid mineral complex, applied topically to the teeth, can help reverse "soft teeth."

■ **For dry mouth:** we recommend the product Salix SST, a natural saliva substitute that helps relieve dry mouth immediately and promotes the production of natural saliva.

■ **For gingivitis:** applying chlorophyll directly to the gums, rinsing with diluted hydrogen peroxide, or using a toothpaste containing tea tree oil, citrus seed extract, or hydrogen peroxide can aid in reversing gingivitis.

■ **For inflammation:** we often recommend an aloe vera juice gargle or rinse in cases of mouth and throat tissue inflammation; Herbal Aloe Force, which contains herbal extracts as well, is one liquid product we have used with success.

■ **For tooth and gum pain relief:** clove oil applied to the problem area can provide temporary relief; dilute the oil for gum application.

Products for Mouth and Dental Conditions

Belladonna: Homeopathic remedy. Helpful for toothache, sore throat, fever, headache, earache, and colic.
STANDARD HOMEOPATHIC CO., 201 West 131st, Los Angeles, CA 90061; tel: 800-624-9659 or 310-768-0700.

Breath Fresh: Mints. Contains sorbitol and natural flavoring.
NATURE'S WAY PRODUCTS, INC., 10 Mountain Springs Parkway, Springville, UT 84663; tel: 801-489-1500.

Breath Freshener: Liquid. Blends organic peppermint, antiseptic tea tree oil, and herbs for fresh breath.
DESERT ESSENCE, 9700 Topanga Canyon Boulevard, Chatsworth, CA 91311; tel: 800-848-7331 or 818-734-1735.

Broken Cell Chlorella: Tablets. Contains chlorella, a microscopic green freshwater plant that has a concentrated supply of vitamins, minerals, proteins, and fatty acids. Chlorella contains a form of chlorophyll that supports the bloodstream, bowels, kidneys, and liver, and helps provide support for normal cellular growth and metabolic balance. Chlorella also supports the immune system and absorbs toxins and heavy metals.
SOLAR GREENS, NUTRACEUTICAL CORP., P.O. Box 681869, Park City, UT 84068; tel: 800-669-8877.

Chamomilla: Homeopathic remedy. Helpful for toothache, teething difficulties, pain, fever, earache, colic, and temper.
STANDARD HOMEOPATHIC CO., 201 West 131st, Los Angeles, CA 90061; tel: 800-624-9659 or 310-768-0700.

Chloraid: Capsules. Natural chlorophyll to reduce offensive body odors originating in the digestive and urinary tracts.

NATURE'S HERBS, 600 East Quality Drive, American Fork, UT 84003; tel: 800-437-2257 or 801-763-0700.

Chlorella: Tablets. Contains concentrated chlorophyll, or "green energy," combined with rich levels of blood-building iron, folic acid, and vitamin B12. Recent Japanese research demonstrates that Chlorella also offers a protective shield against toxic influences.

NEW CHAPTER, 22 High Street, Brattleboro, VT 05301; tel: 800-543-7279 or 802-257-9345.

Chlorophyll Caps. Water-soluble chlorophyll derived from organically grown alfalfa.

NATURE'S PLUS, 548 Broadhollow Road, Melville, NY 11747-3708; tel: 800-645-9500 or 516-293-0030.

Concentrated Mineral Drop Complex: Liquid. Contains complete, soluble, liquid ionic minerals and trace minerals in the proper balance needed for overall health and the functioning of the body's electrical system.

BIO NATIVUS, P.O. Box 3281, Ogden, UT 84401; tel: 888-628-4887 or 801-732-1294.

Dental Floss: Naturally waxed and saturated with pure tea tree oil; removes food particles between teeth.

COUNTRY LIFE, 101 Corporate Drive, Hauppauge, NY 11788; tel: 800-645-5768 or 516-231-1031.

DentalGel. Promotes healthy gums and freshens the mouth; contains aloe vera, vitamin C, baking soda, sanguinaria, vitamin E, and grapefruit seed extract.

NUTRIBIOTIC, NUTRITION RESOURCES, INC., P.O. Box 238, Lakeport, CA 95453; tel: 800-225-4345 or 707-263-0411.

Dental Pics: For after-meal cleaning.

DESERT ESSENCE, 9700 Topanga Canyon Boulevard, Chatsworth, CA 91311; tel: 800-848-7331 or 818-734-1735.

Dental Tape: Thicker thread for flossing wider spaces between teeth.

DESERT ESSENCE, 9700 Topanga Canyon Boulevard, Chatsworth, CA 91311; tel: 800-848-7331 or 818-734-1735.

E • GEM Lip Care: Lip balm. Helps heal dry, chapped, sunburned, or windburned lips; contains vitamin E, vitamin A, and aloe vera.

J.R. CARLSON LABS, INC., 15 College Drive, Arlington Heights, IL 60004-1985; tel: 800-323-4141 or 708-255-1600.

Fresh Breath Rx: Softgels. Contains concentrated herbal extracts to help neutralize and eliminate bad breath, morning breath, and halitosis.
PHYTO-THERAPY, INC., OPTIMUM HEALTH, 483 West Middle Turnpike, Manchester, CT 06040; tel: 800-228-1507 or 860-647-9729.

Fresh n' Free: Softgels. Contains chlorophyll complex, an anti-odor compound from plants, for the elimination of breath and body odors commonly found in people with fecal or urinary incontinence and odors associated with colostomies and ileostomies; prophylactic use may reduce the need for expensive sprays or deodorized protective briefs.
PHILLIPS NUTRITIONALS, 27071 Cabot Road #122, Laguna Hills, CA 92653; tel: 800-514-5115 or 702-898-8141.

FoliCare: Liquid. Oral rinse with folic acid, B complex vitamin, aloe vera, vitamin C, and zinc.
AMNI, 2247 National Avenue, Hayward, CA 94540-5012; tel: 800-437-8888 or 510-783-6969.

Healthy Gums: Liquid. Contains grapefruit seed extract with herbal extracts of plantain, white oak bark, witch hazel bark, and calendula to help maintain healthy gums.
IMHOTEP, P.O. Box 183, Ruby, NJ 12475; tel: 800-677-8577 or 914-336-2070.

Hempola Hempseed Oil Lip Balm. High in essential fatty acids for absorption and moisturization.
HEMPOLA, 3405 American Drive #5, Mississauga, Ontario, Canada L4V1T6; tel: 800-240-9215.

Herbal Aloe Force: Juice or topical gel. Processed aloe vera juice containing vitamins, minerals, enzymes, amino acids, essential fatty acids, growth factors, glycoproteins, sterols, bioflavonoids, polysaccharides (complex sugars), ionized colloidal silver, and herbal extracts (cat's claw, chamomile, burdock root, hawthorn berry, *Astragalus membranaceus* root, sheep sorrel, pau d'arco bark, slippery elm bark, and rhubarb root).
HERBAL ANSWERS, INC., P.O. Box 1110, Saratoga Springs, NY 12866; tel: 888-256-3367 or 518-581-1968.

Herbal Mouth and Gum Therapy: Liquid. Oral rinse to reduce and prevent swollen gums, soothe bleeding gums, and fight plaque; contains echinacea, goldenseal, calendula, aloe vera, bloodroot, grapefruit seed extract, and essential oils for flavoring.

WOODSTOCK NATURAL PRODUCTS, 140 Sylvan Avenue, Englewood Cliffs, NJ 07632; tel: 800-615-6895 or 201-944-0123.

Herbal Toothpaste and Gum Therapy. Fights gingivitis and plaque, helps prevent cavities, and whitens teeth naturally; contains natural fluoride (derived from fluoride ore, a naturally occurring element) and baking soda.

WOODSTOCK NATURAL PRODUCTS, 140 Sylvan Avenue, Englewood Cliffs, NJ 07632; tel: 800-615-6895 or 201-944-0123.

Jojoba Oil Lip Rescue: Lip balm. Softens and protects lips during everyday exposure to sun and wind contains jojoba oil, aloe vera, and vitamin E.

COUNTRY LIFE, 101 Corporate Drive, Hauppauge, NY 11788; tel: 800-645-5768 or 516-231-1031.

Salix SST: Lozenges. Stimulates saliva for relief of dry mouth discomfort and helps prevent tooth decay.

SCANDINAVIAN NATURAL HEALTH & BEAUTY PRODUCTS, INC., 13 North 7th Street, Perkasie, PA 18944; tel: 800-688-2276.

Tea Tree Chap-Mate: Lip balm. Moisturizes and protects lips with tea tree and safflower oils and botanical extracts.

THURSDAY PLANTATION, INC., NATURE'S PLUS, 548 Broadhol- low Road, Melville, NY 11747-3708; tel: 800-645-9500.

Tea Tree Lip-Clear: Lip balm. Accelerates the natural healing process of sore, damaged lips with the natural antiseptic properties of therapeutic-grade tea tree oil and herbal extracts of vitamins A and E, aloe vera, chamomile, calendula, and pure shea butter.

THURSDAY PLANTATION, INC., NATURE'S PLUS, 548 Broadhol- low Road, Melville, NY 11747-3708; tel: 800-645-9500.

Tea Tree Lozenges. Breath freshener and sore throat aid; combines the antiseptic qualities of tea tree oil with a blend of wild cherry, horehound, and lemon balm.

THURSDAY PLANTATION, INC., NATURE'S PLUS, 548 Broadhol- low Road, Melville, NY 11747-3708; tel: 800-645-9500.

Tea Tree Mouth Drops. Contains extracts of tea tree, cassia, menthol, peppermint, and sweet oil of fennel.

THURSDAY PLANTATION, INC., NATURE'S PLUS, 548 Broadhol- low Road, Melville, NY 11747-3708; tel: 800-645-9500.

Tea Tree Mouthwash. Cleans and refreshes the mouth and gums with antiseptic tea tree oil and essential oil of spearmint.

DESERT ESSENCE, 9700 Topanga Canyon Boulevard, Chatsworth, CA 91311; tel: 800-848-7331 or 818-734-1735.

Tea Tree Mouthwash. Cleanses with tea tree oil without disrupting the delicate environment of the mouth.

THURSDAY PLANTATION, INC., NATURE'S PLUS, 548 Broadhol- low Road, Melville, NY 11747-3708; tel: 800-645-9500.

Tea Tree Oil Lip Rescue: Lip balm. Combines tea tree oil and vitamin E to protect the lips from the effects of extreme weather conditions.

DESERT ESSENCE, 9700 Topanga Canyon Boulevard, Chatsworth, CA 91311; tel: 800-848-7331 or 818-734-1735.

Tea Tree Oil Toothpaste. Contains the antiseptic properties of tea tree oil and the plaque-fighting properties of baking soda.

DESERT ESSENCE, 9700 Topanga Canyon Boulevard, Chatsworth, CA 91311; tel: 800-848-7331 or 818-734-1735.

Tea Tree Toothpaste. Controls bacteria with therapeutic-grade tea tree oil.

THURSDAY PLANTATION, INC., NATURE'S PLUS, 548 Broadhol- low Road, Melville, NY 11747-3708; tel: 800-645-9500.

Tea Tree Toothpicks. Made from birchwood trees and infused with tea tree oil and extracts of peppermint, spearmint, cinnamon, fennel, and menthol.

THURSDAY PLANTATION, INC., NATURE'S PLUS, 548 Broadhol- low Road, Melville, NY 11747-3708; tel: 800-645-9500.

Nail Problems

As the nails and nail beds are the last areas of the body to receive oxygen and nutrients, they will often be the area where signs of deficiencies first appear. The condition and color of the nails and nail beds are useful as a gauge of underlying health.

Dangers of Nail Polish

Nails are porous and allow chemicals such as the acetone used in nail polish and polish remover to travel directly into the highly vascular (having many blood vessels) nail beds. Acetone is the source of the numb fingertips women often experience after removing nail polish. Repeated exposure to acetone can cause such symptoms and conditions as blood poisoning, coma, dizziness, drowsiness, gastritis, headaches, increased heart rate, loss of sensation, nausea, and respiratory problems.[139]

Acetone and other harmful chemicals can be found in a variety of cosmetics. We advise using nonchemical brands of cosmetics, nail polish, and remover. Aveda, Ecobella, Earth Science, Paul Penders, and Real Purity are some of the companies who offer such products.

Nutrients and Herbs for Nail Problems

To strengthen weak or brittle nails, we recommend the following: biotin (a B vitamin) and cysteine, an amino acid component of the primary protein comprising the nails.[140]

Products for Nail Problems

Fundamental Sulfur: Tablets. Contains biologically active sulfur, a mineral that is indispensable as a structural component of nails, connective tissues, hair, skin, and other body proteins.

AMNI, 2247 National Avenue, Hayward, CA 94540-5012; tel: 800-437-8888 or 510-783-6969.

See also
Fungal Infections,
pp. 190-197, for
information about
**fungal nail
infections**.

Hair & Nail Formula With Vegetal Silica: Capsules. Formula of horsetail, which contains silica to help fortify the hair and nails, plus oatstraw and gotu kola.

What Your Nails Can Tell You

The appearance and quality of your nails are indicators of your health. The following are nail characteristics and some of the underlying conditions with which they may be associated:[141]

Nail Characteristics	Underlying Condition
Black bands on nails	Poor adrenal function
Blue nails	Heart or lung problems, copper or silver toxicity, drug reaction
Brittle or splitting nails	Vitamin A, vitamin D, iron, calcium, or HCl deficiency
Dark and/or spoon-shaped nails	Vitamin B12 deficiency or anemia
Fungal infections	Deficient *acidophilus* or *B.bifidum*
Hangnails	Vitamin C, folic acid, or protein deficiency
Ridges or no half moons	Vitamin A or protein deficiency, kidney problems
Thick nails	Poor circulation, thyroid problems
Weak nails with horizontal ridges	Hypothyroidism
White bands/lines	Protein deficiency, heart or liver disease
White nails	Mineral deficiency, liver problems, anemia
White spots	Zinc or HCl deficiency, thyroid problems
Yellow nails	Vitamin E deficiency, lymph or circulatory problems

NATROL INC., 21411 Prairie Street, Chatsworth, CA 91311; tel: 818-739-6000.

Hair, Skin & Nails: Tablets. Contains 24 vitamins, minerals, herbs, and other nutrients to build thicker hair, stronger nails, and well-nourished skin.

FUTUREBIOTICS, 145 Ricefield Lane, Hauppauge, NY 11788; tel: 800-FOR-LIFE (367-5433) or 516-273-6300.

Hair, Skin & Nails: Tablets. Combination of vitamins A, B complex, and E, zinc, and calcium to help create an environment for the formation of healthy nails, hair, and skin; also contains butcher's broom, bilberry, horsetail, and nettles.

OPTIMAL NUTRIENTS, 1163 Chess Drive #F, Foster City, CA 94404; tel: 800-966-8874 or 650-525-0112.

Inner Beauty: Tablets. Blends nourishing herbs with well-balanced vitamins to produce strong and healthy nails, hair, and skin.

BIO NATIVUS, P.O. Box 3281, Ogden, UT 84401; tel: 888-628-4887 or 801-732-1294.

Lustre: Tablets. Targets common deficiencies in American diets and the effects of pollution to provide nutrition for nails, hair, and skin; ingredients include silicon, vitamins A, B1, B2, B3, B5, B6, B12, and E, beta carotene, L-proline, manganese, copper, zinc, folic acid, biotin, inositol, and silica.

SOURCE NATURALS, THRESHOLD ENTERPRISES, 23 Janis Way, Scotts Valley, CA 95066; tel: 800-777-5677 or 831-438-1144.

MSM (Methylsulfonylmethane): Capsules, eye and ear drops, lotion, or powder. Contains sulfur, which is a major component of the human body; MSM provides the body with building materials for healthy, flexible cells.

RICH DISTRIBUTING, P.O. Box 33830, Portland, OR 97292; tel: 877-245-5742 or 503-761-7450.

Vitesse Natural Nail Polish Remover. Contains a solvent derived from milk that is gentle to the nails, cuticles, and skin; supports dried-out, yellow, or fragile nails and contains no harsh chemical (acetone) odors.

SCANDINAVIAN NATURAL HEALTH & BEAUTY PRODUCTS, INC., 13 North 7th Street, Perkasie, PA 18944; tel: 800-688-2276.

Osteoporosis

A condition of decreased bone mass and density resulting in porous spaces in the bones and loss of supporting structure, osteoporosis affects mostly women—80% of the estimated 28 million Americans who have either low bone mass or full-fledged osteoporosis.

Symptoms and Causes of Osteoporosis

Symptoms include weight and height loss, and thin, brittle bones which break easily.

Contrary to the common myth that menopausal estrogen deficiency is behind osteoporosis, the condition is usually under way long before menopause. In addition, the universal estrogen deficiency of menopause is itself a myth. The ratio of estrogen to progesterone is more often the problem; it is a deficiency of progesterone that has the greater impact on osteoporosis because, while estrogen slows bone loss, only progesterone can rebuild bone.[142]

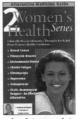

Another myth of osteoporosis is that insufficient calcium intake is a major contributing factor. The diets of the majority of women contain plenty of calcium, important for bone health. The problem is rather that the calcium is not being absorbed or their bones are losing calcium at a rate that calcium intake cannot keep up with.[143] Calcium absorption is complex and involves many nutritional cofactors. Poor absorption can be caused by deficiencies or improper ratios of any of the nutrients required for calcium assimilation.

See **Osteoporosis** in *Alternative Medicine Guide to Women's Health 2* (Future Medicine Publishing, 1998); ISBN 1-887299-30-0); to order, call 800-333-HEAL.

A high caffeine intake, excessive consumption of carbonated soft drinks, and a diet primarily of protein, salt, sugar, and processed foods can all cause the body to excrete calcium. When the condition is chronic, it leads to loss of bone mass as the body pulls calcium from the bones to correct the imbalance.

Other factors that can contribute to osteoporosis include protein or collagen deficiencies, corticosteroid use, cigarettes, alcohol consumption, heavy metals, environmental pollutants (especially cadmium), sedentary lifestyle, and stress.[144]

For information on **bone-loss testing,** see Appendix: Great Smokies Diagnostic Laboratory, pp. 484-485. See Menopausal Symptoms, pp. 268-274, for information about **rebalancing hormone levels.**

Nutrients for Osteoporosis

By altering the lifestyle risk factors discussed above and eliminating what may be contributing to loss of calcium or interfering with calcium absorption, you can take important steps to maintain the health of your bones.

Supplementing with an easily assimilated form of calcium can help offset the imbalance between calcium uptake and loss. We recommend calcium citrate, calcium lactate, calcium aspartate, and calcium gluconate. All of these are more easily absorbed by the body than calcium carbonate or oyster-shell calcium. We also use calcium hydroxyapatite with boron. Another important mineral for bone health, boron is recommended for the prevention of osteoporosis.[145] Calcium should be taken with magnesium as these two minerals function in ratio to each other. Note that taking antacids as a source of calcium is misguided. Calcium must be in an acidic environment in order to be properly assimilated. Antacids provide an alkaline environment which prevents the uptake of calcium.[146]

We often recommend the product OsteoPrime Forte to people with osteoporosis, because it contains the proper ratios of nutrients needed to prevent and even reverse existing osteoporitic symptoms.

Products for Osteoporosis

Bone Builder: Chewable tablets. Contains MCHC (microcrystalline hydroxyapatite, the core matrix substance of bones), vitamin D, and the essential minerals magnesium, zinc, copper, and manganese for additional bone support

ETHICAL NUTRIENTS, 971 Calle Negocio, San Clemente, CA 92673; tel: 800-668-8743 or 949-366-0818.

Bone Builder With Boron: Tablets. Contains MCHC (microcrystalline hydroxyapatite) and boron, a trace mineral that may play a role in maintaining bone health.

ETHICAL NUTRIENTS, 971 Calle Negocio, San Clemente, CA 92673; tel: 800-668-8743 or 949-366-0818.

Bone Density Factors With Boron: Tablets. Calcium is necessary for the prevention of osteoporosis; contains 1,000 mg of calcium from hydroxyapatite (raw bone matrix of organically fed cattle), calcium citrate, and citrate malate, plus vitamins and minerals as a nutritional aid for skeletal and periodontal support; according to clinical trials, hydroxyapatite is an effective form of calcium for re-calcifying bone. COUNTRY LIFE, 101 Corporate Drive, Hauppauge, NY 11788; tel: 800-645-5768 or 516-231-1031.

Calcium/Minerals Plus: Tablets. Contains calcium (from eggshell and dicalcium phosphate) in a base of seaweed and chamomile. NATURAL ENERGY PRODUCTS, 21101 Welch Road, Snohomish, WA 98296; tel: 206-486-5956.

Calcium 900: Softgels. Contains calcium without the fat and calories of calcium-rich foods; calcium is essential in reducing the risk of osteoporosis and in the development of healthy bones and teeth. IVC, 500 Halls Mill Road, Freehold, NJ 07728; tel: 800-666-8482 or 732-308-3000.

Calcium Plus: Tablets. Daily supplement of calcium, magnesium, essential minerals (which support the skeletal and muscular systems) co-nutrients, superfoods, and a blend of seven Chinese herbs considered supportive of skeletal health; for diets high in dairy products and low in magnesium-rich foods (grains and legumes). RAINBOW LIGHT, P.O. Box 600, Santa Cruz, CA 95061; tel: 800-635-1233 or 408-429-9089.

Cal-10 Plus: Capsules. Contains ten forms of calcium with added magnesium and vitamin D; for women of all ages. WGI, 35008 Emerald Coast Parkway, 5th Floor, Destin, FL 32541; tel: 800-854-8353 or 850-654-4744.

Liquid Calcium Rx Calcium 1000 Complex: Softgels. Contains six sources of calcium, two sources of magnesium, herbs, vitamins, and minerals for optimum bioavailability. PHYTO-THERAPY, INC., OPTIMUM HEALTH, 483 West Middle Turnpike, Manchester, CT 06040; tel: 800-228-1507 or 860-647-9729.

Osteo Formula: Capsules. Multi-vitamin containing easily absorbable magnesium and calcium, other essential vitamins and minerals, and the pure plant enzyme phytase, which has been shown to increase the release of dietary minerals from fiber-rich foods. PREVAIL CORP., 2204-8 Northwest Birdsdale, Gresham, OR 97030; tel: 800-248-0885 or 503-667-5527.

Osteo-Gest: Capsules. Bone mineralization formula containing microcrystalline hydroxyapatite, the most absorbable form of calcium, and seven other vitamins and minerals important for proper bone nutrition.

BIO-NUTRITIONAL FORMULAS, 106 East Jericho Turnpike, Mineola, NY 11501; tel: 800-950-8484.

Osteo-guard: Tablets. Calcium source for those at risk of osteoporosis; reduces calcium loss and puts calcium back into the bones, which helps make them stronger and more resistant to breaking with age; contains calcium source from whole bone, boron, and vitamin K, as well as other natural bone minerals and organic constituents, such as collagens.

AMNI, 2247 National Avenue, Hayward, CA 94540-5012; tel: 800-437-8888 or 510-783-6969.

OsteoPrime Forte: Tablets. Provides a balanced combination of nutrients to support and maintain healthy bones.

ENZYMATIC THERAPY, 825 Challenger Drive, Green Bay, WI 54311-8328; tel: 800-558-7372 or 920-469-1313.

OsteoPro: Capsules. Bone-building formula that strengthens bones and the skeletal framework.

PHOENIX BIOLOGICS, 2794 Loker Avenue West #104, Carlsbad, CA 92008; tel: 800-947-8482 or 760-631-7729.

OsteoProCare: Liquid. Combines calcium with 15 essential minerals, 45 trace minerals, and vitamin D3 in a colloidal suspension for better absorption.

LIFE FORCE, INTL., 2731 Via Orange Way #106, Spring Valley, CA 91978; tel: 800-531-4877.

Osteo-Support: Tablets. Contains a blend of vitamins and minerals to promote healthy strong bones.

HVL INC., 600 Boyce Road, Pittsburgh, PA 15205; tel: 800-245-4441.

PhytoGest: Cream. Natural progesterone cream containing wild yam, aloe vera, and AHA (alpha-hydroxy acid); natural progesterone is an estrogen antagonist, stimulates bone building, helps protect against breast and endometrial cancers, enhances energy and fat utilization, enhances thyroid hormone function, normalizes blood-sugar levels, restores libido, and acts as a natural antidepressant and diuretic (increases urine flow).

KARUNA CORP., 42 Digital Drive # 7, Novato, CA 94949; tel: 800-826-7225 or 415-382-0147.

Super Absorbeze Calcium Magnesium Phosphorus: Liquid. Complete mineral formula to build and maintain strong and healthy bones and teeth; contains calcium source that is easily absorbable, natural vitamin D3 to improve calcium absorption, milk, lactose, and sucrose; available in natural orange flavor.

NATURE'S LIFE, 7180 Lampson Avenue, Garden Grove, CA 92841-3914; tel: 800-854-6837 or 714-379-6500.

Vegetarian Balanced Calcium Formula: Caplets. Provides support for women with osteoporosis or who are post-menopausal; contains calcium, an important mineral for maintaining the body, as well as magnesium, vitamin D, boron, silicon, and vitamin K.

PHILLIPS NUTRITIONALS, 27071 Cabot Road #122, Laguna Hills, CA 92653; tel: 800-514-5115 or 702-898-8141.

Parasitic Infections

Although technically a parasite is any organism that lives off of a host organism, the term *parasite* typically refers to protozoa (single-cell organisms such as *Giardia lamblia*) or worms (such as tapeworms) which infect the intestines. As with all infections, the parasite's ability to infest depends on the general health, nutritional competence, and immune vitality of its host. Although there are exceptions of a healthy person succumbing to parasitic infection due to consumption of contaminated food or other concentrated exposure, in most cases a healthy body will fight off infestation.

Symptoms of Parasitic Infections

The most common symptom of intestinal parasites is explosive and watery diarrhea, typically occuring three to five days after exposure. The diarrhea may alternate with constipation, and other symptoms include indigestion, gas, fatigue, allergic reactions to food, nausea, vomiting, night sweats, and fever. Acute cases can produce compromised immunity, nutritional deficiencies, and severe weight loss. If left untreated, rheumatoid and arthritic symptoms may emerge.

Intestinal parasitic infection can be asymptomatic (without symptoms) or only produce symptoms at one stage in the life of the parasite, and so remain undetected for many years. The infection can also resemble other gastrointestinal conditions; for example, an amoebic infection can be difficult to distinguish from ulcerative colitis. The only way to definitively diagnose parasites is to get a comprehensive fecal parasitology test, which must be ordered by your medical doctor or other qualified health-care professional.

Nutrients and Herbs for Parasitic Infections

There are numerous natural formulations that work well to eliminate parasites in most people. Those who cannot tolerate the toxicity of conventional antiparasitic drugs or those for whom these drugs have failed will find the alternatives particularly useful. Generally, antiparasitic herbs are used on a daily basis for approximately two months to rid the body of parasites. The goal is to create an internal environment that is disagreeable to the parasite so that it will die or leave, without making you sick in the process.

In addition to mugwort, sarsaparilla, chapparal, barberry, myrrh extract, and cat's claw, the following nutrients are known to have beneficial effects on parasitic conditions.

■ **Dietary fiber and bentonite clay:** taking bentonite clay orally and increasing fiber in the diet are recommended to help cleanse the intestines and thus aid in the elimination of worms and parasites from the intestinal tract. (Note: Although there is no specific contraindication regarding the use of bentonite or psyllium by pregnant or lactating women, we always recommend that pregnant or lactating women consult their health-care professional before taking any nutritional or dietary supplement.)

■ **Probiotics:** *Lactobacillus acidophilus, Bifidobacteria,* and other beneficial intestinal bacteria are recommended in cases of intestinal parasites. A deficiency of beneficial intestinal bacteria is frequently associated with parasitic conditions.

■ **Berberine (goldenseal):** the plant alkaloid berberine is found in several plants, but that derived from goldenseal seems to be the strongest intestinal antimicrobial. It is particularly effective in cases of giardiasis (*Giardia* infection) and can clear up the ailment in as little as ten days without the side effects of its conventional counterpart, Flagyl (metronidazole). Children respond well to berberine.[147]

■ **Black walnut bark:** used externally, black walnut can kill ringworm; taken orally, it can kill tapeworms.[148]

■ **Garlic extract:** this potent herb can destroy common intestinal parasites including hookworms, pinworms, roundworms, and tapeworms; garlic oil can be used topically for ringworm infections.[149]

■ **Grapefruit seed extract and Chinese wormwood (*Artemisia annua*):** these are two nutrients we often recommend to eliminate intestinal parasites.

■ **Pumpkin seed:** pumpkin seed has a long history of use against intestinal parasites.

Products for Parasitic Infections

Acidophilus Chewable: Wafers. Blend of the beneficial bacteria *B. bifidum* and *L. acidophilus* for intestinal health; for children or adults who prefer a chewable *acidophilus* product.
PHILLIPS NUTRITIONALS, 27071 Cabot Road #122, Laguna Hills, CA 92653; tel: 800-514-5115 or 702-898-8141.

All-Flora: Capsules or powder. Supplies billions of friendly flora, vitamins, and detoxifying and supportive enzymes to the digestive system.

NEW CHAPTER, 22 High Street, Brattleboro, VT 05301; tel: 800-543-7279 or 802-257-9345.

Biocidin: Tablets. Herbal antimicrobial for intestinal dysbiosis (imbalance in the intestinal flora) in which parasitic, fungal, or bacterial pathogens have been identified. *In vitro* testing by Great Smokies Diagnostic Laboratory has shown that all strains of bacteria and yeast tested show high levels of sensitivity to this combination of medicinal plants. According to Dr. Martin Lee, Ph.D., Great Smokies' laboratory director, "The herbal mixture Biocidin has been the most broadly acting and powerful natural or nonprescriptive substance evaluated. In separate experiments, we have found that Biocidin was a potent inhibitor of growth for *Candida albicans*, as well as other *Candida* species." When used for an extended period of time, the cold nature of the herbs in Biocidin may weaken digestive energy, causing nausea or loss of appetite. In this case, appropriate tonic formulations can be chosen.

BIO-BOTANICAL RESEARCH, INC., 144 Pioneer Road, Corralitos, CA 95076; distributed by WELLNESS HEALTH PHARMACY, 2800 South 18th Street, Homewood, AL 35209; tel: 800-227-2627 or 205-879-6551.

Garlic-Black Walnut: Capsules. Herbal formula traditionally used for animals with parasites; contains odorless garlic, black walnut, fennel seed, and cascara sagrada bark.

NATURE'S HERBS, 600 East Quality Drive, American Fork, UT 84003; tel: 800-437-2257 or 801-763-0700.

Garlic-Power: Tablets. Concentrated garlic extract from a Chinese formula of red and white garlic equivalent to 1,200 mg of fresh garlic; contains higher allicin potential (minimum 3 mg of total allicin potential calculated as allicin content and relative allinase enzyme activity per tablet) than any other garlic supplement; odor-controlled.

NATURE'S HERBS, 600 East Quality Drive, American Fork, UT 84003; tel: 800-437-2257 or 801-763-0700.

Garlic Power Rx: Softgels. Contains organic garlic that is five times more potent than fresh garlic, vitamin E, hawthorn berry, and parsley.

PHYTO-THERAPY, INC., OPTIMUM HEALTH, 483 West Middle Turnpike, Manchester, CT 06040; tel: 800-228-1507.

Garlinase 4000: Tablets. Daily supplement that contains beneficial allicin (the active component of garlic) while promising odor-free breath.

ENZYMATIC THERAPY, 825 Challenger Drive, Green Bay, WI 54311-8328; tel: 800-558-7372 or 920-469-1313.

Grapefruit Extract Liquid Concentrate. Contains Citricidal®, a powerful antimicrobial compound from grapefruit seed and pulp; useful for parasites, bacteria, viruses, and fungi.

NUTRIBIOTIC, NUTRITION RESOURCES, INC., P.O. Box 238, Lakeport, CA 95453; tel: 800-225-4345 or 707-263-0411.

Katsu Herbal Garlic Complex: Tablets. Concentrated extract of garlic, coix, and rice bran with shark cartilage and vitamin C. Garlic is well known for its ability to inhibit parasites (protozoa and worms), bacteria, fungi, and yeast (including *Candida*), promote immune functions, lower cholesterol, reduce platelet aggregation, and aid digestion.

KENSHIN TRADING CORP., P.O. Box 7511, Torrance, CA 90504; tel: 800-766-1313 or 310-212-3199.

Kyo-Dophilus: Capsules or tablets. Tablets contain one strain of the beneficial bacteria *L. acidophilus*; capsules contain three strains of beneficial bacteria (*L. acidophilus*, *B. bifidum*, and *B. longum*) that are prevalent in the intestines; this probiotic supplement helps to normalize the intestinal flora.

WAKUNAGA OF AMERICA, 23501 Madero, Mission Viejo, CA 92691; tel: 800-421-2998 or 949-855-2776.

Liquid Bentonite. Bentonite clay has been used for centuries as an internal and external purification aid; it is known for its highly absorptive properties, drawing out metals, drugs, and toxins for release from the body.

ARISE AND SHINE, P.O. Box 1439, Mount Shasta, CA 96067; tel: 800-688-2444 or 530-926-0891.

MSM (Methylsulfonylmethane): Capsules, eye and ear drops, lotion, or powder. Contains sulfur, which is a major component of the human body; MSM provides the body with building materials for healthy, flexible cells.

RICH DISTRIBUTING, P.O. Box 33830, Portland, OR 97292; tel: 877-245-5742 or 503-761-7450.

Oregamax: Capsules. Contains crushed wild oregano, *Rhus cariaria*, garlic, and onion; wild oregano contains carvacrol (antimicrobial), flavonoids (antiseptic), and terpenes (anti-inflammatory).

PURITY PRODUCTS, 1804 Plaza Avenue, New Hyde Park, NY 11040; tel: 800-769-7873.

ProSeed Grapefruit Seed Extract: Liquid. Multi-purpose concentrate containing grapefruit seed extract; useful for numerous stomach, intestinal, skin, and scalp conditions; also can be used as a sore throat gargle, dental rinse, and as a broad spectrum cleanser for food.

IMHOTEP, P.O. Box 183, Ruby, NJ 12475; tel: 800-677-8577 or 914-336-2070.

Vermex Caps. Cleansing combination with black walnut hulls and pumpkin seeds.

CRYSTAL STAR HERBAL NUTRITION, 4069 Wedgeway Court, Earth City, MO 63045; tel: 800-736-6015 or 314-739-7551.

Pregnancy and Side Effects

For the health of the mother and child, giving special attention to nutrition is essential before, during, and after pregnancy.

Prenatal—A critical factor in a healthy pregnancy and baby is the pre-pregnancy nutritional condition of both parents. If a woman enters into pregnancy with nutritional deficiencies, a poor diet, unhealthy addictions or habits, or illnesses such as iron-deficient anemia, she risks not being able to provide the necessary nutritional building blocks to create a healthy baby. She also increases her likelihood of a difficult pregnancy and potential long-term health problems.

During Pregnancy—While pregnant, the mother needs more of everything, especially protein, B vitamins, calcium, magnesium, phosphates, iron, and zinc. Sufficient amounts of folic acid are especially important during pregnancy. Folic acid is vital to the formation of red blood cells, the growth of new cells, and the development of the baby's nervous system. Supplementation during pregnancy may help prevent spina bifida or a cleft lip in the baby.[150] Vitamin E and citrus bioflavonoids can help prevent miscarriage or premature labor.[151]

Many doctors advise pregnant women to drink a quart of milk per day or consume large amounts of dairy products to increase their calcium and protein intake. If the woman is lactose-intolerant, however, she will not fully digest these foods and so her body will not assimilate the calcium or protein. She will also experience gastrointestinal disturbances such as gas, bloating, and cramping. Many babies whose mothers followed the increased-dairy diet during pregnancy are born lactose-intolerant and therefore have digestive difficulties from the very beginning if they are given cow's milk or formula containing milk products. For these children, we recommend food allergy blood tests for cow's milk, goat milk, rice milk, and soy milk to determine the one best tolerated.

After Pregnancy—Following pregnancy, we recommend that women keep their protein intake high, although not as high as during pregnancy. While iron, calcium, and magnesium supplementation needs remain the same as during pregnancy, the need for iodine, zinc, and

Nutrients to Avoid During Pregnancy

While many herbs and nutritional supplements are useful during pregnancy, some should definitely be avoided.

Herbs—When pregnant, use herbs only under the guidance of a professional and do not take the following:

• Autumn crocus, barberry, concentrated aloe vera, cotton root, ginseng, goldenseal, *dong quai*, lobelia, mandrake, marsh tea, pennyroyal, poke root, rue, sage, shepherd's purse, southernwood, tansy, thuja, wahoo bark, wormwood, and yohimbe: can trigger miscarriage.

• Berberine (found in goldenseal, barberry, and Oregon grape root): causes strong uterine contractions.

• Licorice: contains estrogen-like substances which can interfere with hormonal balance.

• Juniper: can harm the fetus and possibly induce miscarriage.

• Senna and cascara: laxatives found in both herbal preparations and over-the-counter drugs; senna encourages menstruation and may promote miscarriage, while cascara can cause abnormal development of the fetus.

Nutritional Supplements—Use caution in taking vitamins and minerals during pregnancy; take only those that are necessary. Vitamin A should be treated with special caution. Doses as low as 15,000 IU have been associated with birth defects such as microcephaly (a congenital abnormal smallness of the head often seen in mental retardation).[152] Beta carotene, which is converted by the body into vitamin A, is relatively nontoxic, but it is best to err on the side of caution and not take high doses of beta carotene either, especially early in the pregnancy.

vitamins A and C are higher. Folic acid requirements decrease approximately 25%.

Side Effects of Pregnancy

Anemia—Iron-deficiency anemia, which can be due to dietary factors or loss of iron during menses or previous pregnancies, is common during pregnancy. Symptoms include fatigue, loss of stamina, and, in extreme cases, a craving for dirt, paint, or ice. Anemic pregnant women may also experience inflammation of the tongue, dryness and cracking at the corners of the mouth, and fingernails becoming thin and concave with raised edges.

Constipation—Another common ailment, constipation during pregnancy can be caused by a sedentary lifestyle, increased progesterone, a diet low in fiber, and the baby pressing on the intestines. Pregnant women should avoid over-the-counter laxatives, with the exception of natural psyllium fiber products. Taking psyllium, increasing intake of high-fiber foods, and walking daily (consult your physician before beginning any new exercise program) can all help ease constipation.

Heartburn—This condition occurs often during pregnancy due to the reflux (re-entry) of stomach fluids into the throat and mouth because of pressure on the stomach from the growing baby. Avoid spicy and greasy foods, alcohol, and caffeine. We do not recommend that anyone use over-the-counter antacids to ease heartburn, but pregnant women in particular should avoid using them, as antacids can stunt the development of the fetus.[153]

Mood Swings—Mood swings and emotional changes during pregnancy are believed to be related to hormonal changes and a deficiency of B vitamins.

Nausea/Morning Sickness—Acute, transient nausea associated with pregnancy is thought to be caused by increased levels of estrogen.

Decreased Lactation—Diminished ability of the mother to produce milk can be caused by nutritional deficiencies, vitamin B6 in particular. Approximately 50% of pregnant women are deficient in B6.[154] Supplementation is delicate, however, as too much B6 can actually reduce lactation.[155] A safe dose of vitamin B6 for lactating women is 20-30 mg daily.[156] Emotional factors can also affect lactation. Activation of the sympathetic nervous system (the "fight-or-flight" instinct), as occurs when one is nervous or jumpy, can inhibit the release of oxytocin (the hormone responsible for milk production) and diminish milk production.[157]

Nutrients and Herbs for Pregnancy and Side Effects

■ **For support before and during pregnancy:** we often recommend to prospective mothers a product called Complete Prenatal, which contains the full complement of nutrients needed by women who want to get pregnant or who are pregnant.

■ **For constipation:** a diet high in fiber along with supplementation with psyllium husks or other fiber product helps improve bowel regularity.

■ **For heartburn:** taking digestive enzymes can help ease heartburn.

■ **For leg cramps during pregnancy:** to avoid muscle cramps, maintain the proper calcium-magnesium levels by using a supplement containing a 2:1 ratio of magnesium to calcium.

■ **For lactation support:** if a lactating woman's protein intake is low, we recommend protein powders or free-form amino acids. The herbs fenugreek and chasteberry can help increase lactation.[158]

■ **For morning sickness:** vitamin B6 and ginger reduce nausea and morning sickness. Acidic foods such as sugar, alcohol, caffeine, citrus fruits and juices, supplemental iron medications, and dairy products contribute to nausea and vomiting and should be avoided.

Products for Pregnancy and Side Effects

Amino Acids: Capsules, powder, or tablets. Contains only the natural (L) forms of the amino acids as it naturally occurs in plants and animals.

NOW, 550 Mitchell Road, Glendale Heights, IL 60139; tel: 800-283-3500 or 630-545-9098.

AminoHealth: Capsules. Contains a balanced complex of 18 isolated L-crystalline amino acids for maximum utilization during times of intense mental and physical stress; ingredients include sulfur-bearing amino acids, which constitute a high percentage of the amino acids found in hair, skin and nails.

NUTRI-SOURCE, 3290 Cessna Drive, Cameron Park, CA 95682; tel: 800-293-1683 or 530-676-8838.

Complete PreNatal System: Tablets. Multivitamin for pregnant and lactating women; contains essential nutrients such as folic acid and calcium, *acidophilus*, supportive herbs, and a range of plant-source enzymes.

RAINBOW LIGHT, P.O. Box 600, Santa Cruz, CA 95061; tel: 800-635-1233 or 408-429-9089.

Folic Acid: Tablets. Adequate daily amounts of folic acid throughout the childbearing years can help reduce the risk of having a child with brain and spinal-cord birth defects.

BRONSON LABORATORIES, INC., 600 East Quality Drive, American Fork, UT 84003; tel: 800-235-3200 or 801-756-5670.

Ginger-Peppermint Combination: Capsules. For relief of stomach and intestinal distress, bloating, fullness, pressure, and cramps after eating; contains ginger root, peppermint leaves, cramp bark, wild yam root, spearmint leaves, fennel seed, catnip herb, and papaya leaves.

NATURE'S HERBS, 600 East Quality Drive, American Fork, UT 84003; tel: 800-437-2257 or 801-763-0700.

Great Mother's Belly Butter: Salve. For the skin; contains cocoa butter, olive oil, coconut oil, wheat germ oil, calendula, marshmallow root, white oak bark, comfrey root, hawthorn berry, passionflower, red raspberry leaves, vitamin E, and pure essential oils.

GREAT MOTHER'S GOODS, 501 West Fayette Street, Suite #214-215, Syracuse, NY 13204; tel: 800-984-4848.

Great Mother's Sitz Bath: Muslin bags. For soaking the pelvic area (sitz bath) or compresses; contains comfrey leaf, plantain, calendula, yarrow, marshmallow root, and sea salt; these herbs are known for their protective and demulcent (membrane-soothing) properties.

GREAT MOTHER'S GOODS, 501 West Fayette Street, Suite #214-215, Syracuse, NY 13204; tel: 800-984-4848.

Great Mother's Quiet Herbal Soak. Blend of lavender, chamomile, rose petals, comfrey leaf, calendula, and oatmeal.

GREAT MOTHER'S GOODS, 501 West Fayette Street, Suite #214-215, Syracuse, NY 13204; tel: 800-984-4848.

Ocean Nutrition Canada Mother's Gift: Capsules. For pregnant and lactating mothers; contains DHA (docosahexaenoic acid) and arachidonic acid, which are essential nutrients for the baby in the womb and during the first months of life because the baby cannot produce sufficient amounts of DHA from linoleic and alpha-linolenic acid.

OCEAN NUTRITION CANADA LTD., 757 Bedford Highway, Bedford, Nova Scotia, Canada B2A3Z7; tel: 888-980-8889 or 902-457-2399.

Perfect Prenatal: Tablets. Dietary supplement to help with a healthy and comfortable pregnancy.

NEW CHAPTER, 22 High Street, Brattleboro, VT 05301; tel: 800-543-7279 or 802-257-9345.

PN-6 Formula: Capsules. For last six weeks of pregnancy; ingredients include squaw vine, red raspberry leaves, blessed thistle, black cohosh root, pennyroyal, and false unicorn root. Caution: Should not be taken prior to last six weeks of pregnancy.

NATURE'S WAY PRODUCTS, Inc., 10 Mountain Springs Parkway, Springville, UT 84663; tel: 800-962-8873 or 801-489-1500.

Pre-Natal: Tablets. Natural source of vitamins and minerals, especially high in calcium and iron.

J.R. CARLSON LABS, INC., 15 College Drive, Arlington Heights, IL 60004-1985; tel: 800-323-4141 or 708-255-1600.

Prenatal Forte: Tablets. Vegetarian daily multivitamin/mineral supplement high in calcium, magnesium, bioflavonoids, minerals (citrate and amino acid–chelate forms), iron, and folic acid; also includes digestive enzymes from plant sources, alfalfa, dandelion, nettle, raspberry leaf, yellowdock, cranberry, and papaya.

NF FORMULAS, INC., 9755 Southwest Commerce Circle, C-5, Wilsonville, OR 97070; tel: 800-547-4891 or 503-682-9755.

Psyllium Husk Powder. Fibrous bulking agent that gels and thickens when mixed with water or juice and helps detoxify the alimentary canal.

ARISE AND SHINE, P.O. Box 1439, Mount Shasta, CA 96067; tel: 800-688-2444 or 530-926-0891.

Ultra Prenatal Complex: Tablets. Prenatal formula containing increased doses of calcium and other major minerals, vitamins A, C, D, and E, amino acids, and a complete B complex.

NATURE'S PLUS, 548 Broadhollow Road, Melville, NY 11747-3708; tel: 800-645-9500 or 516-293-0030.

Premenstrual Syndrome (PMS)

For ten days to two weeks before menstruation, many women experience a range of symptoms, from uncomfortable to painful, the cluster of which is referred to as premenstrual syndrome, or PMS. The symptoms may continue through part or sometimes all of menstruation.

Symptoms and Causes of PMS

PMS encompasses such emotional symptoms as anxiety, panic attacks, mood swings, irritability, depression, and hostility. Physical manifestations include abdominal bloating, swelling and water retention in the hands and feet, weight gain, intestinal disturbance (constipation or diarrhea), headaches, lower back pain, cramps, tender or swollen breasts, fatigue, acne, and food cravings (notably for salt and sugar).

Poor diet (especially low in B vitamins and high in sugar) and estrogen dominance (excess estrogen in relation to progesterone) are two of the main causes of PMS. Other contributing factors are low thyroid function (hypothyroidism), exhausted adrenal glands, candidiasis (*Candida* yeast overgrowth), stress, high caffeine consumption, and lack of exercise.

Environmental estrogens (SEE QUICK DEFINITION) are a common source of excess estrogen in the body. A concentrated source of these estrogen-mimicking chemicals is meat and dairy products from cows that have been injected with growth or other hormones and been given feed grown or treated with herbicides and pesticides. These hormones and chemicals are stored in fat cells. For this reason, we strongly recommend eating only organically raised meats and organic dairy products. Eating only organically grown fruits and vegetables

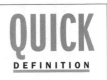

QUICK
DEFINITION

Environmental estrogens are foreign compounds and/or chemical toxins that mimic the effects of estrogen. Environmental estrogens, also called xenoestrogens, are present primarily in man-made chemicals (herbicides and pesticides such as DDT) and industrial by-products (from manufacture of plastics, paper, and the incineration of hazardous wastes). Environmental estrogens often cause an imbalance of estrogen relative to progesterone, another key hormone. When a woman's body has too much estrogen (a condition called estrogen dominance), a variety of health problems can result, including breast cancer, fibroids, and endometriosis, among others. According to some researchers, environmental estrogens also affect men and may contribute to testicular cancer, urinary tract disorders, and low sperm count.

is also a good idea due to the environmental estrogens used in conventional agriculture.

Chlorine-based chemicals, called organochlorines, found in over 11,000 agricultural and industrial products also have the ability to disrupt human hormonal balance by mimicking estrogen in the body.[159] It is advisable to reduce your exposure to these harmful chemicals wherever possible.

As the liver is the organ that processes excessive estrogen for elimination from the body, liver toxicity or liver overload can also be a factor in estrogen dominance. Nutritionally supporting the liver enables it to better fulfill its function of getting rid of excess estrogen and synthetic chemicals.

Nutrients and Herbs for PMS

■ **Vitamin B6:** numerous studies have demonstrated the ability of vitamin B6 to alleviate symptoms of PMS.[160]

■ **Magnesium and calcium:** supplementation with magnesium can ease PMS symptoms such as nervousness, mood changes, weight gain, breast tenderness, and headaches.[161] As magnesium and calcium function interactively, these minerals should be taken together in the proper ratio.

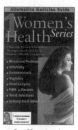

See **Menstrual Problems** in *Alternative Medicine Guide to Women's Health 1* (Future Medicine Publishing, 1998); ISBN 1-887299-12-2); to order, call 800-333-HEAL.

For a **home test for hormone levels,** see Appendix: Great Smokies Diagnostic Laboratory, pp. 484-485.

■ **Gamma-linolenic acid (GLA):** a deficiency of this essential fatty acid has been linked to PMS; supplementation can reduce symptoms.[162]

■ **Natural progesterone cream:** applied topically to soft tissue areas such as the abdomen and inside the upper arm, natural progesterone cream can alleviate the estrogen dominance often present with PMS.

■ **Thyroid support:** a significant number of women who suffer from PMS have some sort of thyroid gland imbalance or dysfunction. After performing standard thyroid blood tests to rule out underlying disease, we usually recommend supporting the thyroid gland with mineral products or Katsu Kelp (high in natural iodine) and organic thyroid glandular extracts.

■ **Chasteberry:** this herb helps to correct estrogen dominance and diminish PMS symptoms.[163] Chasteberry *(Vitex agnus-castus)* is one of the active ingredients in Fema-Gen, a good overall tonic for the female system.

■ **Hawthorn, dandelion, and corn silk:** by promoting the elimination of excess fluids from the tissues, these diuretic herbs can relieve the water-retention symptoms of PMS.

■ **Milk thistle (silymarin):** this herb cleanses the liver, improves its function, and protects it from damage by toxins and free radicals.[164] A healthy liver is better able to process excess estrogen, the elimination of which helps diminish symptoms of PMS. We recommend Liver Guard, a product containing milk thistle.

Products for PMS

Amino-Mag 200: Tablets. Supplies 200 mg of elemental magnesium per tablet as a patented amino acid–chelate, which can be absorbed intact; no gastrointestinal side effects.

AMNI, 2247 National Avenue, Hayward, CA 94540-5012; tel: 800-437-8888 or 510-783-6969.

Aqua-Trim: Capsules. Gentle diuretic with potassium for relief of the bloating, puffiness, and fatigue associated with periods; ingredients include uva ursi, natural caffeine, potassium, and the extracts of buchu leaf, juniper berry, and horse chestnut seed.

NATURE'S HERBS, 600 East Quality Drive, American Fork, UT 84003; tel: 800-437-2257 or 801-763-0700.

BHI Calming: Homeopathic tablets. For temporary relief of insomnia, restlessness, anxiety, and symptoms of PMS.

HEEL/BHI, INC., 11600 Cochiti Road Southeast, Albuquerque, NM 87123-3376; tel: 800-621-7644 or 505-293-3843.

Calcium Plus: Tablets. Daily supplement of calcium, magnesium, essential minerals (which support the skeletal and muscular systems), co-nutrients, superfoods, and a blend of seven Chinese herbs important for skeletal health; for diets high in dairy products and low in magnesium-rich foods (grains and legumes).

RAINBOW LIGHT, P.O. Box 600, Santa Cruz, CA 95061; tel: 800-635-1233 or 408-429-9089.

Chasteberry-Power: Capsules. Contains standardized extract of chasteberry, in a base of wild countryside *dong quai* root and Siberian ginseng; chasteberry has been used since ancient times by women, especially in Europe.

NATURE'S HERBS, 600 East Quality Drive, American Fork, UT 84003; tel: 800-437-2257 or 801-763-0700.

For information about supporting the liver, see Liver Disorders, pp. 257-262. For information about detoxifying the liver, see Detoxification in Part III, pp. 446-461.

Concentrated Mineral Drop Complex: Liquid. Complete, soluble, liquid ionic minerals necessary for developing and maintaining good health and conducting and generating the body's electrical system; also an excellent way to remineralize distilled water.

BIO NATIVUS, P.O. Box 3281, Ogden, UT 84401; tel: 888-628-4887 or 801-732-1294.

Cramp-Prin: Capsules. Relieves cramp pains, premenstrual tension, irritability, headache, and backache associated with the menstrual cycle; ingredients include magnesium salicylate, white willow, *dong quai*, peppermint, cnidium, pleurisy root, and uva ursi.

RIDGECREST HERBALS, 1151 South Redwood Road #106, Salt Lake City, UT 84104-3729; tel: 800-242-4649 or 801-978-9633.

Easy Change for Women Caps. Contains black cohosh, *dong quai*, cramp bark, and Ayurvedic herbs to encourage normality and balance in the female system.

CRYSTAL STAR HERBAL NUTRITION, 4069 Wedgeway Court, Earth City, MO 63045; tel: 800-736-6015 or 314-739-7551.

Emotional Balance-Chaste Berry Extract: Liquid. For promoting hormonal balance.

PLANETARY FORMULAS, 23 Janis Way, Scotts Valley, CA 95066; tel: 800-606-6226.

Evening Primrose Oil: Capsules or liquid. Good source of omega-6 essential fatty acids necessary for optimal health, maintaining cell structure, and producing energy. Contains about 72% (1.1 g) omega-6 or linoleic acid and about 9% (135 mg) gamma-linolenic acid (GLA, a derivative of omega-6), which help improve circulation and hormonal balance.

SPECTRUM NATURALS, 133 Copeland Street, Petaluma, CA 94952; tel: 800-995-2705 or 707-778-8900.

Evening Primrose Oil Extract: Capsules. Evening primrose oil with vitamin E (a source of polyunsaturated fatty acids) is used for premenstrual conditions such as irritability, breast tenderness, and water retention and bloating.

NATURE'S SOURCE, 15451 San Fernando Mission Boulevard, Mission Hills, CA 91345; tel: 800-423-2405 or 818-837-3633.

Fema-Gen: Caplets or liquid. Blend of herbs traditionally used for women needing balancing support, especially as it applies to the female cycle; contains chasteberry, dandelion root, blue cohosh, valerian, prickly ash bark, cramp bark, and lavender.

RAINBOW LIGHT, P.O. Box 600, Santa Cruz, CA 95061; tel: 800-635-1233 or 408-429-9089.

Female Balance: Capsules. Combination of herbal extracts and borage oil (a source of essential fatty acids) for general hormone support.

NOW, 550 Mitchell Road, Glendale Heights, IL 60139; tel: 800-283-3500 or 630-545-9098.

Female Balance: Tablets. Helps support a woman's natural balance for a healthy monthly cycle by utilizing herbal combinations created by Ayurvedic physicians. These formulas are in harmony with the science of Ayurveda, which incorporates a holistic view of health by balancing the body's mechanisms and organs.

VEDA HEALTH INC., P.O. Box 1535, Soquel, CA 95073; tel: 888-856-8334 or 408-465-9084.

Female Formula: Tablets. Herbal/glandular formula; supports the endocrine system and the female hormones for hormonal and glandular balance; contains the raw glandulars DHEA, heart, kidney, pancreas, thymus, adrenal, ovarian, RNA powder, whole pituitary, and spleen in a base including blue cohosh, catnip, chamomile, seaweed, and hawthorn berry.

NATURAL ENERGY PRODUCTS, 21101 Welch Road, Snohomish, WA 98296; tel: 425-486-5956.

Female Harmony Caps. PMS monthly balancer and female system toner.

CRYSTAL STAR HERBAL NUTRITION, 4069 Wedgeway Court, Earth City, MO 63045; tel: 800-736-6015 or 314-739-7551.

Fem-Gest: Cream. Natural progesterone cream (900 mg of progesterone per two-ounce jar) used topically to relieve PMS and menopausal symptoms, improve bone density, and help restore balance in hypothyroidism (an underactive thyroid gland); comes with a free educational booklet outlining proper cycling and transdermal application.

BIO-NUTRITIONAL FORMULAS, 106 East Jericho Turnpike, Mineola, NY 11501; tel: 800-950-8484.

Katsu Kelp Root: Tablets. Contains extract and powder of kelp root, a source of iodine, potassium, calcium, amino acids, and plant fiber; supports proper thyroid function.

KENSHIN TRADING CORP., P.O. Box 7511, Torrance, CA 90504; tel: 800-766-1313 or 310-212-3199.

Liver Guard: Tablets. Nutritional supplement for the liver providing nutrients and related substances identified in scientific studies as nourishing or protecting the liver; contains dandelion root and extract, turmeric, silymarin (from milk thistle seed extract), N-acetyl-cysteine, vitamins, minerals, and coenzyme Q10.

SOURCE NATURALS, THRESHOLD ENTERPRISES, 23 Janis Way, Scotts Valley, CA 95066; tel: 800-777-5677 or 831-438-1144.

Mega Primrose: Softgels. Contains gamma-linolenic acid (GLA), a precursor to prostaglandin E1, a compound that may help reduce the discomforts of breast tenderness and irritability that accompany fluctuating estrogen levels.

SOURCE NATURALS, THRESHOLD ENTERPRISES, 23 Janis Way, Scotts Valley, CA 95066; tel: 800-777-5677 or 831-438-1144.

Phyto Estrogen-Power: Capsules. Nutritional supplement for the needs of women. Contains soy germ isoflavone concentrate, the extracts of kudzu root, Mexican wild yam, and *dong quai*, Korean ginseng, boron, and natural vitamin E in a base of chasteberry (*Vitex agnus-castus*) powder and arrowroot.

NATURE'S HERBS, 600 East Quality Drive, American Fork, UT 84003; tel: 800-437-2257 or 801-763-0700.

PhytoGest: Cream. Natural progesterone cream containing wild yam, aloe vera, and AHA (alpha-hydroxy acid); natural progesterone is an estrogen antagonist, stimulates bone building, helps protect against breast and endometrial cancers, enhances energy and fat utilization, enhances thyroid hormone function, normalizes blood-sugar levels, restores libido, and acts as a natural antidepressant and diuretic.

KARUNA CORP., 42 Digital Drive # 7, Novato, CA 94949; tel: 800-826-7225 or 415-382-0147.

PhytoGyn: Liquid. Phytoestrogen (plant-derived) nutritional support for women with hormone-related complaints including dysmenorrhea, amenorrhea, PMS, and the symptoms of menopause. Contains concentrated extracts of chasteberry, *dong quai*, black cohosh, and licorice in a fluid for improved absorption.

KARUNA CORP., 42 Digital Drive # 7, Novato, CA 94949; tel: 800-826-7225 or 415-382-0147.

PMS by Jade: Tablets. Chinese herbal menstrual stress relief.

EAST EARTH HERB, INC., P.O. Box 2802, Eugene, OR 97402; tel: 800-827-HERB (4372) or 541-687-0155.

PMS Formulae: Homeopathic liquid. Relieves fluid retention, cramping, headache, and irritability associated with the menstrual period.

LIDDELL LABORATORIES, 1036 Country Club Drive, Moraga, CA 94556; tel: 800-460-7733 or 925-631-0257.

PMS.O.S: Capsules. Helps support nutritional needs and maintain good health during premenstrual syndrome; contains vitamins B6 and E, the extracts of uva ursi, valerian root, white willow, and chasteberry, ginger root, and *dong quai* root.

NATURE'S HERBS, 600 East Quality Drive, American Fork, UT 84003; tel: 800-437-2257 or 801-763-0700.

PMT Support: Capsules. Multiple vitamin/mineral in a base of herbals that possess phytoestrogenic properties to minimize the stress of a woman's monthly cycle.

HVL INC., 600 Boyce Road, Pittsburgh, PA 15205; tel: 800-245-4441.

Positive Menstrual Support: Tablets. For problems that often accompany the female cycle; contains B vitamins, calcium and potassium, and a combination of herbal extracts such as chasteberry and *dong quai*, both used as hormonal balancers and tonifiers.

RAINBOW LIGHT, P.O. Box 600, Santa Cruz, CA 95061; tel: 800-635-1233 or or 408-429-9089.

Pregnenolone: Tablets. Pregnenolone, a hormone balancer, can help increase the levels of steroid hormones that are deficient in our bodies and reduce the levels of excess circulating hormones; cells may only convert pregnenolone into other hormones when needed, pregnenolone may correct imbalances in the levels of some hormones, without affecting others.

SOURCE NATURALS, THRESHOLD ENTERPRISES, 23 Janis Way, Scotts Valley, CA 95066; tel: 800-777-5677 or 831-438-1144.

Pre-Menses (Formula VI): Vegitabs. Nutritional aid for menstrual support.
COUNTRY LIFE, 101 Corporate Drive, Hauppauge, NY 11788; tel: 800-645-5768 or 516-231-1031.

Premenstrual Harmony: Liquid or tablets. Alleviates breast tenderness, irritability, and premenstrual tension, which normally dissipate with the onset of menstruation; also helps with irregular menstruation, headache, dizziness, and mental weariness.
FLORA INC., 805 East Badger Road, Lynden, WA 98264; tel: 800-446-2110 or 360-354-2110.

Premenstrual Relief: Homeopathic remedy. For relief of temporary water weight gain, bloating, swelling and/or the full feeling associated with the premenstrual period; ingredients include *Calcarea carbonica* 12X, *Natrom muriaticum* 12X, *Thuja occidentalis* 12X, *Sepia* 12X, *Lac caninum* 12X, pyridoxine HCl, vitamin B6, buchu, couch grass, juniper berries, *dong quai*, black haw, ginger, licorice and pleurisy root.
RIDGECREST HERBALS, 1151 South Redwood Road #106, Salt Lake City, UT 84104-3729; tel: 800-242-4649 or 801-978-9633.

Pre-Menstrual Support: Tablets. Contains vitamins, minerals, trace minerals, and herbs for nourishing the female system during the premenstrual time.
BIO NATIVUS, P.O. Box 3281, Ogden, UT 84401; tel: 888-628-4887 or 801-732-1294.

Premium North American Ginseng Women's Formula: Capsules. Builds stamina, assists in balancing the body cycles, tonifies, and regulates; contains a blend of damiana, cranberry, North American ginseng *(Panax quinquefolius)*, and chasteberry.
CHAINATA CORP., 5965 205 A Street, Langley, British Columbia, Canada V3A8C4; tel: 800-406-7668 or 604-533-8883.

Progesterone Transdermal: Cream. Contains natural progesterone identical to what the body produces to balance the effects of estrogen. If you suffer from PMS or hormonal migraines, these can be due to estrogen dominance. Progesterone helps alleviate symptoms of PMS, build new bones, reduce the risk for uterine cancer, and restore vascular tone by counteracting the dilation.
LIFEENHANCEMENT PRODUCTS, INC., P.O. Box 751390, Petaluma, CA 94975-1390; tel: 800-543-3873 or 707-762-6144.

Soy Isoflavones: Capsules. Helps balance hormones, particularly in women suffering menstrual or menopausal difficulties.

SCHIFF, WEIDER NUTRITION GROUP, 2002 South 5070 West, Salt Lake City, UT 84104; tel: 800-439-8042 or 801-975-5000.

Vitex Black Cohosh: Capsules or liquid. Female monthly balancing blend containing chasteberry, motherwort, partridge berry, and black cohosh to balance the reproductive system; cramp bark to relax pelvic muscles and release cyclic tension; licorice for its soothing and supportive effects on the reproductive system; nettle for nourishment; and ginger for its warming quality. Caution: Do not use during pregnancy.

FRONTIER COOPERATIVE HERBS, 3021 78th Street, Norway, IA 52318; tel: 800-669-3275 or 319-227-7996.

Viva-Lift: Tablets. Isolated, singular, amino acid formula of L-tyrosine and pyridoxal-5-phosphate (the active form of vitamin B6); helps alleviate moodiness due to stress or PMS.

THURSDAY PLANTATION, INC., NATURE'S PLUS, 548 Broadhollow Road, Melville, NY 11747-3708; tel: 800-645-9500 or 516-293-0030.

Woman: Tablets. Helps women maintain a natural estrogen balance and provides nutritional support for the heart and bones; combines natural estrogens from soy and black cohosh with essential vitamins and minerals including magnesium, folic acid, iron, and vitamin B6.

AMERIFIT, 166 Highland Park Drive, Bloomfield, CT 06002; tel: 800-990- FIRM (3476) or 860-242-3476.

Woman's Select by Earth's Bounty: Tablets. Herbal formula used for over ten years by naturopathic doctors; contains herbs selected for their traditional ability to safely balance and harmonize a woman's body; ingredients include holy thistle, *dong quai*, red raspberry, squaw vine, false unicorn, echinacea, cramp bark, bearberry, black cohosh, Oregon grape, ginger, sarsaparilla, and licorice.

MATRIX HEALTH PRODUCTS, 8400 Magnolia Avenue, Suite N, Santee, CA 92071; tel: 800-736-5609 or 619-448-7550.

Women's Best Friend: Capsules. Herbal balancing formula for women.

CRYSTAL STAR HERBAL NUTRITION, 4069 Wedgeway Court, Earth City, MO 63045 tel: 800-736-6015 or 314-739-7551.

Women's Comfort: Tablets. Combines herbs that help balance and ease women through premenstrual and menstrual cycles, including *dong quai* extract, European chasteberry, and cramp bark.

PLANETARY FORMULAS, 23 Janis Way, Scotts Valley, CA 95066; tel: 800-606-6226.

Women's Essence by Jade: Tablets. Helps regulate the menstrual cycle, nourish the blood, liver, and heart.

EAST EARTH HERB, INC., P.O. Box 2802, Eugene, OR 97402; tel: 800-827-HERB (4372) or 541-687-0155.

Women's Ginseng Formula: Capsules or liquid. Herbal combination for the energy needs of women; supports the adrenals, builds depleted blood after menstruation, and balances the hormonal system; contains American and Siberian ginseng, *dong quai*, and chasteberry; for women of all ages for one to three weeks a month (do not use during menstruation).

ZAND HERBAL FORMULAS, 1722 14th Street #230, Boulder, CO 80302; tel: 800-800-0405 or 303-786-8558.

Women's Nutritional System: Tablets. Multiple for women of all ages, especially those who are active or concerned with supporting the delicate balance of the female system; ingredients include amino acids, enzymes, and extracts of herbs supportive of the female system (including the balancing herb *vitex agnus-castus*) in a base of superfoods and herbs.

RAINBOW LIGHT, P.O. Box 600, Santa Cruz, CA 95061; tel: 800-635-1233 or 408-429-9089.

Women's Treasure: Tablets. Modified version of a classical Chinese herbal formula (Dong Quai Four) to tonify and normalize the female cycle; contains the Chinese herbs *dong quai*, lingusticum, rehmannia, and peony along with Native American "female" herbs (cramp bark, false unicorn, and blue cohosh).

PLANETARY FORMULAS, 23 Janis Way, Scotts Valley, CA 95066; tel: 800-606-6226.

The prostate gland is the most common source of disorders of the male genitourinary system, which is made up of the kidneys, ureter, bladder, urethra, prostate gland, male genitals, and associated tissues. The prostate is a doughnut-shaped male sex gland located directly below the bladder at the base of the penis.

Causes of Prostate Problems

Causes of prostate problems include lack of dietary fiber, excessive consumption of acid-forming foods and beverages (sugar, red meats, animal fats, dairy, alcohol), essential fatty acid or zinc deficiency, lack of exercise, venereal disease, and addictive use of alcohol, caffeine, or antihistamines.[165]

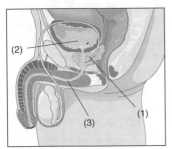

(2)

(3)   (1)

The prostate (1), a male sex gland, is located below the bladder (2) and encompasses the urethra (3). Typically in older men, the prostate tends to enlarge resulting in restricted urinary flow, bladder infections, or kidney damage.

Types of Prostate Problems

The most common prostate problems are prostatitis and benign prostatic hypertrophy.

Prostatitis—An inflammation or infection of the prostate, prostatitis occurs in men of all ages (most often between the ages of 20 and 50). Acute prostatitis is usually bacterial. Chronic prostatitis can be bacterial or nonbacterial (the latter is more common). Symptoms include difficulty, frequency, and urgency of urination and a burning sensation while urinating. Chills, fever, fatigue, and radiating pain near the prostate can accompany acute prostatitis. Symptoms of chronic prostatitis are similar, but milder. Weakening of the bladder, bladder obstruction, and prostate stones may occur if the condition is left untreated.

For information on **prostate cancer treatment,** see *Alternative Medicine Definitive Guide to Cancer* (Future Medicine Publishing, 1997; ISBN 1-887299-01-7); to order, call 800-333-HEAL.

Benign Prostatic Hypertrophy (BPH)—Advancing age often results in an enlarged prostate gland, a condition known as BPH; 50% to 60% of men between the ages of 40 and 60 have BPH. The enlargement can restrict urinary flow; symptoms include increased frequency of urination, urgency to urinate during the night, difficulty starting and stopping urine flow, and decreased pressure behind the urine stream. If BPH becomes severe enough, it can completely block the flow of urine, which can lead to kidney damage. Urinary bladder infections are common in men with BPH.

Nutrients and Herbs for Prostate Problems

In our clinical practice, we've found that more than 75% of men with prostate problems experience long-lasting relief with nutritional supplement and herbal protocols.

The following nutrients are helpful for general prostate health and specific prostate problems:

■ **Zinc:** this mineral is important for general prostate and gonadal function, sperm production, and reproductive system health. Zinc deficiency has been linked to BPH and supplementation can reduce symptoms.[166] As copper and zinc levels are interdependent in the body, when taking a zinc supplement, it is important to take copper as well. Our recommended daily dose is 50 mg of zinc and 3 mg of copper.

■ **Essential fatty acids (EFAs):** these dietary oils have been shown to promote prostate health. A deficiency can contribute to prostatic swelling, because EFAs (SEE QUICK DEFINITION) are vital to the formation of prostaglandins, hormone-like compounds which regulate inflammatory processes. Supplementation may inhibit prostate cell growth.[167]

■ **Saw palmetto:** extract from saw palmetto berries has proven effective in the treatment of BPH. In one study of 1,000 BPH sufferers, those who took saw palmetto twice daily for one to three months reported significant improvement in both urinary function and subjective symptoms. In comparison studies, saw palmetto was found to be as effective as Finasteride, a conventional BPH medication, without the side effects.[168]

■ *Pygeum africanum:* an extract from the bark of this African evergreen tree can both significantly reduce BPH symptoms and improve sexual function.[169] We have found pygeum to work well in reversing urinary frequency, weak urine stream, dribbling, and interruption of the urine flow. There are no known side effects or toxicity.

■ **Stinging nettle:** extracts of this herb have been shown to help

BPH. Research indicates that it may work by preventing testosterone, which is involved in prostate cell growth, from binding to receptor sites on prostate cells and by interfering with enzyme activity also necessary for the growth of prostate cells.[170]

■ **Pumpkin seed:** a source of essential fatty acids and zinc, pumpkin seed appears to help reverse the age-related decline of the prostate gland's health. Helpful for BPH, it can increase urinary flow and decrease urinary frequency.[171]

■ **Parsley, cornsilk, and buchu leaf:** diuretics (increase urine output), these herbs can help alleviate painful and incomplete urination and are more effective taken in combination. They also provide nutritional support to the prostate.[172]

■ **Cernilton extract and bromelain:** an extract of flower pollen, cernilton has a history of success in Europe as a treatment for prostatitis.[173] Taken on an empty stomach, bromelain (an enzyme compound from pineapple) enters the bloodstream and travels to sites of inflammation where it helps "digest" the by-products of inflammation.

■ **Wild oat extract, kelp, and watermelon seed:** these nutrients provide general nutritional support in prostate conditions.

Products for Prostate Problems

BioE Prostatic: Homeopathic liquid. For temporary relief of frequent/difficult urination, pain in the low back, and a heavy feeling in the pelvis.
BIOENERGETICS, INC., P.O. Box 127, Sandy, OR 97055; tel: 800-334-4043 or 503-668-7478.

Formula 3/6/9: Softgels. Contains natural essential oils that provide essential fatty acids (EFAs) necessary for maintenance of energy and health. Ingredients include borage oil, fish oil, and flaxseed oil.
PHILLIPS NUTRITIONALS, 27071 Cabot Road #122, Laguna Hills, CA 92653; tel: 800-514-5115 or 702-898-8141.

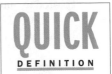

QUICK DEFINITION

Essential fatty acids (EFAs) are unsaturated fats required in the diet. Omega-3 and omega-6 oils are the two principal types. The primary omega-3 oil is alpha-linolenic acid (ALA), found in flaxseed (58%) and canola oils, as well as pumpkins, walnuts, and soybeans. Fish oils, such as salmon, cod, and mackerel, contain the other important omega-3 oils, DHA (docosa-hexaenoic acid) and EPA (eicosapentaenoic acid). Linoleic acid or cis-linoleic acid is the main omega-6 oil and is found in most plants and vegetable oils, including safflower (73%), corn, peanut, and sesame. The most therapeutic form of omega-6 oil is gamma-linolenic acid (GLA), found in evening prim-rose, black currant, and borage oils. Once in the body, omega-3 and omega-6 are converted to prostaglandins, hor-mone-like substances that regulate many meta-bolic functions, particu-larly inflammatory processes.

Lycopene: Softgels. Contains the phytonutrient lycopene (derived from tomato), which is the most plentiful carotenoid in the prostate gland and has powerful influences on the human body; studies have explored the link between diets high in lycopene and prostate function.

SOURCE NATURALS, THRESHOLD ENTERPRISES, 23 Janis Way, Scotts Valley, CA 95066; tel: 800-777-5677 or 831-438-1144.

Max Omega: Oil. Black currant seed oil is the most complete source of essential fatty acids (EFAs); contains linoleic acid (an omega-6 EFA) and, unlike primrose or borage oil, alpha linolenic acid (ALA, an omega-3 EFA). Also, unlike flaxseed, black currant seed oil contains 18% gamma-linolenic acid (GLA), twice the amount in primrose oil.

BIO-NUTRITIONAL FORMULAS, 106 East Jericho Turnpike, Mineola, NY 11501; tel: 800-950-8484.

Men's Formula 800+ Prostate Support: Softgels. Formula with herbs and nutrients to improve prostate gland function, increase urine flow, and maintain normal prostate gland size.

NATURE'S LIFE, 7180 Lampson Avenue, Garden Grove, CA 92841-3914; tel: 800-854-6837 or 714-379-6500.

Premium North America Ginseng Men's Formula: Capsules. Provides nutritional support for healthy prostate function, assists the body's ability to adapt to stress and fatigue, and acts as an overall tonifier; contains saw palmetto, smilax, North American ginseng *(Panax quinquefolius)*, oatstraw *(Avena sativa)*, horsetail, stinging nettle, pumpkin seed, Siberian ginseng, pygeum, and an enzyme blend.

CHAINATA CORP., 5965 205 A Street, Langley, British Columbia, Canada V3A8C4; tel: 800-406-7668 or 604-533-8883.

Pro • Essence: Vegicaps. Nontoxic treatment to help eliminate male problems and other ailments associated with aging; contains five herbs that have been effective in helping men or women with urinary discomfort, including aqueous extracts from burdock root, slippery elm bark, prickly ash bark, juniper berry, and bearberry.

FLORA INC., 805 East Badger Road, Lynden, WA 98264; tel: 800-446-2110 or 360-354-2110.

Pro-Sanoa Plus: Softgels. Formula of standardized saw palmetto extract similar to the formula used in the European clinical trials for benign prostatic hyperplasia; also contains pumpkin seed oil extract, pygeum extract, uva ursi, zinc, and vitamin B6.

BIO-NUTRITIONAL FORMULAS, 106 East Jericho Turnpike, Mineola, NY 11501; tel: 800-950-8484.

Pros-Power: Capsules. Nutritional supplement combining extract of saw palmetto and kudzu root with vitamin E and zinc.
NATURE'S HERBS, 600 East Quality Drive, American Fork, UT 84003; tel: 800-437-2257 or 801-763-0700.

ProstActin: Softgels. Nutritionally supports a healthy prostate gland; contains standardized saw palmetto, pygeum, pumpkin seed oil, OptiZinc (a patented yeast-derived zinc), and vitamin E.
NATURE'S PLUS, 548 Broadhollow Road, Melville, NY 11747-3708; tel: 800-645-9500 or 516-293-0030.

Prosta-Forte by Earth's Bounty: Tablets. Prostate support formula that contains saw palmetto berries, juniper berries, bearberry, parsley, cuceb berries, marshmallow root, gravel root, licorice, and kelp.
MATRIX HEALTH PRODUCTS, 8400 Magnolia Avenue, Suite N, Santee, CA 92071; tel: 800-736-5609 or 619-448-7550.

ProstaLife: Capsules. Contains standardized extracts of saw palmetto and *Pygeum africanum*, plus stinging nettle and phytosterols, which have demonstrated the ability to reduce symptoms of prostate dysfunction in cases of BPH (prostate enlargement); several double-blind clinical studies with standardized extracts of saw palmetto have demonstrated significant improvement in urological function, including bladder stability, increased urinary flow and output, and decreased urgency and frequency.
KARUNA CORP., 42 Digital Drive # 7, Novato, CA 94949; tel: 800-826-7225 or 415-382-0147.

Prosta-Max: Vegitabs. Nutritional aid for the health and function of the prostate gland and urinary tract; contains the amino acids glycine, L-glutamic acid, and L-alanine, anti-inflammatory nutrients, zinc, pygeum, and herbs traditionally used for urogenital function.
COUNTRY LIFE, 101 Corporate Drive, Hauppauge, NY 11788; tel: 800-645-5768 or 516-231-1031.

ProstaMed: Softgels. Contains saw palmetto berry extract standardized to 85% to 95% fatty acids and sterols, which are important for prostate function.

ENZYMATIC THERAPY, 825 Challenger Drive, Green Bay, WI 54311-8328; tel: 800-558-7372 or 920-469-1313.

Prosta Plus: Tablets. Prostate function formula containing the extracts of saw palmetto berry, pumpkin seed, and stinging nettle root; also contains the amino acids alanine, glycine, and glutamic acid, which provide anti-inflammatory action.

HEALTH PRODUCTS DISTRIBUTORS, INC., 23847 Peaceful Ridge Road, Smithsburg, MD 21783; tel: 800-228-4265 or 301-416-0500.

Prostasure: Liquid. Contains extracts of saw palmetto, ginger, hops, licorice, Siberian ginseng, horsetail, and the support herbs sarsaparilla, cayenne, kelp, buchu, white atractylodes, goldenrod, poria, aconite, peony, rehmannia, and pipisissewa in a base of purified water, brown rice syrup, honey, natural licorice flavor, and 18% USP alcohol.

NATURE'S APOTHECARY, P.O. Box 17970, Boulder, CO 80308; tel: 800-999-7422 or 303-664-1600.

Prostate Control Rx System: Softgels. Blend of herbs, antioxidant vitamins, and minerals that have been shown to help promote and support the health and function of the prostate.

PHYTO-THERAPY, INC., OPTIMUM HEALTH, 483 West Middle Turnpike, Manchester, CT 06040; tel: 800-228-1507 or 860-647-9729.

Prostate Enzyme Formula: Capsules. Dietary supplement for men; contains concentrated extracts of saw palmetto and pygeum, OptiZinc (a patented source of bioavailable zinc), which fights free radicals and provides nutritional support of prostate function and overall health.

PREVAIL CORP., 2204-8 Northwest Birdsdale, Gresham, OR 97030; tel: 800-248-0885 or 503-667-5527.

Prostate Preventive Support Rx System: Caplets. Blend of minerals, amino acids, and herbs to support the health and function of the prostate.

PHYTO-THERAPY, INC., OPTIMUM HEALTH, 483 West Middle Turnpike, Manchester, CT 06040; tel: 800-228-1507 or 860-647-9729.

Prostease: Capsules. Provides nutrition for the prostate gland; ingredients include glutamic acid, alanine, and glycine (clinical studies conducted in the 1950s showed the combination of these three amino acids to be effective in providing relief from the symptoms of enlarged prostate), saw palmetto berries, Siberian ginseng, echinacea root, watermelon seed, and sandalwood.

RIDGECREST HERBALS, 1151 South Redwood Road #106, Salt Lake City, UT 84104-3729; tel: 800-242-4649 or 801-978-9633.

ProstFX: Tablets. Helps promote a healthy prostate without side effects; provides saw palmetto extract, pumpkin seed, nettle root, pygeum bark, and zinc.

SYNERGY PLUS, IVC, 500 Halls Mill Road, Freehold, NJ 07728; tel: 800-666-8482.

Pygeum and Saw Palmetto: Capsules. Contains wild saw palmetto berry and pygeum bark extracts, which are intended to provide nutritive support to help maintain a normal, healthy prostate; also includes zinc, vitamin B6, pumpkin seeds, and amino acids.

SOLARAY, NUTRACEUTICAL CORP., P.O. Box 681869, Park City, UT 84068; tel: 800-669-8877.

Saw Palmetto Classic: Tablets. Contains extracts of saw palmetto berries, pygeum bark, and pumpkin seeds for men's health and ten traditional Chinese and Western herbs to soothe, tonify, and promote circulation to the prostate and related organs (bladder, kidneys, and adrenals).

PLANETARY FORMULAS, 23 Janis Way, Scotts Valley, CA 95066; tel: 800-606-6226.

Saw Palmetto Complex: Softgels. Combines the extract of saw palmetto with natural pygeum, bearberry, and pumpkin seed oil.

AMERICAN HEALTH, 4320 Veterans Memorial Highway, Holbrook, NY 11741; tel: 800-445-7137.

Saw Palmetto and Pygeum-Power: Softgels. Blend of saw palmetto extract and pygeum extract to support healthy prostate function.

NATURE'S HERBS, 600 East Quality Drive, American Fork, UT 84003; tel: 800-437-2257 or 801-763-0700.

SRF Forte: Capsules. Contains saw palmetto, pumpkin seed, sarsaparilla, and pygeum, combined with zinc, ginseng, amino acids, gamma-oryzanol, and other supportive herbs.

NF FORMULAS, INC., 9755 Southwest Commerce Circle, C-5, Wilsonville, OR 97070; tel: 800-547-4891 or 503-682-9755.

Uro Pro: Capsules. Contains herbs that promote healthy prostate function for men over the age of 30.

HVL INC., 600 Boyce Road, Pittsburgh, PA 15205; tel: 800-245-4441.

Vitality: Caplets. Combination of 13 herbs to support the male body and promote a healthy prostate and hormone levels.

NUPRO, 735-L Park Street, Castle Rock, CO 80104; tel: 800-704-8910 or 303-660-0562.

Skin Problems

The skin is a major organ, acting as a protective barrier between the body and millions of foreign environmental organisms and substances. It is also one of the body's detoxification mechanisms; toxins are eliminated from the body through the skin's pores.

Symptoms and Causes of Skin Problems

In response to the foreign substances it protects against or is excreting, the skin may exhibit allergic reactions, bumps, rashes, redness, scales, and other eruptions. Skin irritations are characterized by color changes, cracking, dryness, flaking, scaling, and thickening.

A deficiency of vitamin A or essential fatty acids (SEE QUICK DEFINITION), both of which are necessary for skin health, can lead to skin problems. Skin problems can also result from reactions to drugs, plants such as poison oak or ivy, insect bites and stings, excess wind or sun, or perfumes, cosmetics, soaps, and detergents. The use of skin lotions can block the pores and hair follicles, producing skin ailments.

Less obviously, food allergies are frequently behind skin problems, especially eczema, psoriasis, rashes, and acne. Certain foods have been linked to each of these conditions, so if you suffer from one of them, it is a good idea to eliminate those foods from your diet. For eczema, the problem foods tend to be wheat, dairy products (especially cow's milk), eggs, soy, peanuts, chocolate, and potatoes. Ceasing to give cow's milk to an infant with eczema is often all that is needed to clear up the condition.

People suffering from psoriasis should try giving up fruits (especially citrus), nuts, corn, milk, and acid-forming foods and beverages such as tomatoes, pineapple, coffee, and cola. Seasonal rashes are frequently linked to eating strawberries or tomatoes. Acne is often helped by eliminating cow's milk, chocolate, cola, nuts, and eggs from the diet.

Another common source of skin conditions is toxic overload. When too many toxins pass through the skin, problems such as acne, dermatitis, or psoriasis develop. We usually find that the skin condition clears up after we detoxify and nutritionally support the colon, liver, and kidneys, the body's other organs of detoxification. Water is essential for flushing out toxins, assisting the passage of nutrients throughout the body, and rehydrating the tissues. Drinking six to eight 8-ounce glasses of pure, filtered water every day helps improve and prevent skin problems.

The use of conventional topical medications (especially cortisone cream) to treat skin problems suppresses symptoms without addressing the underlying causes. This often leads to recurring symptoms or more serious health conditions, as the suppressed problem surfaces in another body system. For this reason, a more holistic approach to skin problems is advisable. By correcting nutritional deficiencies, cleansing the organs of detoxification, and supporting the body with herbs and nutrients, skin conditions can be permanently reversed.

Types of Skin Problems

Acne, eczema, and psoriasis are among the most common skin problems.

Acne—When the sebaceous (oil-secreting) glands in hair follicles become inflamed and the follicles impacted with oil (sebum) and dead skin cells, the raised bumps and pustules known as acne develop on the skin. Acne can be caused by poor diet or digestion, food allergies, stress, hormonal stimulation or imbalances, a toxic colon, and certain bacterial infections.

Eczema—Also called dermatitis, eczema is inflammation of the outermost layer of the skin involving blisters, red bumps, swelling, oozing, scaling, crusting, and itching. Causes include allergies, allergies secondary to digestive disorders such as hydrochloric acid (stomach acid) deficiency, rashes secondary to immune diseases, and nutritional deficiencies, especially in vitamins B3 and B6.

Psoriasis—A chronic skin condition most common between the ages of 15 and 30, psoriasis consists of reddish and thickened patches of skin that may be covered with silvery scales, but which usually do not itch. Psoriasis can appear anywhere on the body, but the areas most frequently affected are the arms, elbows, behind the ears, scalp, back, legs, and knees. Causes of psoriasis are hereditary predisposition, deficiency or malabsorption of essential fatty acids, food allergies, low digestive enzymes, vitamin B-complex deficiencies, stress, and excessive consumption of meat, alcohol, and refined foods. Psoriasis attacks can be triggered by anxiety, illness, bacterial or viral infections, sunburn, surgery, and certain drugs (nonsteroidal anti-inflammatory drugs, lithium, antibiotics, and beta-blockers which are used for hypertension and heart disease).[174]

Nutrients and Herbs for Skin Problems

■ **For general skin health:** essential fatty acids (EFAs) are the dietary oils which promote skin health, so supplementation can be useful for any skin condition or as a preventive measure. Kelp is a good source of the trace minerals needed for maintenance of the skin. Copper is necessary for the formation of the connective tissue proteins elastin and collagen, which keep the skin firm and supple (resulting in fewer wrinkles).[175] Beta carotene and vitamin A act as antioxidants and help reduce the effects of aging caused by chemicals and smoke. Silica is a vital component for healthy skin.[176] Selenium and vitamin E help reduce the risk of skin and other cancers.[177]

■ **For acne or pimples:** increase water intake, decrease consumption of sugar, oils, fats, fried foods and junk foods, and support the body nutritionally with vitamin A, vitamin B complex (especially B5 and folic acid), and zinc. Zinc helps prevent acne by regulating the oil glands.[178] Vitamin A and tea tree oil can be used topically to decrease skin outbreaks. Women who get premenstrual acne should take vitamin B6 and the herbs burdock root and chastetree berry.

■ **For eczema:** vitamin A and GLA (gamma-linolenic acid), an omega-6 essential fatty acid found in high quantities in evening primrose oil, have been shown to improve the symptoms of eczema.[179] Ginkgo and licorice root extract (applied topically) demonstrate similar benefits.[180]

■ **For psoriasis:** increase pure water intake, cleanse the colon (and sometimes the liver and/or kidneys), decrease stress with adaptogenic (aid the body in dealing with stress) herbs such as Siberian ginseng, improve the assimilation of essential fatty acids by taking digestive enzymes, and support the body nutritionally with vitamins A and C, beta carotene, bioflavonoids, liquid lecithin, and zinc. Supplementing with

See also
Fungal Infections, pp. 190-197,
Herpes, pp. 238-240,
Stress, pp. 369-384,
and Detoxification in Part III, pp. 446-461.

fish oil, a source of omega-3 EFAs, can help heal the skin lesions of psoriasis.[181] Topical capsaicin cream can reduce the scaling, thickness, redness, and itching. Silymarin is beneficial for psoriasis due to its positive effects on liver function.[182]

■ **For dry, scaly skin:** vitamin A, beta carotene, B vitamins, folic acid, zinc, and essential fatty acids are useful supplements for this condition. EFAs are especially helpful as dry, scaly skin is common in people who do not digest fats well and are lacking the dietary fatty acids needed to produce lubricating oils for the skin. Deficiencies of biotin, a member of the vitamin-B family, can cause dry, scaly skin and seborrhea (excessive secretion of sebum).

■ **For disinfecting the skin:** tea tree oil is one of the best skin disinfectants; we recommend it for acne, canker (cold) sores, boils, burns, insect bites, psoriasis, and other skin infections. Colloidal silver, a natural disinfectant with antibacterial, antiviral, and antifungal properties, is also useful for topical application.

■ **For skin tissue repair:** amino acid (protein) supplements aid in rebuilding skin tissue.

■ **For wrinkles:** lotions and creams that block the harmful effects of the sun can help prevent wrinkles and other skin conditions. Antioxidant nutrients can prevent the damage caused by exposure to cigarette smoke, environmental pollution, or excessive stress. A diet rich in essential fatty acids and vitamin C can prolong the youthful appearance of skin. Supporting the liver, the primary organ of detoxification, can also benefit skin health.

Products for Skin Problems

Acne Formulae: Liquid. Helps relieve symptoms associated with acne, such as pimples, redness, itching, and inflammation; safe for children.
LIDDELL LABORATORIES, 1036 Country Club Drive, Moraga, CA 94556; tel: 800-460-7733 or 925-377-3000.

Acneteen: Phyto-homeopathic gel. Helps heal pimples and soothe inflamed skin; ingredients include homeopathic ingredients in a base of marigold flower extract, Australian tea tree leaf oil, and echinacea root extract; does not interfere with any other medicine.
SUPHERB LTD., P.O. Box 1135, Nahariya 22100, Israel; tel: 800-409-HERB (4372).

Alkyrol: Capsules. Purified and standardized shark liver oil, which clinical studies have proven to be an immune stimulant; helps reduce

symptoms of psoriasis and asthma, prevent colds and other infections, and lessen the side effects of chemotherapy and radiation treatments.
SCANDINAVIAN NATURAL HEALTH & BEAUTY PRODUCTS, INC., 13 North 7th Street, Perkasie, PA 18944; tel: 800-688-2276.

Angel Skin: Drops. Contains plant collagen, which helps make wrinkles disappear.
OLYMPIC BOTANICALS, 231 Otto Street, Port Townsend, WA 98368; tel: 800-310-6924 or 360-385-9468.

Anti-Inflammatory Cell Signal Enhancer CSE-3 (TGF Beta 1): Homeopathic liquid. For relief from skin irritations and inflammations associated with minor injuries.
BIOMED COMM, INC., 2 Nickerson Street, Suite 102, Seattle, WA 98109; tel: 888-637-3516 or 206-284-3433.

Apis Mellifica: Sublingual tablets. Helpful for bee stings, insect bites, and puffy swelling.
STANDARD HOMEOPATHIC CO., 201 West 131st, Los Angeles, CA 90061; tel: 800-624-9659 or 310-768-0700.

Bug Ban Spray. Herbal insect repellent that contains essential oils of citronella, lavender, pennyroyal, eucalyptus, and jojoba oil.
NATURE'S APOTHECARY, P.O. Box 17970, Boulder, CO 80308; tel: 800-999-7422 or 303-664-1600

Burn Ease: Phyto-homeopathic gel. Relieves the pain, burning sensation, irritation, blistering, and skin inflammation of first degree burns; contains active homeopathic ingredients in a base of aloe leaf and marigold flower extracts.
SUPHERB LTD., P.O. Box 1135, Nahariya 22100, Israel; tel: 800-409-HERB (4372).

Burn Relief Spray. Contains aloe, calendula, comfrey, and lavender essential oil.
NATURE'S APOTHECARY, P.O. Box 17970, Boulder, CO 80308; tel: 800-999-7422 or 303-664-1600.

Clear-AC Cleanser: Liquid. Cleansing, healing lotion for teenage acne.
P & S LABS, 210 West 131st Street, Los Angeles, CA 90061; tel: 800-624-9659 or 310-768-0700.

Clear Up: Tablets. Herbal formula for acne; contains vitamin A, to reduce sebum production and the overgrowth of sebaceous follicles, and zinc, to control inflammation and promote tissue regeneration.

UNIVERSAL, 3 Terminal Road, New Brunswick, NJ 08901; tel: 800-872-0101 or 732-545-3130.

DermaComplex: Caplets or liquid. Blend of herbs to support a healthy complexion.

RAINBOW LIGHT, P.O. Box 600, Santa Cruz, CA 95061; tel: 800-635-1233 or 408-429-9089.

Desert Essence 100% Pure Jojoba Oil. Plant extract that moisturizes without an oily residue; can be used as a makeup remover, massage oil, skin softener, or an aftershave moisturizer for all skin types.

DESERT ESSENCE, 9700 Topanga Canyon Boulevard, Chatsworth, CA 91311; tel: 800-848-7331 or 818-734-1735.

Dr. Bronner's Castile Soap: Liquid.

MAGIC CHAIN, 2598 Fortune Way, Suite K, Vista, CA 92083; tel: 800-622-6648 or 760-598-6050.

E • GEM Skin Care Soap. Each glycerin bar contains 100 IU of vitamin E (d-alpha tocopheryl acetate) with 1,000 IU of vitamin A and a lemon oil fragrance.

J.R. CARLSON LABS, INC., 15 College Drive, Arlington Heights, IL 60004-1985; tel: 800-323-4141 or 708-255-1600.

Essential Fatty Acid Complex: Softgels. Contains evening primrose and flaxseed oils, vitamin E, and plant antioxidants from rosemary and sage. The essential fatty acids linoleic acid and alpha linolenic acid found in evening primrose and flaxseed oils are converted to eicosanoids in all human cells. Eicosanoids control a variety of body functions including pain, inflammation, blood pressure, and skin softness.

SCHIFF, WEIDER NUTRITION GROUP, 2002 South 5070 West, Salt Lake City, UT 84104; tel: 800-439-8042 or 801-975-5000.

Essential Oils Formula: Softgels. Contains flaxseed, borage, and fish oils, which are sources of essential fatty acids; also contains vitamin E.

ATKINS NUTRITIONALS, INC., 185 Oser Avenue, Hauppauge, NY 11788; tel: 800-628-5467 or 516-951-7171; or CANADIAN AMERICAN RESOURCES, 327 West Fayette Street, Suite 211, Syracuse, NY 13202; tel: 315-476-4944.

Fazit: Drops. Combination of tea tree oil and salicylic acid (active ingredient of tea tree oil), which helps control acne, pimples, blackheads, whiteheads, and skin blemishes.

THURSDAY PLANTATION, INC., NATURE'S PLUS, 548 Broadhollow Road, Melville, NY 11747-3708; tel: 800-645-9500 or 516-293-0030.

Foot Powder. Contains grapefruit extract and tea tree oil in a base of absorbent vegetable starch.

NUTRIBIOTIC, NUTRITION RESOURCES, INC., P.O. Box 238, Lakeport, CA 95453; tel: 800-225-4345 or 707-263-0411.

Formula 3/6/9: Softgels. Contains natural essential oils that provide essential fatty acids (EFAs) necessary for maintenance of energy and health. Humans cannot synthesize EFAs and must obtain them from their diet. By reducing saturated fat intake or consumption of meat, dairy products, and bread, the intake of EFAs are reduced as well; ingredients include borage, fish, and flaxseed oils.

PHILLIPS NUTRITIONALS, 27071 Cabot Road #122, Laguna Hills, CA 92653; tel: 800-514-5115 or 702-898-8141.

Fundamental Sulfur: Tablets. Supplies biologically active sulfur (a mineral missing from many diets) that supports connective tissues, immune function, and detoxification; the liver also depends on sulfur to detoxify food or airborne compounds that are foreign to the body.

AMNI, 2247 National Avenue, Hayward, CA 94540-5012; tel: 800-437-8888 or 510-783-6969.

Garden Fresh: Soap. Contains a palm-and-coconut-oil base with aloe vera gel and a collection of oils from avocados, cucumbers, carrots, and olives; does not contain animal products, artificial fragrances, or detergents, and is biodegradable.

J.R. CARLSON LABS, INC., 15 College Drive, Arlington Heights, IL 60004-1985; tel: 800-323-4141 or 708-255-1600.

Hair, Skin & Nails: Tablets. Contains 24 vitamins, minerals, herbs, and other nutrients to build well-nourished skin and strengthen hair and nails.

FUTUREBIOTICS, 145 Ricefield Lane, Hauppauge, NY 11788; tel: 800-FOR-LIFE (367-5433) or 516-273-6300.

Hair, Skin & Nails: Tablets. Combination of vitamins A, B complex, and E, zinc, and calcium to help create an environment for the formation of healthy skin, nails, and hair; also contains butcher's broom, bilberry, horsetail, and nettle, which provide nutritional support.

OPTIMAL NUTRIENTS, 1163 Chess Drive #F, Foster City, CA 94404; tel: 800-966-8874 or 650-525-0112.

Hemp Oil. Source of essential fatty acids for health and longevity, maintaining cell structure, and producing energy; contains a 3:1 balance of omega-6 to omega 3; also rich in active phospholipids and sterols, which promote cell membrane regeneration and improve immunity; does not contain active THC (tetrahydrocannabinol).

SPECTRUM NATURALS, 133 Copeland Street, Petaluma, CA 94952; tel: 800-995-2705 or 707-778-8900.

Hempola Hempseed Oil for Massage. High in EFAs (essential fatty acids) for better skin absorption and rejuvenation without oil residue; also good as a natural moisturizer.

HEMPOLA, 3405 American Drive #5, Mississauga, Ontario, Canada L4V1T6; tel: 800-240-9215.

Hempola Hempseed Oil Soap With Hempseed Kernel. Contains crushed hempseed, which stimulates, exfoliates, and moisturizes the skin.

HEMPOLA, 3405 American Drive #5, Mississauga, Ontario, Canada L4V1T6; tel: 800-240-9215.

Hempola Hempseed Oil Soap With Tea Tree Oil. Contains tea tree oil and helps heal skin irritations.

HEMPOLA, 3405 American Drive #5, Mississauga, Ontario, Canada L4V1T6; tel: 800-240-9215.

Herbal Aloe Force: Juice or topical gel. Processed aloe vera juice containing vitamins, minerals, enzymes, amino acids, essential fatty acids, growth factors, glycoproteins, sterols, bioflavonoids and polysaccharides (complex sugars), ionized colloidal silver, and herbal extracts (cat's claw, chamomile, burdock root, hawthorn berry, astragalus root, sheep sorrel, pau d'arco bark, slippery elm bark, and rhubarb root); effective for all skin needs.

HERBAL ANSWERS, INC., P.O. Box 1110, Saratoga Springs, NY 12866; tel: 888-256-3367 or 518-581-1968.

Hypericum: Homeopathic remedy. Helpful in puncture wounds, splinters, bites, cuts, burns, dental surgery, post-operative pain, and eye, nerve, and tailbone injury.

STANDARD HOMEOPATHIC CO., 201 West 131st Street, Los Angeles, CA 90061; tel: 800-624-9659 or 310-768-0700.

Inner Beauty: Tablets. Blends nourishing herbs with well-balanced vitamins to produce strong and healthy skin, hair, and nails.

BIO NATIVUS, P.O. Box 3281, Ogden, UT 84401; tel: 888-628-4887 or 801-732-1294.

Insect Bite: Phyto-homeopathic gel. Soothes the pain and reduces the swelling caused by insect bites and stings and local skin rashes caused by poison oak; contains active homeopathic ingredients in a base of witch hazel leaf, marigold flower, aloe leaf, and chickweed extracts.

SUPHERB LTD., P.O. Box 1135, Nahariya 22100, Israel; tel: 800-409-HERB (4372).

Jungle Juice: Spray. Insect repellent; contains essential oils of clove, peppermint, and lemon in a base of plant wax; effective for up to six hours against mosquitoes, flies, ticks, and gnats; available with or without SPF-18 sunblock.

NUTRIBIOTIC, NUTRITION RESOURCES, INC., P.O. Box 238, Lakeport, CA 95453; tel: 800-225-4345 or 707-263-0411.

Lilly of the Desert Suncare Products: Sunblock and lip balm. Sunblocks contain aloe vera, which relieves minor cuts and burns, abrasions, bites, chafing, rashes, skin irritation, and sunburn; sunblocks available in SPF-16 for two hours of protection or SPF-40 for eight hours, both are waterproof. Lip balm contains aloe vera and provides SPF-16 protection to moisturize dry, chapped lips.

LILY OF THE DESERT, 1887 Geesling Road, Denton, TX 76208; tel: 800-229-5459 or 940-566-9914.

Liquid Castile Soap. From Castile, Spain, where rich coconut and olive oils were first used as skin softeners; also includes the antiseptic tea tree oil.

DESERT ESSENCE, 9700 Topanga Canyon Boulevard, Chatsworth, CA 91311; tel: 800-848-7331 or 818-734-1735.

Lustre: Tablets. Targets common deficiencies in American diets and the effects of pollution to provide nutrition for skin, hair, and nails;

ingredients include silicon, vitamins A, B1, B2, B3, B5, B6, B12, and E, beta carotene, manganese, copper, zinc, magnesium, L-proline, folic acid, biotin, and inositol.

SOURCE NATURALS, THRESHOLD ENTERPRISES, 23 Janis Way, Scotts Valley, CA 95066; tel: 800-777-5677 or 831-438-1144.

ProSeed Grapefruit Seed Extract: Liquid. Multi-purpose liquid concentrate containing grapefruit seed extract; useful for numerous skin and scalp conditions and as a sore throat gargle, dental rinse, or broad spectrum cleanser for food.

IMHOTEP, P.O. Box 183, Ruby, NJ 12475; tel: 800-677-8577 or 914-336-2070.

Maui Babe I: Lotion. Natural tanning accelerator with moisturizing benefits; contains light mineral oil, kukui nut oil, vitamins A, C, and E, knoa coffee plant extract, and aloe; water resistant. *Author's note: This is a natural alternative to chemical-based tanning products.*

MAUI BABE, INC., P.O. Box 238, Wailuku, HI 96793; tel: 800-250-3581 or 808-244-2102.

Max Omega: Oil. Contains black currant seed oil, which is the most complete source of essential fatty acids; also contains linoleic acid (an omega-6 EFA) and, unlike primrose or borage oil, alpha linolenic acid (ALA, an omega-3 EFA). Also, unlike flaxseed, black currant seed oil contains 18% gamma-linolenic acid (GLA), twice the amount in primrose oil.

BIO-NUTRITIONAL FORMULAS, 106 East Jericho Turnpike, Mineola, NY 11501; tel: 800 950-8484.

MSM (Methylsulfonylmethane): Capsules, eye and ear drops, lotion, or powder. Contains sulfur, which is a major component of the human body. Diet is normally a source of sulfur, but food processing has resulted in a depletion of sulfur from foods. MSM provides the body with building materials for healthy, flexible cells.

RICH DISTRIBUTING, P.O. Box 33830, Portland, OR 97292; tel: 877-245-5742 or 503-761-7450.

Natural Cleansing Pads. With antiseptic tea tree oil and herbal extracts to remove dirt from pores and improve the texture and clarity of the skin.

DESERT ESSENCE, 9700 Topanga Canyon Boulevard, Chatsworth, CA 91311; tel: 800-848-7331 or 818-734-1735.

Natural Roll-On Deodorant. Contains essential oil of sage and baking powder, which is effective in controlling underarm odor.

DESERT ESSENCE, 9700 Topanga Canyon Boulevard, Chatsworth, CA 91311; tel: 800-848-7331 or 818-734-1735.

New Feeling: Lotion. Formula of alpha-hydroxy acids (fruit acids), vitamins, antioxidants, amino acids, essential growth hormone regulators, moisturizers, penetration aids, skin protectors, antimicrobials, and other skin care ingredients.

LIFEENHANCEMENT PRODUCTS INC., P.O. Box 751390, Petaluma, CA 94975-1390; tel: 800-543-3873 or 707-762-6144.

100% Pure Tea Tree Oil. Antiseptic first aid treatment for minor cuts, burns, abrasions, bites, and stings.

THURSDAY PLANTATION, INC., NATURE'S PLUS, 548 Broadhollow Road, Melville, NY 11747-3708; tel: 800-645-9500 or 516-293-0030.

OptiZinc: Tablets. Contains zinc combined with the essential amino acid methionine. Zinc is necessary for enzyme function, maintaining healthy skin, wound healing, and carbohydrate metabolism.

SOURCE NATURALS, THRESHOLD ENTERPRISES, 23 Janis Way, Scotts Valley, CA 95066; tel: 800-777-5677 or 831-438-1144.

Ouch & Itch Spray: Liquid. Dries out poison ivy and poison oak lesions and helps heal scrapes and scratches; contains grapefruit seed extract, aloe vera, goldenseal, and calendula.

IMHOTEP, P.O. Box 183, Ruby, NJ 12475; tel: 800-677-8577 or 914-336-2070.

Oxy-Screen SPF-15 Sunscreen: Lotion. Waterproof sunscreen that protects the skin from ultraviolet light; does not contain waxes, film-forming polymers, PABA, or oil-in-water emulsions.

ECOLOGICAL FORMULAS, 1061-B Shary Circle, Concord, CA 94518; tel: 800-888-4585 or 925-827-2636.

Perfect Woman With Alpha Hydroxy and Yamcon: Cream. Face moisturizer with yamcon (wild Mexican yam extract), softening ingredients, and sunblock to reduce the appearances of lines due to sun damage and aging.

PHILLIPS NUTRITIONALS, 27071 Cabot Road #122, Laguna Hills, CA 92653; tel: 800-514-5115 or 702-898-8141.

Poison Ivy/Oak: Tablets. Antidote for poison ivy and poison oak; can also be used to desensitize the allergic reaction to poison ivy and poison oak.

P & S LABS, 210 West 131st Street, Los Angeles, CA 90061; tel: 800-624-9659 or 310-768-0700.

Propolis: Cream. Bee propolis has been used for centuries for topical cosmetic purposes.

CC POLLEN CO., 3627 East Indian School Road #209, Phoenix, AZ 85018-5126; tel: 800-875-0096 or 602-957-0096.

Psoractin: Cream. Emollient (softening) cream with fumaric acid esters and monolaurin that retards the overproduction of short-lived cells, a characteristic of psoriasis.

ECOLOGICAL FORMULAS, 1061-B Shary Circle, Concord, CA 94518; tel: 800-888-4585 or 925-827-2636.

Psorex: Capsules. Supplement containing fumaric acid esters and other nutrients; fumaric acid is derived from malic acid and retards the overproduction of short-lived cells, prevalent in psoriasis. *Authors' note: Our patients with psoriasis have had good success with this product. For best results, we recommend using Psorex oral capsules in combination with Psoractin topical cream.*

ECOLOGICAL FORMULAS, 1061-B Shary Circle, Concord, CA 94518; tel: 800-888-4585 or 925-827-2636.

Pycnogenol Plus: Cream and tablets. Fights the appearance of wrinkles, helps neutralize the free radicals that can accelerate aging, and nourishes collagen fibers that are important to the skin's firmness and elasticity.

QUANTUM, INC., 754 Washington Street, Eugene, OR 97401; tel: 800-448-1448 or 541-345-5556.

Royal Jelly: Cream. For topical cosmetic applications.

CC POLLEN CO., 3627 East Indian School Road #209, Phoenix, AZ 85018-5126; tel: 800- 875-0096 or 602-957-0096.

Sincera Skin Survival System. Contains tablets that nourish the skin, a cleanser, a day/night cream, and eye gel.

SCANDINAVIAN NATURAL HEALTH & BEAUTY PRODUCTS, INC., 13 North 7th Street, Perkasie, PA 18944; tel: 800-688-2276 or 215-453-2505.

Skin and Hair Nutrients: Tablets. Contains vitamins, minerals, and concentrated herbal extracts for healthier-looking skin and hair.
NEW CHAPTER, 22 High Street, Brattleboro, VT 05301; tel: 800-543-7279 or 802-257-9345.

Skin Ointment. First aid ointment that contains 2% grapefruit extract.
NUTRIBIOTIC, NUTRITION RESOURCES, INC., P.O. Box 238, Lakeport, CA 95453; tel: 800-225-4345 or 707-263-0411.

Skin-Power: Capsules. Vitamin and herbal antioxidant formula for healthy skin; contains vitamins A, B2, B6, C, and E, beta carotene, selenium, zinc, and biotin in a base of horsetail, burdock root, green tea extract, turmeric extract, gingko extract, red clover, pycnogenol, and arrowroot.
NATURE'S HERBS, 600 East Quality Drive, American Fork, UT 84003; tel: 800-437-2257 or 801-763-0700.

Skin Spray. Topical first aid spray that contains 1% grapefruit extract.
NUTRIBIOTIC, NUTRITION RESOURCES, INC., P.O. Box 238, Lakeport, CA 95453; tel: 800-225-4345 or 707-263-0411.

Squalene (Shark Liver Oil): Softgels. Squalene is an extract from the liver of the Aizame shark; increases new tissue growth (granulation which covers wounds), supports the activity of the liver, acts as an adaptogen similar to ginseng and antioxidants, stimulates the defensive forces of the body, and enhances the resistance to immune system disorders.
OPTIMAL NUTRIENTS, 1163 Chess Drive #F, Foster City, CA 94404; tel: 800-966-8874 or 650-525-0112.

Sting Soothe: Lotion. Relieves pain and helps prevent infection of common bites and stings without lidocaine or other drugs.
QUANTUM, INC., 754 Washington Street, Eugene, OR 97401; tel: 800-448-1448 or 541-345-5556.

Sulphur. Helpful for unhealthy skin, eczema, acne, and styes.
STANDARD HOMEOPATHIC CO., 201 West 131st Street, Los Angeles, CA 90061; tel: 800-624-9659 or 310-768-0700.

Sweet Dreams DHEA Day Cream With Vitamin E. Non-greasy cream that contains the anti-aging hormone DHEA, which stimulates oil secretion to soften skin; vitamin E and beta carotene, which protect skin; and retinyl palmetate (a form of vitamin A found in fish liver oils), which helps prevent wrinkles.

EMERALD LABORATORIES, 5933 Sea Lion Place #105, Carlsbad, CA 92008; tel: 800-775-1112 or 760-930-8091.

Sweet Dreams Melatonin Night Cream With Vitamins C and E.
Contains the antioxidant melatonin plus the anti-wrinkle agents vitamin C and retinyl palmitate (a form of vitamin A found in fish liver oils).

EMERALD LABORATORIES, 5933 Sea Lion Place #105, Carlsbad, CA 92008; tel: 800-775-1112 or 760-930-8091.

Tea Tree Antiseptic Cream.
Herbal antiseptic for relief of sunburn, windburn, chafing, minor skin irritations, and burns.

THURSDAY PLANTATION, INC., NATURE'S PLUS, 548 Broadhollow Road, Melville, NY 11747-3708; tel: 800-645-9500 or 516-293-0030.

Tea Tree Foot Powder and Foot Spray.
Talc-free formula designed to keep feet dry and refreshed with the odor-fighting benefits of tea tree oil, the mildly astringent properties of zinc, and the cooling sensations of menthol and camphor.

THURSDAY PLANTATION, INC., NATURE'S PLUS, 548 Broadhollow Road, Melville, NY 11747-3708; tel: 800-645-9500 or 516-293-0030.

Tea Tree Herbal Skin Wash:
Liquid. Cleansing formula containing tea tree oil with the moisturizing benefits of nettle, chamomile, birch, coltsfoot, horsetail, yarrow, rosemary, and trefoil; pH-balanced for all skin types.

THURSDAY PLANTATION, INC., NATURE'S PLUS, 548 Broadhollow Road, Melville, NY 11747-3708; tel: 800-645-9500 or 516-293-0030.

Tea Tree Oil Deodorant With Lavender Oil.
Contains tea tree oil, chamomile, aloe vera, and farnesol, a natural deodorizer that helps eliminate body odor without inhibiting perspiration.

DESERT ESSENCE, 9700 Topanga Canyon Boulevard, Chatsworth, CA 91311; tel: 800-848-7331 or 818-734-1735.

Tea Tree Oil Skincare Bar Soap.
Contains tea tree oil and natural moisturizers; pH-balanced for all skin types.

THURSDAY PLANTATION, INC., NATURE'S PLUS, 548 Broadhollow Road, Melville, NY 11747-3708; tel: 800-645-9500 or 516-293-0030.

Tea Tree Oil Skin Ointment. Skin moisturizer that relieves irritations from waxing or other treatments.

DESERT ESSENCE, 9700 Topanga Canyon Boulevard, Chatsworth, CA 91311; tel: 800-848-7331 or 818-734-1735.

Wheat Germ Oil: Softgels. Contains 73% wheat germ oil, which is recognized as an excellent source of vitamin E (alpha-tocopherol) complex, and 27% flaxseed oil concentrate, which is a rich source of the omega-3 essential fatty acids. Vitamin E functions as an antioxidant that stabilizes cell membranes and protects cells and tissues from damage. It protects the tissues of the eyes, liver, skin, nerves, and muscles and protects red blood cells from cell damage.

SONNE'S ORGANIC FOODS, INC., P.O. Box 2160, Cottonwood, CA 96022; tel: 800-544-8147 or 530-347-5868.

Wild West Manuka Honey: Ointment. Manuka plant was a treatment used by the Maoris (native people of New Zealand) as a topical ointment when treating bacterial infections of the skin, athlete's foot, scrapes, cuts, and boils.

WGI, 35008 Emerald Coast Parkway, 5th Floor, Destin, FL 32541; tel: 800-854-8353 or 850-654-474

Sleep Disorders

Sleep is a restorative process for physical and psychological replenishment. Sufficient, restful sleep is essential to health; chronic disturbances in the quantity and quality of sleep can be both a reflection of and a contributing factor in disease.

Types of Sleep Disorders

Insomnia, nightmares, and restless leg syndrome are common types of sleep disturbance.

Insomnia—The sleep disorder known as insomnia is divided into three main types: sleep-onset insomnia (difficulty falling asleep), sleep-maintenance insomnia (difficulty staying asleep), and early morning awakening. Insomnia can result from asthma, frequent drug use (prescription or recreational), low blood sugar (hypoglycemia), muscle aches, indigestion, pain, and stress. Deficiencies of calcium and magnesium can also result in insomnia.[183]

Nightmares—Nightmares occur mostly during deep sleep and are more common during fever, with excess fatigue, after eating sugar or spicy food, or consuming alcohol before bed. Eating sugar before bed results in high blood sugar (hyperglycemia) for a short time, followed by a drop in blood sugar during sleep, which is thought to contribute to nightmares.

Restless Leg Syndrome—In this disorder, sleep is disturbed by periodic involuntary leg movements and uncomfortable sensations in the legs described as tingling or "pins-and-needles" sensations. As magnesium is the muscle-relaxant nutrient, a person with restless leg syndrome should be evaluated for calcium/magnesium deficiency.

Causes of Sleep Disorders

In addition to the causes cited above, sleep disorders can be the result of chronic stress or psychological/emotional stress such as fear or anxiety, inappropriate use of sleeping pills or other drugs, poor diet, lack of exercise, prolonged illness, nutritional deficiencies, environmental disturbances such as noises or lights, disturbed wake/sleep patterns due to night-shift work or jet lag, and sleeping in or near electromagnetic fields (emitted by any electrical product such as a bedside clock) or over geopathic stress zones (areas of harmful earth radiation). In addition, many prescription drugs are associated with a higher incidence of sleeplessness; check the list of side effects of any medication you are taking.

Stress is perhaps the most common underlying cause of sleep problems. In a stress response, which many people have repeatedly in the course of a day, the adrenal glands release the hormone adrenaline into the bloodstream. This hormone contributes to nervous and anxious feelings and inhibits regular sleep patterns. If chronic stress is behind your sleep disorder, we recommend that you implement techniques of stress management and nutritionally support your adrenal glands with adaptogenic (assist the body in dealing with stress) herbal formulas or organically raised adrenal glandular extracts.

See **Stress**, pp. 369-384.

Another common factor in sleep disorders is diet. Overeating, excess salt, excess copper levels or copper/iron deficiencies in women, vitamin B-complex deficiencies, and food allergies can all contribute to problems with sleep. People who have trouble sleeping should avoid (especially near bedtime) foods that contain tyramine, which increases levels of the brain stimulant norepinephrine. These include bacon, ham, sausage, cheese, eggplant, potatoes, sauerkraut, spinach, tomatoes, sugar, and chocolate.[184] Caffeine and tobacco are stimulants and can interfere with sleep. Although alcohol in small amounts is a sleeping aid, habitual use can upset sleep patterns.

Nutrients and Herbs for Sleep Disorders

For Insomnia—A deficiency of calcium and magnesium in the body makes it difficult to relax and fall asleep. As sufficient amino acids (proteins) are necessary to transport calcium and magnesium into the tissues, we recommend taking free-form amino acids with calcium/magnesium supplements; this is especially important for people who don't digest proteins well. Take these nutrients a half hour before trying to go to sleep. Inositol (a member of the B-complex family) is another useful nutrient, as it enhances the important stage of sleep called REM (rapid eye movement) sleep or dream sleep.

Melatonin, a hormone produced by the pineal gland, is involved in the regulation of the sleep/wake cycle. Although it has become a popular sleep-aid supplement, we recommend that melatonin only be taken when a hormonal test reveals a low level of melatonin.

Valerian root is one of the best herbal tonics for insomnia and calming the nervous system. It is particularly recommended for people with sleep disorders that are the result of anxiety, nervousness, hysteria, and exhaustion.[185] The herb balm also calms the nerves and promotes relaxation and sleep. Hops, kava-kava, passionflower, skullcap, and St. John's wort exert a mild sedative effect on anxiety, depression, and restlessness and thereby can improve the ability to sleep.

For information on a **home test for hormone levels,** see Appendix: Great Smokies Diagnostic Laboratory, pp. 484-485.

For Nightmares—Avoid eating sugar and high-carbohydrate foods before bedtime. Before going to bed and upon waking during the night, take vitamin B complex, especially B1 and niacinamide, and free-form amino acids to assist in keeping the body's blood sugar balanced all night.

For Restless Leg Syndrome—Before bed, take vitamin B complex (especially B5, inositol, and folic acid), vitamin E, calcium, magnesium, potassium, and amino acids. Melatonin and herbal relaxants (see insomnia above) may also help.

Products for Sleep Disorders

BHI Calming: Homeopathic tablets. For temporary relief of insomnia, restlessness, anxiety, and symptoms of PMS.

HEEL/BHI INC., 11600 Cochiti Road Southeast, Albuquerque, NM 87123-3376; tel: 800-621-7644 or 505-293-3843.

Biotonin: Tablets. Remedy for sleep disorders and jetlag; ingredients include melatonin along with sleep-enhancing herbal extracts, vitamins, and minerals.

SCANDINAVIAN NATURAL HEALTH & BEAUTY PRODUCTS INC., 13 North 7th Street, Perkasie, PA 18944; tel: 800-688-2276.

Calcium Plus: Tablets. Daily supplement of calcium, magnesium, essential minerals (which support the skeletal and muscular systems), co-nutrients, superfoods, and a blend of seven Chinese herbs important for skeletal health; for diets high in dairy products and low in magnesium-rich foods (grains and legumes).

RAINBOW LIGHT, P.O. Box 600, Santa Cruz, CA 95061; tel: 800-635-1233 or 408-429-9089.

Calming Formulae: Homeopathic liquid. Helps relieve hyperactivity, apprehension, and nightmares resulting from physiological imbalance.

LIDDELL LABORATORIES, 1036 Country Club Drive, Moraga, CA 94556; tel: 800-460-7733 or 925-377-3000.

Calms: Tablets. Composed of four botanicals (passionflower, hops, wild oats, and chamomile) long used by the homeopathic medical profession to soothe and quiet irritated nerves and edginess without sedatives or tranquilizers; no side effects or drug hangover.

P & S LABS, 210 West 131st Street, Los Angeles, CA 90061; tel: 800-624-9659 or 310-768-0700.

Calms Forté: Tablets. Contains the botanicals passionflower, hops, wild oats, and chamomile plus five biochemic phosphates in three times the potency; helps feed and strengthen the nerves of the body to withstand everyday stress and strain.

P & S LABS, 210 West 131st Street, Los Angeles, CA 90061; tel: 800-624-9659 or 310-768-0700.

Dream On: Capsules. Nutritionally strengthens the nervous system so the body can sleep; ingredients include passionflower, valerian root, black cohosh, German chamomile flowers, lupulin, and lemon balm.

RIDGECREST HERBALS, 1151 South Redwood Road #106, Salt Lake City, UT 84104-3729; tel: 800-242-4649 or 801-978-9633.

Echinacea PM: Liquid. Sedating, nighttime herbal syrup that stimulates the immune system to reduce the active symptoms of a cold or flu while promoting sleep; features antiviral and antibacterial herbs to reduce irritating symptoms, and nervine herbs to relax the nervous system and facilitate recovery.

ZAND HERBAL FORMULAS, 1722 14th Street #230, Boulder, CO 80302; tel: 800-800-0405 or 303-786-8558.

EuroCalm Valerian Special Formula: Capsules. Contains valerian extract with a guaranteed potency of 0.8% valeric acid, chamomile, passionflower, and hawthorn; valerian root helps provide nutritive support for restful sleep.

SOLARAY, NUTRACEUTICAL CORP., P.O. Box 681869, Park City, UT 84068; tel: 800-669-8877.

5HTP SeroTonic: Capsules. Scientists have discovered that conditions of sleeplessness, depression, carbohydrate cravings (with resultant weight gain), anxiety, obsessions, and compulsions are all connected to reduced levels of serotonin in the brain. If serotonin levels are restored, these conditions often disappear. The amino acid 5-HTP is a precursor of serotonin that increases its production and availability; 5-HTP SeroTonic contains 50 mg of 5-HTP per capsule with St. John's wort (10 mg) and pyridoxal-5-phosphate (15 mg), plus magnesium hydroxide, inositol hexanicotinate, and calcium citrate.

LIFEENHANCEMENT PRODUCTS, INC., P.O. Box 751390, Petaluma, CA 94975-1390; tel: 800-543-3873 or 707-762-6144.

Good-Nite: Capsules. Contains valerian root, chamomile extract, skullcap, passionflower, kava-kava, hops, and catnip.

NATURE'S HERBS, 600 East Quality Drive, American Fork, UT 84003; tel: 800-437-2257 or 801-763-0700.

Herbal Calm: Capsules. Contains valerian, passionflower, skullcap, hops, and kava-kava.

NATURE'S HERBS, 600 East Quality Drive, American Fork, UT 84003; tel: 800-437-2257 or 801-763-0700.

Herbal Rest (Salusan): Liquid. Tonic that aids relaxation and encourages sleep; can be used during the day without drowsiness.

FLORA INC., 805 East Badger Road, Lynden, WA 98264; tel: 800-446-2110 or 360-354-2110.

Horse Chestnut Seed Extract: Capsules. Helps to reduce swelling of legs caused by nighttime leg cramps (especially in the calves) or standing too long; horse chestnut is an anti-inflammatory that protects arteries, veins, and capillaries from damage and is a free-radical scavenger that improves blood circulation in the legs.

NATURE'S LIFE, 7180 Lampson Avenue, Garden Grove, CA 92841-3914; tel: 800-854-6837 or 714-379-6500.

Hyland's Insomnia: Ointment. For relief of insomnia due to nervousness, worry, grief, stress, or excitement.

P & S LABS, 210 West 131st Street, Los Angeles, CA 90061; tel: 800-624-9659 or 310-768-0700.

Insomnia by Jade: Tablets. Calming formula for conditions of stress or the inability to sleep; contains valerian root and Chinese herbs to relax the mind and body.

EAST EARTH HERB INC., P.O. Box 2802, Eugene, OR 97402; tel: 800-827-HERB (4372) or 541-687-0155.

KavaMax: Capsules or liquid. Contains 100 mg of kava-kava with 100 mg of valerian to provide nutritional support for relaxed muscles and restful sleep.
NATURAL MAX, NUTRACEUTICAL CORP., P.O. Box 681869, Park City, UT 84068; tel: 800-669-8877.

Knock-Out: Tablets. Contains 3 mg of synthetic melatonin with the natural sedatives valerian and kava-kava (in a 2:1 extract); other ingredients include GABA (gamma-aminobutyric acid), pyridoxal-5-phosphate, and the amino acid glycine, which enhance relaxation by normalizing nerve impulses.
SCHIFF, WEIDER NUTRITION GROUP, 2002 South 5070 West, Salt Lake City, UT 84104; tel: 800-439-8042 or 801-975-5000.

L-5-HTP: Capsules. Contains the amino acid L-5-HTP, vitamins B6 and C, and bioflavonoids. Clinical studies indicate that administration of L-5-HTP enhances the synthesis of serotonin in the brain; vitamin B6 is the cofactor for enzymes that convert L-tryptophan to serotonin, while vitamin C is a catalyzer for the hydroxylation of tryptophan to serotonin.
SOLARAY, NUTRACEUTICAL CORP., P.O. Box 681869, Park City, UT 84068; tel: 800-669-8877.

Melatol Sublingual: Tablets. Contains vitamin B6 combined with melatonin to induce relaxation.
PHILLIPS NUTRITIONALS, 27071 Cabot Road #122, Laguna Hills, CA 92653; tel: 800-514-5115 or 702-898-8141.

Melatonin Dual-Release: Tablets. Sleep supplement that releases half of its potency immediately to induce sleep quickly and the remainder is gradually released over six to eight hours to provide sound, undisturbed sleep throughout the night.
NUTRIMEDIKA CORP., 101 Newport Street, Bayport, NY 11705-2224; tel: 800-688-7462 or 516-472-5761.

MetaRest: Capsules or liquid. Contains melatonin, which helps the body's natural resting rhythms, and kava-kava root extract, which is used for its relaxing and calming effect.

NUTRIBIOTIC, NUTRITION RESOURCES, INC., P.O. Box 238, Lakeport, CA 95453; tel: 800-225-4345 or 707-263-0411.

NervaHerb With Valerian Root Extract: Capsules. Contains valerian combined with kava-kava and the soothing herbs hops, skullcap, catnip, and lemon balm.

NATROL, INC., 21411 Prairie Street, Chatsworth, CA 91311; tel: 818-739-6000.

NiteNite: Tablets. Regular strength formula contains a potent herbal blend with the extract equivalent of 750 mg of valerian; NiteNite Plus Melatonin formula additionally contains 500 mcg of this sleep-cycle regulating hormone.

IVC, 500 Halls Mill Road, Freehold, NJ 07728; tel: 800-666-8482 or 732-308-3000.

NutraSleep: Tablets. Helps occasional sleeping difficulties; contains GABA (gamma-aminobutyric acid, a normal constituent of the human brain), which plugs into and activates anti-anxiety brain receptors; taurine, the most plentiful amino acid in the brain; inositol, reported to have a calming, sedative effect; the minerals calcium and magnesium, which are essential for muscle relaxation; and the "nervine" herbs, including chamomile, skullcap, valerian root, and passionflower.

SOURCE NATURALS, THRESHOLD ENTERPRISES, 23 Janis Way, Scotts Valley, CA 95066; tel: 800-777-5677 or 831-438-1144.

Quietude: Tablets. For temporary relief of occasional sleeplessness, and/or restless sleep.

BOIRON, 6 Campus Boulevard, Building A, Newtown Square, PA 19073; tel: 800-264-7661 or 610-325-7464.

Relax and Sleep: Capsules. For relief of occasional sleeplessness and fatigue due to nervous tension, stress, and exhaustion from mental conflicts; contains valerian root and catnip (which are known to help sustain relaxation), hops, strobile, and passionflower.

PHILLIPS NUTRITIONALS, 27071 Cabot Road #122, Laguna Hills, CA 92653; tel: 800-514-5115 or 702-898-8141.

Restful: Capsules. Vitamins, minerals, and herbs to support restful sleep and relaxation without side effects; ingredients include kava-kava root extract, chamomile, passionflower, calcium, and magnesium.

BIODYNAMAX, 6525 Gunpark Drive #150-507, Boulder, CO 80301; tel: 800-926-7525 or 303-530-4665.

RollaDream: Lotion. Ayurvedic aromatherapy containing mild, herbal aromatics to encourage rest and relaxation for the body and mind.
VEDA HEALTH, INC. P.O. Box 1535, Soquel, CA 95073; tel: 888-856-8334 or 408-465-9084.

Sleep and Tranquility: Capsules. Helps soothe and calm the over-stimulated mind, relieve anxiety and nervous tension, and relax tense muscles; ingredients include valerian root extract, passionflower, chamomile, kava-kava, GABA (gamma-aminobutyric acid), calcium glycerophosphate, magnesium citrate, vitamin B6, and digestive enzyme complex.
ALTERNATIVE THERAPY INC., 1664 Fairlawn Avenue, San Jose, CA 95125; tel: 800-311-7922.

SleepRelax by Farmacopia: Capsules. Dietary supplement with pure kava-kava herbal extract traditionally used in the Pacific Islands for calming restless or anxious children and inducing sleep.
BOTANICAL PRODUCTS INTERNATIONAL, P.O. Box 174, Hakalau, HI 96710; tel: 808-963-6771.

Sleep-Rite: Phyto-homeopathic lozenges. For mild cases of restless sleep and difficulty falling asleep due to anxiety or excitement; contains the active homeopathic ingredients that relieve mild stress and sleeplessness in a base of passionflower and hops fruit extracts; less physical disruption than tranquilizers; no bad dreams, next-day drowsiness, or side effects.
SUPHERB LTD., P.O. Box 1135, Nahariya 22100, Israel; tel: 800-409-HERB (4372).

SlumberActin: Capsules. Supports normal sleep patterns and contains the herbs chamomile, valerian, kava-kava, and passionflower, plus the nutrients magnesium and calcium.
NATURE'S PLUS, 548 Broadhollow Road, Melville, NY 11747-3708; tel: 800-645-9500 or 516-293-0030.

SnoreStop: Tablets. For the conditions that contribute to nighttime snoring, including post-nasal drip, swollen membranes, or tonsil spasms; clinical studies found that 81% of the people tested reported a significant improvement in their condition and demonstrated no incidents of allergic or hypersensitive reactions, or side effects.

NUTRITION NOW, 501 Southeast Columbia Shore Boulevard #350, Vancouver, WA 98661; tel: 800-929-0418 or 360-737-6800.

St. John's Wort • Kava Compound: Liquid. Mild relaxing sedative, antispasmodic, and muscle relaxant; indicated in depression and despondency, and associated anxiety, nervous agitation, stress, restlessness, and sleeplessness; ingredients include St. John's wort flower and bud, kavakava lateral root, skullcap flowering herb, and prickly ash bark.

HERB PHARM, 20260 Williams Highway, Williams, OR 97544; tel: 800-348-4372 or 541-846-6262.

St. John's Wort • Melissa SuperComplex: Liquid. Blend of herbs, containing St. John's wort with lemon balm and wild indigo.

RAINBOW LIGHT, P.O. Box 600, Santa Cruz, CA 95061; tel: 800-635-1233 or 408-429-9089.

Sweet Dreams Melatonin: Capsules or liquid. Recent studies have demonstrated that melatonin plays a role in facilitating the onset of natural sleep.

EMERALD LABORATORIES, 5933 Sea Lion Place #105, Carlsbad, CA 92008; tel: 800-775-1112 or 760-930-8091.

TranQaCalm: Tablets. Contains herbs for support of nervous system and a balance of minerals and digestive enzymes.

BIO NATIVUS, P.O. Box 3281, Ogden, UT 84401; tel: 888-628-4887 or 801-732-1294.

T-Slumber: Capsules. Sleep aid that contains melatonin, valerian, skullcap, peppermint, rose hips, wild lettuce, shave grass, and sage.

WGI, 35008 Emerald Coast Parkway, 5th Floor, Destin, FL 32541; tel: 800-854-8353 or 850-654-4744.

Valerian and Chamomile Plus Calcium: Softgels. Standardized extracts of valerian and chamomile plus calcium.

J.R. CARLSON LABS INC., 15 College Drive, Arlington Heights, IL 60004-1985; tel: 800-323-4141 or 708-255-1600.

Valerian Combination: Capsules. Contains valerian (*Valeriana officinalis*) root, hops, wood betony, skullcap, black cohosh root, passionflower, and cayenne.

NATURE'S HERBS, 600 East Quality Drive, American Fork, UT 84003; tel: 800-437-2257 or 801-763-0700.

Valerian Hops: Capsules or liquid. Scientific studies confirm valerian's effects in supporting restful sleep.

FRONTIER COOPERATIVE HERBS, 3021 78th Street, Norway, IA 52318; tel: 800-669-3275 or 319-227-7996.

Valerian • Kava PM: Liquid. Blend of herbs traditionally used to relax the body and mind for a restful night's sleep.

RAINBOW LIGHT, P.O. Box 600, Santa Cruz, CA 95061; tel: 800-635-1233 or 408-429-9089.

Valerian • Passionflower Compound: Liquid. Gentle, non-narcotic sedative, which is indicated in insomnia, nervous excitement and hysteria, mental depression due to worry or imagined wrongs, nervous headache, and in nervousness associated with menopause.

HERB PHARM, 20260 Williams Highway, Williams, OR 97544; tel: 800-348-4372 or 541-846-6262.

Valerian Power: Capsules. Nutritionally promotes restful sleep.

NATURE'S HERBS, 600 East Quality Drive, American Fork, UT 84003; tel: 800-437-2257 or 801-763-0700.

Sports Injuries

Sports injuries include sprains and strains, shin splints, bruises, torn ligaments, inflammation, tendonitis, shooting pains in the muscles, tendons, or ligaments, and wrenched, twisted, or hyperextended joints. Muscle fibers are composed mainly of proteins (amino acids) while the fluid between muscle fibers contains high amounts of calcium, potassium, magnesium, phosphate, phosphocreatine, and sodium. Skeletal muscles are usually connected to a bone by a tendon, or cord of fibrous connective tissue. Ligaments are bands of fibrous tissue that connect bones or cartilage and support and strengthen joints in the body.

Types of Sports Injuries

Acute Inflammation–A protective tissue response to injury or destruction of tissues, acute inflammation serves to destroy the injurious agent or contain the affected area. Symptoms of inflammation are pain, heat, redness, swelling, and loss of function.

Muscle Fatigue–Sustained muscle contraction results in an accumulation of potassium and increased nerve activity, which in turn produces fatigue in the muscle. Fatigue during moderate, rhythmic exercise that would not normally produce muscle fatigue is caused either by the accumulation of lactic acid, which increases acidity and limits energy production in the muscle, or from the cellular loss of calcium, which inhibits the contraction of the muscle.

Sprain/Strain/Torn Ligaments–A sprain in a joint results from strain of the ligaments and/or tendons due to wrenching, twisting, or hyperextension of the joint. Symptoms are swelling, heat, and motion restriction. If the trauma to the joint is severe enough, it can tear ligaments. Shin splints involve pain along the front of the lower leg caused by minute tears in the tissues, usually from strenuous exercises.

Nutrients and Herbs for Sports Injuries

Proper nutrition is essential for athletes for optimum healing of various sports-related, soft-tissue injuries. Even minor deficiencies of antioxidants, enzymes, minerals, proteins, and vitamins have been documented to delay the time of repair and recovery. Carbohydrates, fats, and proteins provide the fuel for physical exercise. Vitamins and minerals are required for the body's metabolic (energy-producing) and enzymatic reactions, while enzymes are the biological catalysts in nerve transmission and muscle activity.

Drinking six to eight 8-ounce glasses of pure, filtered water daily is crucial for the athlete. Dehydration can lead to diminished delivery of oxygen and nutrients to tissues, leading in turn to fatigue and poor performance. We have found that most athletes do not drink enough water or are still drinking tap water. One out of four public water systems has violated federal standards for tap water and the chemical additives may be hazardous to your health.[186]

Producing energy at an increased rate during heavy exercise generates a large amount of free radicals (destructive molecules released naturally during metabolism) in the muscle tissues. Free-radical damage is now believed to cause some of the muscle soreness felt after a workout. Nutrients with antioxidant properties can help prevent free-radical damage; these include vitamins A, C, and E, selenium, the amino acids cysteine and glutathione, coenzyme Q10, ginkgo, Siberian and *Panax* ginseng, chlorella, spirulina, and green tea.

■ **For muscle fatigue:** through perspiration and energy expenditure at the cellular level, the mineral supply in the athlete's body can become depleted and compromise performance. A deficiency of potassium chloride, for example, can result in reduced endurance and muscle cramping or spasms. Chromium is essential for glucose metabolism and energy production; increased amounts of chromium are used by the body during exercise. Iron aids in transporting oxygen in the blood to muscles, lungs, and other tissues; if the iron supply is inadequate, energy levels and physical performance diminish.[187]

Concentrated Liquid Ionic Minerals is one of our favorite mineral products. We recommend that athletes place drops of liquid minerals into their water bottles (10-20 drops per quart) so that these crucial nutrients are replaced as they are used up.

Coenzyme Q10, ginkgo, dimethyl glycine (DMG), and germanium sesquoxide support oxygen delivery to the cells and tissues of the body, which is an essential component of athletic endurance and performance. OxyNutrients, which contains malic acid, magnesium, coenzyme Q10, and other nutrients, is another product we often recommend to athletes.

■ **For muscle spasms:** valerian root, a sedative and tranquilizer, is a muscle relaxant, effective for cramps and spasm. Topical application of liquid ionic minerals, lobelia extract, or arnica tincture helps reduce these muscle afflictions. Passionflower, another sedative and nervine (supports the nervous system), can also aid in easing muscle spasms.

■ **For pain and imflammation:** plant-based digestive enzymes, taken between meals, help reduce the pain and inflammation in muscles, tendons, ligaments, and other soft tissues, caused by sports injuries such as a sprained ankle or pulled muscle. Papain, trypsin, and SOD (superoxide dismutase) are other anti-inflammatory enzymes. Pycnogenol (pine park or grape seed extract), bromelain (enzyme compound from the pineapple plant), vitamin E, and evening primrose oil also help reduce inflammation.

White willow bark, which is high in salicylates (the active ingredient of aspirin) possesses anti-inflammatory and analgesic (pain-relieving) properties. Feverfew also reduces both pain and inflammation. Turmeric and boswellia decrease inflammation and boswellia additionally improves blood supply to the joints.[188]

■ **For rebuilding muscles and preventing tissue loss:** stress or injury from endurance training increases the body's uptake and utilization of amino acids (SEE QUICK DEFINITION) by three to four times the normal amount. Easily digested and assimilated by the body, free-form amino acids are important for athletes who are trying to increase muscle mass and decrease fat. We recommend the amino acid formula Aminoform and Cell Guard for rebuilding muscles and preventing tissue loss.

Branched-chain amino acids (BCAAs), which include leucine, isoleucine, and valine, are important for energy production and the formation and repair of muscles. Whey protein (derived from dairy) is a good source of BCAAs. There are non-dairy formulas containing BCAAs available for people who do not eat dairy products.

Creatine monohydrate, an amino acid nutrient, is a precursor, or building block, of phosphocreatine, the form of creatine stored in muscle cells. Muscle creatine is used by the body to replace ATP (adenosine triphosphate), which is involved in the production of energy. Phosphocreatine acts as a source of energy for muscle contraction and is involved in the formation of new muscle cells.

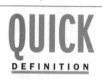

DEFINITION

Amino acids are the basic building blocks of the 40,000 different proteins in the body, including enzymes, hormones, the key brain chemical messenger molecules called neurotransmitters, and the proteins that compose muscle. The basic process of building muscle involves stretching and contracting the muscle until there are actually microscopic tears in the muscle tissue fibers. This is partially why muscles ache after a hard workout. Within one to two days the body will repair these tissues, using amino acids to rebuild the protein that make up the muscle.

■ **For repair of soft tissue injuries:** taken on an empty stomach, protease enzymes enter the bloodstream and digest cellular debris and toxins in the blood. They also travel to sites of inflammation where they break down excessive intracellular proteins (found in swollen tissues). These functions relieve the immune system of some of its workload.

Taking vitamin C is advisable with any kind of injury; it both promotes tissue repair and neutralizes free radicals, which are naturally generated during repair of injuries. The mineral silica, which contributes to the health of skin, bone, and connective tissue, can assist in healing sprains, strains, and joint and other soft tissue injuries; horsetail is an excellent herbal source of silica.

For muscle and connective tissue injuries, comfrey root is both soothing and stimulates tissue repair.[189] When used topically, comfrey root soothes and stimulates repair of injured muscles and connective tissues. Comfrey should be used internally only under the supervision of a qualified health-care professional.

■ **For sore muscles after working out:** calcium and magnesium are vital minerals for muscle relaxation; taking these as well as vitamin E can ease soreness.

■ **For joint support:** glucosamine sulfate or NAG (N-acetyl glucosamine) are useful supplements to support the joints of the body and prevent the breakdown of cartilage; glucosamine is used often in sports medicine for ligament or tendon repair, fracture repair, recovery from traumatic injury, and degenerative joint conditions.

Products for Sports Injuries

Ache-Prin: Capsules. Provides relief of headaches and other body aches and pains; also effective in reducing fever; ingredients include magnesium salicylate, feverfew, white willow bark, and lupulin (hops).

RIDGECREST HERBALS, 1151 South Redwood Road #106, Salt Lake City, UT 84104-3729; tel: 800-242-4649 or 801-978-9633.

Advanced Enzyme System: Vegicaps. Formula of plant-source enzymes for breaking down protein, fiber, fats, and carbohydrates; contains green papaya, apple pectin, sea vegetables, ginger, and peppermint.

RAINBOW LIGHT, P.O. Box 600, Santa Cruz, CA 95061; tel: 800-635-1233 or 408-429-9089.

After Max: Powder. Post-workout recovery formula that replenishes depleted glycogen (the storage form of glucose) stores and nitrogen;

contains 30-40 g of protein, 30-40 g of high glycemic-index carbohydrates, 5 g of creatine monophosphate and taurine, 2 g of L-glutamine, and the proper ratio of electrolytes.

OPTIMUM NUTRITION, 600 North Commerce Street, Aurora, IL 60504; tel: 800-705-5226 or 630-236-0993.

Amino Acids: Capsules, powder, or tablets. Protein supplement containing only the natural form of the amino acids naturally occurring in plants and animals; amino acids are the building blocks of protein, which is used to make muscle.

NOW, 550 Mitchell Road, Glendale Heights, IL 60139; tel: 800-283-3500 or 630-545-9098.

AminoForm: Capsules. Concentrated source of branched-chain amino acids, containing 11 L-crystalline amino acids designed to assist in the development of muscle growth and fat reduction. Indicated for beginner and intermediate body builders with body fat exceeding 15% to 23%, anyone who exercises four or less times per week with muscle growth as the goal, and aerobic enthusiasts training to tone, firm, and reduce body fat.

NUTRI-SOURCE, 3290 Cessna Drive, Cameron Park, CA 95682; tel: 800-293-1683 or 530-676-8838.

Amino Fuel: Powder. Nutritionally complete, highly potent anabolic amino acid drink to help speed recuperation and recovery, build muscle tissue, and increase lean body mass; contains 20 g of peptide-bonded and free-form amino acids from whey and egg-white protein and 50 g of protein-sparing carbohydrates predominantly from glucose polymers for optimum exercise performance and recovery.

TWIN LABS, 150 Motor Parkway, Hauppauge, NY 11788; tel: 800-645-5626.

Amino-Mag 200: Tablets. Supplies 200 mg of elemental magnesium per tablet as a patented amino acid-chelate, which can be absorbed intact; no gastrointestinal side effects.

AMNI, 2247 National Avenue, Hayward, CA 94540-5012; tel: 800-437-8888 or 510-783-6969.

Amino 1000: Capsules. Combination of amino acids for developing and maintaining solid muscle tissue.

SPORTS ONE INC., 47 Capital Drive, Wallingford, CT 06492; tel: 800-624-8787 or 203-294-6370.

AminoPro: Capsules. Complex of 15 isolated, L-crystalline amino acids designed to nutritionally support highly conditioned athletes; good for body builders with low body fat (6%-13%, male/female), advanced body builders whose tendons/joints need to catch up with their muscles, and athletes on detoxification programs.

NUTRI-SOURCE, 3290 Cessna Drive, Cameron Park, CA 95682; tel: 800-293-1683 or 530-676-8838.

Amino 2222: Capsules or tablets. Protein supplement containing 2,222 mg of a protein blend of amino acids derived from the enzymatic digest of lactalbumin (protein derived from whey), soy protein isolate, whey protein concentrate, L-ornithine HCl, and L-carnitine.

OPTIMUM NUTRITION, 600 North Commerce Street, Aurora, IL 60504; tel: 800-705-5226 or 630-236-0993.

Anti-Flam Caps. Anti-inflammatory herbal formula with white willow bark.

CRYSTAL STAR HERBAL NUTRITION, 4069 Wedgeway Court, Earth City, MO 63045 tel: 800-736-6015 or 314-739-7551.

Anti-Inflammatory Cell Signal Enhancer CSE-3 (TGF Beta 1): Homeopathic liquid. For relief from inflammation associated with minor injuries.

BIOMED COMM, INC., 2 Nickerson Street, Suite 102, Seattle, WA 98109; tel: 888-637-3516 or 206-284-3433.

Antioxidant Formula: Capsules. Protection against free radicals; containing antioxidants and nutrients that enhance the uptake of vitamin C and cellular function; ingredients include vitamins A, C, and E, beta and alpha carotenes, coenzyme forms of vitamins B1, B2, and B6, N-acetyl L-cysteine, ferulic acid, malic acid, lipoic acid, calcium, copper, manganese, magnesium, selenium, zinc, pycnogenol, and green tea catechins.

HEALTH PRODUCTS DISTRIBUTORS INC., 23847 Peaceful Ridge Road, Smithsburg, MD 21783; tel: 800-228-4265 or 301-416-0500.

Antioxidant Formula: Capsules. Contains the beneficial properties of vitamin E and beta carotene (natural, mixed carotenoid complex derived primarily from the sea algae *Dunaliella salina*) in a base of antioxidant-supportive food concentrates, nutrients, and herbs to reduce free-radical formation; sources of carotenoids include alpha carotene, zeazanthin, cryptoxanthin, and lutein, and whole food sources of beta carotene such as broccoli powder, carrot powder, and blue-green algae; also contains powdered extracts of grape seed, green tea, and pine bark, which are all proven antioxidants.

ZAND HERBAL FORMULAS, 1722 14th Street #230, Boulder, CO 80302; tel: 800-800-0405 or 303-786-8558.

Anti-SPZ Caps. Herbal combination for pain relief.

CRYSTAL STAR HERBAL NUTRITION, 4069 Wedgeway Court, Earth City, MO 63045; tel: 800-736-6015 or 314-739-7551.

Anti Stress Enzymes: Capsules. Fitness booster containing live enzymes to enhance endurance for rigorous athletic training.

BIOTEC FOODS, 5152 Borsa Avenue, Suite 101, Huntington Beach, CA 92649; tel: 800-788-1084 or 714-899-3477.

Arnica Montana: Homeopathic liquid, ointment, or tablets. Helpful for sore muscles, tendon injury, shin splints, shock from trauma, bruises, falls, blows, black eyes, and surgery.

STANDARD HOMEOPATHIC CO., 201 West 131st, Los Angeles, CA 90061; tel: 800-624-9659 or 310-768-0700.

Baby Boomer Bone and Joint: Tablets. Helps support healthy joints and strong bones; contains glucosamine (one of the most promising natural substances for joint support), calcium, phosphorus, folic acid, curcumin, and vitamin C.

AMERIFIT, 166 Highland Park Drive, Bloomfield, CT 06002; tel: 800-990-FIRM (3476) or 860-242-3476.

Back-Prin: Capsules. Provides relief of minor muscular back pain; ingredients include magnesium salicylate, white willow, calcium lactate, valerian, bromelain, manganese chelate, and lupulin. (Alternative to Doan's Pills, DeWitt's Pills)

RIDGECREST HERBALS, 1151 South Redwood Road #106, Salt Lake City, UT 84104-3729; tel: 800-242-4649 or 801-978-9633.

BHI RendiMAX: Homeopathic tablets. For temporary relief of symptoms of muscle soreness and cramping, physical exertion, and burning from lactic acid buildup, which may occur during or following physical exertion.

HEEL/BHI INC., 11600 Cochiti Road Southeast, Albuquerque, NM 87123-3376; tel: 800-621-7644 or 505-293-3843.

BHI Traumed: Homeopathic ointment. For temporary relief of mild to moderate pain associated with inflammatory, exudative (oozing of fluids), and degenerative processes due to repetitive and overuse injuries, acute trauma, or arthritic conditions.

HEEL/BHI INC., 11600 Cochiti Road Southeast, Albuquerque, NM 87123-3376; tel: 800-621-7644 or 505-293-3843.

BioE Myalgia: Homeopathic liquid. For the temporary relief of muscle and joint pain, tenderness, and weakness.

BIOENERGETICS, INC., P.O. Box 127, Sandy, OR 97055; tel: 800-334-4043 or 503-668-7478.

Black Belt by Jade: Herbal bar. Power food containing 35 Chinese and Western herbs; when eaten before exercise, enhances endurance and provides energy and muscle support; useful for long-duration exercise such as hiking.

EAST EARTH HERB INC., P.O. Box 2802 Eugene, OR 97402; tel: 800-827-HERB (4372) or 541-687-0155.

Body Mend: Homeopathic liquid. For treatment of minor injuries such as sprains, strains, and bruises, and as an aid in the recovery from surgical procedures.

BIOENERGETICS, INC., P.O. Box 127, Sandy, OR 97055; tel: 800-334-4043 or 503-668-7478.

Boswellin Cream. Contains capsaicin (from cayenne) and methyl salicylate (from wintergreen) in a base of *Boswellia serrata* (standardized for boswellic acids) and vitamin E; for temporary relief of minor aches and pains of muscles and joints; greaseless, stainless, with a pleasant aroma.

NATURE'S HERBS, 600 East Quality Drive, American Fork, UT 84003; tel: 800-437-2257 or 801-763-0700.

Bromelain Joint Ease: Capsules. Ingredients include bromelain, quercetin, vitamin C, and SOD (superoxide dismutase) precursors. Bromelain helps to reduce swelling and inhibit the inflammatory response in joints. Bromelain and vitamin C lessen minor bruising. Quercetin, a potent plant bioflavonoid, reduces painful inflammatory responses.

NATURE'S LIFE, 7180 Lampson Avenue, Garden Grove, CA 92841-3914; tel: 800-854-6837 or 714-379-6500.

Calcium Citrate: Capsules. Contains elemental calcium (from calcium citrate) and elemental magnesium (from magnesium oxide and magnesium aspartate).

TWIN LABS, 150 Motor Parkway, Hauppauge, NY 11788; tel: 800-645-5626.

Calcium Magnesium Phosphorus: Liquid. Lactose-free, sucrose-free mineral formula from calcium sources to build and maintain strong bones and teeth; contains natural vitamin D3 to improve calcium absorption.

NATURE'S LIFE, 7180 Lampson Avenue, Garden Grove, CA 92841-3914; tel: 800-854-6837 or 714-379-6500.

Calcium/Magnesium/Zinc: Tablets. Helps maintain strong bones; contains calcium, magnesium, and zinc, the nutrients that help build bones and teeth and aid in nerve, muscle, and metabolic functions.

NATURE MADE LLC, NATURE'S RESOURCE, P.O. Box 9606, Mission Hills, CA 91346-9606; tel: 800-314-HERB (4372) or 800-423-2405.

Calcium/Minerals Plus: Tablets. Contains eggshell-source calcium (more compatible and assimilable than oystershell) and dicalcium phosphate in a base of seaweed and chamomile.

NATURAL ENERGY PRODUCTS, 21101 Welch Road, Snohomish, WA 98296; tel: 425-486-5956.

Calcium 900: Softgels. Contains calcium without the fat and calories of calcium-rich foods; calcium is essential in the development of healthy bones and teeth.

IVC, 500 Halls Mill Road, Freehold, NJ 07728; tel: 800-666-8482 or 732-308-3000.

Calcium Plus: Tablets. Daily supplement of calcium, magnesium, essential minerals (which support the skeletal and muscular systems), co-nutrients, superfoods, and a blend of seven Chinese herbs considered supportive of skeletal health; for diets high in dairy products and low in magnesium-rich foods (grains and legumes).

RAINBOW LIGHT, P.O. Box 600, Santa Cruz, CA 95061; tel: 800-635-1233 or 408-429-9089.

Carpaltun: Tablets. Contains vitamin B6 and its active coenzyme form (pyridoxal-5-phosphate), bromelain, and serratia peptidase, a proteolytic enzyme with anti-inflammatory properties.

ECOLOGICAL FORMULAS, 1061-B Shary Circle, Concord, CA 94518; tel: 800-888-4585 or 925-827-2636.

Cell Guard: Capsules. Potent combination of dismutase, glutathione peroxidase, and catalase for maximum cellular protection and health.
BIOTEC FOODS, 5152 Borsa Avenue, Suite 101, Huntington Beach, CA 92649; 800-788-1084 or 714-899-3477.

Concentrated Mineral Drop Complex: Liquid. Contains complete, soluble, liquid ionic minerals and trace minerals in the proper balance needed for overall health and the functioning of the body's electrical system.
BIO NATIVUS, P.O. Box 3281, Ogden, UT 84401; tel: 888-628-4887 or 801-732-1294.

Creatine Fuel: Capsules or powder. For athletes who need power and strength.
TWIN LABS, 150 Motor Parkway, Hauppauge, NY 11788; tel: 800-645-5626.

Creatine Monohydrate: Powder. Creatine monohydrate is a precursor to ATP (adenosine triphosphate, the form of energy used by cells), which helps increase the amount of energy available for the body to use and decrease muscle fatigue; may also increase anaerobic exercise capacity for high intensity/low duration activities.
BIODYNAMAX, 6525 Gunpark Drive #150-507, Boulder, CO 80301; tel: 800-926-7525 or 303-530-4665.

Creatine Pump: Powder. Contains pure creatine monohydrate in a glycemic system for efficient and rapid delivery to the muscles; when used in conjunction with a proper exercise program, creatine can help increase strength and muscle mass as well as improve recovery times and energy levels.
CYBERGENICS AMERICA LLC., 417 Fifth Avenue, New York, NY 10016; tel: 800-635-8970 or 212-252-7782.

Creatine 2500 Caps. Creatine monohydrate is converted by the body into phosphocreatine and used to replace ATP (adenosine triphosphate) that has been exhausted for energy production; contains 2,500 mg of creatine monohydrate, to help the transfer of energy into the working muscle; useful for high-intensity/short-duration exercise.

OPTIMUM NUTRITION, 600 North Commerce Street, Aurora, IL 60504; tel: 800-705-5226 or 630-236-0993.

CSE-2 (PDGF BB) Cell Signal Enhancer: Homeopathic liquid. Contains homeopathic PDGF (platelet-derived growth factor BB) for temporary relief of minor muscle aches and pains; aids in faster recovery from strenuous exercise.

BIOMED COMM INC., 2 Nickerson Street, Suite 102, Seattle, WA 98109; tel: 888-637-3516 or 206-284-3433.

DMG: Liquid. DMG (dimethylglycine) appears to enhance performance by buffering lactic acid, a breakdown product of anaerobic metabolism that causes muscle fatigue; helpful for endurance athletes.

ETHICAL NUTRIENTS, 971 Calle Negocio, San Clemente, CA 92673; tel: 800-668-8743 or 949-366-0818.

Electrolyte Vital Support: Tablets. Energy formula for athletes that refreshes the body and replenishes minerals.

BIO NATIVUS, P.O. Box 3281, Ogden, UT 84401; tel: 888-628-4887 or 801-732-1294.

Enada NADH: Tablets. NADH (coenzyme vitamin B3) is involved in production of cellular energy; users report increased energy and sense of well-being. NADH is necessary for the synthesis of neurotransmitters (chemical messengers in the brain), which may explain its beneficial effects on energy, mood, and mental function; human studies in Europe with exercising athletes have shown improvement in exercise performance (better utilization of oxygen) and improved reaction times (better brain function).

SCHIFF, WEIDER NUTRITION GROUP, 2002 South 5070 West, Salt Lake City, UT 84104; tel: 800-439-8042 or 801-975-5000.

Endurox Excel: Caplets. Contains endurox, the standardized extract of the herb ciwujia, plus the antioxidant vitamin E to help build endurance during exercise, raise the lactic-acid threshold, speed workout recovery, and increase cardiac efficiency; has been used extensively without reported side effects.

PACIFIC HEALTH LABS INC., 1480 Route 9 North #204, Woodbridge, NJ 07095; tel: 800-39P-ROVE (7-7683).

Energy/Sports: Tablets. Multiple vitamin/mineral formula with high energy nutrients for active lifestyles.

HVL Inc., 600 Boyce Road, Pittsburgh, PA 15205; tel: 800-245-4441.

Flex: Tablets. For tissue structure and connective tissue support and formation; contains manganese and zinc (important for proper formation of connective tissue), pantothenic and folic acids (B vitamins that enable the body to deal with stress and lessen inflammation), NAG (N-acetyl-glucosamine) and glucosamine sulfate (which are the base of the tissue structure forming joints, ligaments, and tendons), vitamin C (aids in the body's utilization of NAG and glucosamine sulfate and helps form collagen found in connective tissue), calcium, horsetail, magnesium, and potassium.

OPTIMAL NUTRIENTS, 1163 Chess Drive #F, Foster City, CA 94404; tel: 800-966-8874 or 650-525-0112.

Flex-Ability: Liquid. Herbal extracts developed to minimize the discomfort of muscular aches and joint stiffness that may occur before and after strenuous exercise or activity.

PLANETARY FORMULAS, 23 Janis Way, Scotts Valley, CA 95066; tel: 800-606-6226.

GS-500 Glucosamine Sulfate: Capsules. Glucosamine is naturally present in joint cartilage and glucosamine sulfate is the form of supplemental glucosamine recommended by researchers and supported by more than 20 double-blind, placebo-controlled studies.

ENZYMATIC THERAPY, 825 Challenger Drive, Green Bay, WI 54311-8328; tel: 800-558-7372 or 920-469-1313.

Gold Sports: Packets. Helps build and maintain strong bones, heal and repair tired muscles, and increase oxygen flow to the body; also assists the body's natural metabolism; contains L-carnitine, lipotropic fat metabolizers (which hasten removal or decrease fat in the liver), megavitamins, and five mineral complex blends with enzymes to ensure proper use of all nutrients.

SPORTS ONE, INC., 47 Capital Drive, Wallingford, CT 06492; tel: 800-624-8787 or 203-294-6370.

Hyland's Low Back Pain: Homeopathic caplets or tablets. For relief of lower back pain due to strain, cold, or exposure.

P & S LABS, 210 West 131st Street, Los Angeles, CA 90061; tel: 800-624-9659 or 310-768-0700.

InflamActin: Capsules and cream. Supports the body's adaptogenic (dealing with stress) function. Capsules contain boswellin, turmeric, bromelain, feverfew, goldenseal, chamomile, DLPA (DL-phenylala-nine), and vitamin C. Cream is useful for muscle aches, pains, soreness, or stiffness, and contains boswellin, turmeric, and gorgonian extracts in a liposome sphere for greater effectiveness and long-lasting results.

NATURE'S PLUS, 548 Broadhollow Road, Melville, NY 11747-3708; tel: 800-645-9500 or 516-293-0030.

Inflam-Aid: Capsules. Formula of standardized herbal extracts and nutrients including vitamin C, natural vitamin E, ginger root, turmeric and licorice root extracts, quercetin, and selenium in a base of bilberry, odorless garlic, and white willow.

NATURE'S HERBS, 600 East Quality Drive, American Fork, UT 84003; tel: 800-437-2257 or 801-763-0700.

Joint Aid: Capsules. Helps support healthy and smooth functioning of connective tissue; contains glucosamine sulfate, marine lipids, borage oil, chondroitin sulfate A, turmeric, quercetin, zinc, vitamin D3, calcium, magnesium, iron, copper, manganese, vitamins C and E; useful for athletic injuries or protection of joint tissue.

OPTIMUM NUTRITION, 600 North Commerce Street, Aurora, IL 60504; tel: 800-705-5226 or 630-236-0993.

Joint Factors: Capsules. Contains glucosamine sulfate with vitamins A, C, and E, manganese, zinc, and copper.

TWIN LABS, 150 Motor Parkway, Hauppauge, NY 11788; tel: 800-645-5626.

Joint • Ligament • Tendon: Tablets. Herbal combination that helps support the body's natural balance and maintain healthy connective tissue.

VEDA HEALTH INC., P.O. Box 1535, Soquel, CA 95073; tel: 888-856-8334 or 408-465-9084.

Jointment: Tablets. Intensive joint and ligament therapy that helps provide pain-free joint performance.

UNIVERSAL, 3 Terminal Road, New Brunswick, NJ 08901; tel: 800-872-0101 or 732-545-3130.

Joint Modulators: Tablets. Contains the cartilage-protective agents glucosamine sulfate and bovine cartilage, which have been shown to support the health and repair of joint and cartilage tissue.

SOLGAR VITAMIN & HERB COMPANY INC., 500 Willow Tree Road, Leonia, NJ 07605; tel: 800-645-2246 or 201-944-2311.

Joint-Power: Capsules. Herbal, vitamin, and mineral supplement for the joints containing glucosamine sulfate, vitamin C, natural vitamin E, manganese, zinc, copper, turmeric extract, boswellia extract, bromelain, and selenium.

NATURE'S HERBS, 600 East Quality Drive, American Fork, UT 84003; tel: 800-437-2257 or 801-763-0700.

Liga-Tend (Formula III): Tablets. Combination of L-proline, glycine, and mucopolysaccharide complex (cements cells together and lubricates joints and bursae), together with vitamins, minerals, and enzymes for the maintenance of ligaments and tendons.

COUNTRY LIFE, 101 Corporate Drive, Hauppauge, NY 11788; tel: 800-645-5768 or 516-231-1031.

Liquid Calcium-Magnesium. Available in vanilla flavor, which contains calcium and magnesium in a 1:1 ratio, or mint flavor, which contains calcium and magnesium in a 2:1 ratio; both forms also contain vitamin D2 and boron.

NF FORMULAS, INC., 9755 Southwest Commerce Circle, C-5, Wilsonville, OR 97070; tel: 800-547-4891 or 503-682-9755.

Liquid Calcium Rx Calcium 1000 Complex: Softgels. Contains six sources of calcium, two sources of magnesium, herbs, vitamins, and minerals for optimum bioavailability.

PHYTO-THERAPY INC., OPTIMUM HEALTH, 483 West Middle Turnpike, Manchester, CT 06040; tel: 800-228-1507 or 860-647-9729.

MSM (Methylsulfonylmethane): Capsules, eye and ear drops, lotion, or powder. Contains sulfur, which is a major component of the human body; MSM provides the body with building materials for healthy, flexible cells.

RICH DISTRIBUTING, P.O. Box 33830, Portland, OR 97292; tel: 877-245-5742 or 503-761-7450.

Multiplete: Tablets. Joint care component including glucosamine, turmeric, white willow bark, boron, calcium, magnesium, and vitamin

C; also includes green tea, echinacea, grape skin, white willow bark, garlic, peppermint leaves, ginseng root, licorice root, cranberry, schisandra, rosemary, astragalus, sarsaparilla, soy, hops, valerian root, and passionflower.

SYNERGY PLUS, IVC, 500 Halls Mill Road, Freehold, NJ 07728; tel: 800-666-8482.

Orthopedic Rejuvenation System: Tablets. Blend of essential minerals and herbs to benefit joint health.

BIO NATIVUS, P.O. Box 3281, Ogden, UT 84401; tel: 888-628-4887 or 801-732-1294.

OxyNutrients: Capsules. Electron transport nutritional formula; fatigue is a result of many factors, one of which being inadequate energy production on the molecular level; supports aerobic cellular metabolism (molecular energy production). Contains malic acid and magnesium, commonly used to treat chronic fatigue; coenzyme Q10, an important participant in cellular energy production; TTFD (thiamine tetrahydro furfuryl disulfide), essential for the brain and nerves; L-carnitine, contributes to energy production and improves fatty acid and glucose metabolism; DMG (dimethylglycine), for synthesis of energy compounds and liver detoxification; the antioxidants ferulic acid and ascorbyl palmitate; and inosine.

ALLERGY RESEARCH GROUP/NUTRICOLOGY, P.O. Box 55907, Hayward, CA 94544; tel: 800-545-9960 or 510-487-8526.

Pro Complex "The Drink": Liquid. For recovery from workout and for lean muscle gain; contains ion-exchange whey protein, cross-flow microfiltration whey protein, egg-white protein, hydrolyzed lactalbumin, added branched-chain amino acids, a complete vitamin and mineral mix for building muscles, and 2 g of carbohydrates.

OPTIMUM NUTRITION, 600 North Commerce Street, Aurora, IL 60504; tel: 800-705-5226 or 630-236-0993.

Rhus Toxicodendron: Homeopathic remedy. Helps sprains, strains, sore muscles, rheumatic pains, lower back pain, influenza, and restlessness.

STANDARD HOMEOPATHIC CO., 201 West 131st Street, Los Angeles, CA 90061; tel: 800-624-9659 or 310-768-0700.

Runners Edge: Capsules. Live enzyme food with genetically increased methionine reductase, which helps the cells eliminate toxins from heavy exercise and pollution; when the toxins are removed, the body is able to experience peak physical performance.

BIOTEC FOODS, 5152 Borsa Avenue, Suite 101, Huntington Beach, CA 92649; tel: 800-788-1084 or 714-899-3477.

Sports Adaptogen Russian Formula: Capsules. Contains standardized Siberian ginseng and schisandra, which builds resistance to physical stress, delays muscular fatigue, and improves recovery.

NATURE'S HERBS, 600 East Quality Drive, American Fork, UT 84003; tel: 800-437-2257 or 801-763-0700.

Sports Vitamins With Herbs: Capsules. Daily multi-vitamin, mineral, and herbal formula for proper energy metabolism; contains standardized milk thistle extract and special adaptogenic (helping the body adapt to stress) herbs used by Russian athletes; also contains a rich source of antioxidant nutrients to help protect against free radicals and muscle soreness caused by intense training.

NATURE'S HERBS, 600 East Quality Drive, American Fork, UT 84003; tel: 800-437-2257 or 801-763-0700.

Tiger Balm: Ointment. Helps relieve strained muscles, sore shoulders, knotted calves, tightened thighs, aching ankles, and backaches, as well as pain associated with arthritis.

PRINCE OF PEACE ENTERPRISES INC., 3450 Third Street #3G, San Francisco, CA 94124; tel: 800-PEACE2U (732-2328).

Traumed: Homeopathic liquid or ointment. For temporary relief of pain, discomfort, inflammation of various origins, and other symptoms of minor sports injuries, sprains, strains, and bruises.

HEEL/BHI INC., 11600 Cochiti Road Southeast, Albuquerque, NM 87123-3376; tel: 800-621-7644 or 505-293-3843.

Tribestan: Tablets. Body builders use this non-hormonal formula as a safe alternative to anabolic steroids.

SCHIFF, WEIDER NUTRITION GROUP, 2002 South 5070 West, Salt Lake City, UT 84104; tel: 800-439-8042 or 801-975-5000.

Tropical Greens: Powder. Replaces nutrients lost during physical exercise; contains powders of fruits, vegetables, organic barley grass, wheat grass, alfalfa, minerals, added fiber, soy protein, vitamins, and antioxidants.

Solar Greens, Nutraceutical Corp., P.O. Box 681869, Park City, UT 84068; tel: 800-669-8877.

Vita Gold Plus: Tablets. Helps build strong bones, heal and repair tired muscles, and increase oxygen flow to the body; also assists the body's natural metabolism; contains L-carnitine, lipotropic fat metabolizers, megavitamins, and five mineral complex blends with enzymes.

Sports One Inc., 47 Capital Drive, Wallingford, CT 06492; tel: 800-624-8787 or 203-294-6370.

Stress is defined as the reaction of the body to any stimulus or interference that upsets normal functioning and disturbs mental or physical health. Stress can be brought on by internal conditions, such as illness, pain, or emotional conflict, or by external circumstances, such as a death in the family or financial problems. Even a positive experience such as a wedding or job promotion can be a stress-provoking event. Stress is a normal, unavoidable part of everyday life that only becomes harmful to the body when it is prolonged or chronic. Then it can lead to exhaustion, immune suppression, minor illness, and, if left unresolved, more serious health conditions.

Symptoms and Causes of Stress

Typical symptoms associated with chronic stress include anxiety, indigestion, upset stomach, headaches, weight loss or gain (anxiety eating), depression, premenstrual syndrome and menstrual disorders, bad breath, body odor, and muscle spasms.

Causes of stress, in addition to those discussed above, are allergic reactions, poor diet, nutritional deficiencies (especially mineral and B vitamin deficiencies), substance abuse, biochemical imbalances, nerve damage, hypoglycemia, fatigue, glandular problems, environmental pollution, and excessive consumption of caffeine or alcohol.

Types of Stress-Related Conditions

Stress first affects the parts of the body that are involved in the stress reaction—the nervous system, the digestive and intestinal systems, and the adrenal and thyroid glands. Prolonged or chronic stress depletes the body of certain nutrients relatively quickly; those particularly affected are amino acids, B vitamins, and electrolytes. Stress also causes the production of free radicals, the unchecked levels of which can lead to degenerative diseases.

Stress can be a contributing factor in the following health conditions: acidosis (increased body acids), backache, cancer, Crohn's disease (intestinal inflammation), depression, diarrhea, digestive disorders, diverticulitis (inflamed out-pouching of the intestines), hair loss, headaches (including migraine), hypertension (high blood pressure), impotence, insomnia, jaw disorders such as temporomandibular joint (TMJ) syndrome, nervous disorders, obsessive/compulsive disorders, pancreatic problems, ulcers, and various skin conditions.

Stress and the Adrenal Glands

The adrenal glands are responsible for helping the body adjust to stress. They produce the hormones adrenaline and cortisol as part of this function. Chronic stress requires constant production of these hormones and increased levels of these hormones and their metabolites circulating in the blood can leave a person feeling tense, irritable, and anxious. Under the demand of prolonged stress, the adrenal glands grow fatigued which can lead not only to overall exhaustion and lowered immunity, but to disturbances throughout the body, as adreno-cortical hormones act in nearly all body systems. Adrenal gland fatigue and exhaustion, in turn, decreases a person's ability to deal with stress.

See **Fatigue**, pp. 175-183.

In addition to the adrenal exhaustion caused by its continued production, cortisol is known to break down amino acids (proteins) in the muscles. Exercise helps diminish cortisol levels, which is one reason—in addition to the many other physical and psychological benefits—that "stressed-out" people need to exercise regularly.

Nutrients and Herbs for Stress

■ **To support the adrenal glands:** when handling stress, the adrenal glands can be supported nutritionally with vitamins A and E, zinc, and essential fatty acids. Organic adrenal glandular extract and adaptogenic herbal formulas also support the adrenal glands. Adaptogens help organs, glands, and nerves function properly under stressful conditions, and also act as a relaxant without causing drowsiness. One of the best adaptogenic herbal products we have found is Adaptogem, which contains the adaptogenic herbs Siberian ginseng, schisandra fruit, echinacea, wild oats, bladderwrack, and gotu kola. A good adrenal glandular extract formula for times of high stress is Adrenal Glandular Plus.

Panax ginseng strengthens the adrenal glands, protects the body from the negative results of stress, and promotes mental alertness and feelings of well-being. It seems to work best for short-term, episodic stress. Siberian ginseng has similar adaptogenic effects and works specifically by decreasing adrenal response to stress and protecting the thymus gland and lymphatic system (components of the immune system) from damage due to chronic stress.[190]

Licorice root can help reverse adrenal exhaustion and restore normal adrenal function.[191]

■ **For calming:** valerian root has been successfully used by many of our patients to treat stress, nervous tension, anxiety, and insomnia. Passionflower, kava-kava, and hops are also good calming agents. Balm is both invigorating and relaxing to the nervous system and promotes restful sleep as well.

For people who are dealing with constant high-level stress, we recommend Stabilium, a product made from a unique fish oil, which is beneficial for physical or mental exhaustion, extreme fatigue or stress, high-risk professions, public speaking, frequent plane trips, and chronic illness. Stabilium, which is not habit-forming, decreases anxiety and agitation, imparts a general feeling of well-being, and improves physical energy and stamina.[192]

Products for Stress

Adaptogem: Caplets. Combination of adaptogenic herbs traditionally recognized for their ability to help the body adapt to physical and emotional change; particularly recommended after stress, overwork, and overconsumption of sugar and caffeine in order to help the body recover after depletion.

RAINBOW LIGHT, P.O. Box 600, Santa Cruz, CA 95061; tel: 800-635-1233 or 408-429-9089.

Adrenal Glandular Plus: Tablets. Combines bovine adrenal glandular extract and B vitamins involved in hormone production and regulation; nutritional support for adrenal function.

ETHICAL NUTRIENTS, 971 Calle Negocio, San Clemente, CA 92673; tel: 800-668-8743 or 949-366-0818.

Adrn-Active Caps. Herbal combination to increase energy, overcome exhaustion, and nourish the body.

CRYSTAL STAR HERBAL NUTRITION, 4069 Wedgeway Court, Earth City, MO 63045; tel: 800-736-6015 or 314-739-7551.

ADR-NL: Capsules. Ingredients include mullein leaves, licorice root, gotu kola, cayenne, ginger root, Siberian ginseng root, and hawthorn berries; dietary support for an active lifestyle, based on a Dr. John R. Christopher formula.

Nature's Way Products Inc., 10 Mountain Springs Parkway, Springville, UT 84663; tel: 800-962-8873 or 801-489-1500.

Advanced Stress System: Tablets. Contains B-complex vitamins, botanical extracts, and antioxidants to support the body in handling all kinds of stressors, particularly free-radical attack.

Rainbow Light, P.O. Box 600, Santa Cruz, CA 95061; tel: 800-635-1233 or 408-429-9089.

AminoHealth: Capsules. Complex of 18 isolated L-crystalline amino acids for utilization during times of intense mental and physical stress; helpful for busy or stressed-out people, city dwellers exposed to air pollution and contamination, smokers, drinkers, or people on a detoxification program.

Nutri-Source, 3290 Cessna Drive, Cameron Park, CA 95682; tel: 800-293-1683 or 530-676-8838.

B-Complex-50: Capsules. Anti-stress formulation of yeast-free B complex vitamins.

Health Products Distributors Inc., 23847 Peaceful Ridge Road, Smithsburg, MD 21783; tel: 800-228-4265 or 301-416-0500.

Beyond St. John's Wort: Tablets. Contains the active compound hypericin, kava-kava, magnesium, royal jelly concentrate, calcium, vitamin B12, thiamine, and L-tyrosine. St. John's wort can provide nutritive support to help maintain a healthy central nervous system.

KAL, Nutraceutical Corp., P.O. Box 681869, Park City, UT 84068; tel: 800-669-8877.

BHI Calming: Homeopathic tablets. For temporary relief of insomnia, restlessness, anxiety, and symptoms of PMS.

Heel/BHI Inc., 11600 Cochiti Road Southeast, Albuquerque, NM 87123-3376; tel: 800-621-7644 or 505-293-3843.

Brain-Vita With Ginkgo Biloba: Tablets. Combination of vitamins, amino acids, minerals, and herbs to stimulate the brain, which may help improve memory and alertness and decrease feelings of stress.

Health Plus, 13837 Magnolia Avenue, Chino, CA 91710; tel: 800-822-6225 or 909-627-9393.

Bupleurum Calmative Compound (Xiao Yao Wan): Tablets. In traditional Chinese medicine, the liver is considered to be the organ primarily

associated with emotional stability; works to cleanse and tonify the liver to restore a sense of peace and well-being to the entire body.
PLANETARY FORMULAS, 23 Janis Way, Scotts Valley, CA 95066; tel: 800-606-6226.

Calm: Tablets. Calming herbal blend containing kava-kava, chamomile, catnip, valerian root, hops, and passionflower.
AMERIFIT, 166 Highland Park Drive, Bloomfield, CT 06002; tel: 800-990-FIRM (3476) or 860-242-3476.

Calms: Tablets. Composed of four botanicals (passionflower, hops, wild oats, and chamomile) long used by the homeopathic medical profession to soothe and quiet irritated nerves and edginess without sedatives or tranquilizers; no side effects or drug hangover.
P & S LABS, 210 West 131st Street, Los Angeles, CA 90061; tel: 800-624-9659 or 310-768-0700.

Calms Forté: Tablets. Contains the same four botanicals as Calms (see above) plus five biochemic phosphates in three times the potency; helps feed and strengthen the nerves of the body to withstand everyday stress and strain.
P & S LABS, 210 West 131st Street, Los Angeles, CA 90061; tel: 800-624-9659 or 310-768-0700.

Crisis-Relief: Liquid. Useful for stress, fear, trauma, and PMS.
OLYMPIC BOTANICALS, 231 Otto Street, Port Townsend, WA 98368; tel: 888-386-4005.

Depress-Ex Caps. Herbal combination formulated to help maintain peace and calm.
CRYSTAL STAR HERBAL NUTRITION, 4069 Wedgeway Court, Earth City, MO 63045; tel: 800-736-6015 or 314-739-7551.

Eleuthero Chamomile: Capsules or liquid. Herbal adaptogen in a primary base of eleuthero root (Siberian ginseng) with the calming herbs chamomile, valerian, passionflower, skullcap, and oatstraw.
FRONTIER COOPERATIVE HERBS, 3021 78th Street, Norway, IA 52318; tel: 800-669-3275 or 319-227-7996.

Enada NADH: Tablets. NADH (coenzyme vitamin B3) is involved in production of cellular energy; users report increased energy and sense of well-being. NADH is necessary for the synthesis of neurotransmitters (chemical messengers in the brain), which may explain its beneficial effects on mood and mental function.

SCHIFF, WEIDER NUTRITION GROUP, 2002 South 5070 West, Salt Lake City, UT 84104; tel: 800-439-8042 or 801-975-5000.

EuroCalm Valerian Root: Capsules. Contains valerian extract with a potency of 0.8% valeric acid, chamomile, passionflower, and hawthorn.

SOLARAY, NUTRACEUTICAL CORP., P.O. Box 681869, Park City, UT 84068; tel: 800-669-8877.

Executive Stress Formula: Tablets. Supports the body's immune system and overall health and vitality; contains ginkgo extract, coenzyme Q10, lemon bioflavonoids, proanthocyanidins (from red wine grapes), SOD (superoxide dismutase), glutathione peroxidase, L-glutathione, brown rice protein concentrate, NAC (N-acetyl-cysteine), DL-methionine, betain HCl, glutamic acid, and L-glycine.

HVL INC., 600 Boyce Road, Pittsburgh, PA 15205; tel: 800-245-4441.

Ex-Stress Formula: Capsules. Contains skullcap, wood betony, black cohosh root, hops flowers, valerian root, and cayenne.

NATURE'S WAY PRODUCTS INC., 10 Mountain Springs Parkway, Springville, UT 84663; tel: 800-962-8873 or 801-489-1500.

SleepRelax by Farmacopia: Capsules. Dietary supplement with pure kava-kava herbal extract traditionally used in the Pacific Islands for calming restless or anxious children and inducing sleep.

BOTANICAL PRODUCTS INTERNATIONAL, P.O. Box 174, Hakalau, HI 96710; tel: 808-963-6771.

5-HTP SeroTonic: Capsules. Scientists have discovered that conditions of depression, carbohydrate cravings (with resultant weight gain), anxiety, sleeplessness, obsessions, and compulsions are all connected to reduced levels of serotonin in the brain—furthermore, if serotonin levels are restored, these conditions often disappear. The amino acid 5-HTP is a metabolic precursor of serotonin, which increases its production and availability; 5-HTP SeroTonic contains 50 mg of 5-HTP per capsule with St. John's wort (10 mg) and pyridoxal-5-phosphate (15 mg), plus cofactors magnesium hydroxide, inositol hexanicotinate, and calcium citrate.

LifeEnhancement Products Inc., P.O. Box 751390, Petaluma, CA 94975-1390; tel: 800-543-3873 or 707-762-6144.

Formula B-Complex "50": Capsules. Contains high-potency, balanced B complex and the recognized B-complex factors.

Solgar Vitamin & Herb Company Inc., 500 Willow Tree Road, Leonia, NJ 07605; tel: 800-645-2246 or 201-944-2311.

GABA: Capsules. Helps prevent anxiety and stress-related messages from reaching the motor centers of the brain by filling its receptor site and also helps promote better sleep.

Infinity Health, 1519 Contra Costa Boulevard, Pleasant Hill, CA 94523; tel: 800-733-9293 or 925-676-8982.

Ginsana: Capsules. Herbal supplement shown to improve the way the body uses oxygen, which in turn enhances overall physical endurance and well-being; contains no artificial stimulants or caffeine.

Boehringer Ingelheim Pharmaceuticals Inc., 900 Ridgebury Road, Ridgefield, CT 06877; tel: 800-243-0127 or 203-798-9988.

Ginseng-Gotu Kola Combination: Capsules. Dietary product to help supplement the body's increased nutritional needs during periods of increased physical or mental activity; contains Siberian ginseng, gotu kola, cayenne, and bee pollen.

Nature's Herbs, 600 East Quality Drive, American Fork, UT 84003; tel: 800-437-2257 or 801-763-0700.

Ginseng Root-Siberian: Capsules. Siberian ginseng is milder than *Panax ginseng* and is often used to increase the body's resistance to environmental and physical stress.

Nature's Source, 15451 San Fernando Mission Boulevard, Mission Hills, CA 91345; tel: 800-423-2405 or 818-837-3633.

Ginseng Six Super Energy Caps. Herbal combination to revitalize the system.

Crystal Star Herbal Nutrition, 4069 Wedgeway Court, Earth City, MO 63045; tel: 800-736-6015 or 314-739-7551.

Ginsenique: Homeopathic liquid. For relief of symptoms of fatigue; increases energy and mental alertness; contains ginseng, alfalfa, echinacea, and *Avena sativa* (oats), as well as homeopathic dilutions of the plants menyanthese and cyclamen for headaches due to fatigue and the mineral *Kali phosporicum* for mental and physical strain.

BOIRON, Campus Boulevard Building A, Newtown Square, PA 19073; tel: 800-264-7661 or 610-325-7464.

Herbal Calm: Capsules. Contains the soothing natural herbs valerian, passionflower, skullcap, hops, and kava-kava. Caution: May cause drowsiness.

NATURE'S HERBS, 600 East Quality Drive, American Fork, UT 84003; tel: 800-437-2257 or 801-763-0700.

Herbal Relax: Liquid. Contains kava-kava, passionflower, hops, schisandra, skullcap, oatseed, milk thistle, ginger, hawthorn, rose hips, and red clover in a base of purified water, brown rice syrup, honey, natural flavor, and 18% USP alcohol.

NATURE'S APOTHECARY, P.O. Box 17970, Boulder, CO 80308; tel: 800-999-7422 or 303-664-1600.

Herbal Rest (Salusan): Liquid. Tonic that aids relaxation and encourages sleep; can be used during the day without drowsiness.

FLORA INC., 805 East Badger Road, Lynden, WA 98264; tel: 800-446-2110 or 360-354-2110.

Herbal Tranquillity Complex: Vegicaps. Herbal combination for the support and maintenance of the body's normal relaxation process.

SOLGAR VITAMIN & HERB COMPANY, INC., 500 Willow Tree Road, Leonia, NJ 07605; tel: 800-645-2246 or 201-944-2311.

High Performance Stress Relief: Tablets. Stress formula is intended to overcome stress through adaptation, relaxation, nourishment, and replacement.

BIO NATIVUS, P.O. Box 3281, Ogden, UT 84401; tel: 888-628-4887 or 801-732-1294.

Hypericalm: Capsules. Nutritional support containing St. John's wort extract for healthy mental and nervous system function.

ENZYMATIC THERAPY, 825 Challenger Drive, Green Bay, WI 54311-8328; tel: 800-558-7372 or 920-469-1313.

Ignatia Amara: Homeopathic remedy. Helpful in emotional strain, mental stress, grief, hysteria, insomnia, headache, and intolerance of tobacco.

STANDARD HOMEOPATHIC CO., 201 West 131st Street, Los Angeles, CA 90061; tel: 800-624-9659 or 310-768-0700.

L-5-HTP: Capsules. Contains natural L-5-HTP, vitamins B6 and C, and bioflavonoids. Clinical studies indicate that administration of L-5-HTP enhances synthesis of serotonin in the brain; vitamin B6 is the cofactor for enzymes that convert L-tryptophan to serotonin, and vitamin C catalyzes the hydroxylation of tryptophan to serotonin.
SOLARAY, NUTRACEUTICAL CORP., P.O. Box 681869, Park City, UT 84068; tel: 800-669-8877.

Maca: Capsules. Native Peruvians have traditionally used Maca *(Lepidium meyenii)* for its nutritional and adaptogenic properties.
PERUVIAN RAINFOREST BOTANICALS, NUTRAMEDIX, 212 North U.S. Highway 1 #17, Tequesta, FL 33469; tel: 800-730-3130.

Maxi-Energizer: Caplets. For active people who need an energy boost; ingredients include standardized extracts of *ma huang*, green tea, and kola nut, L-pyroglutamic acid (L-PCA), and a Chinese herbal blend extract (epimedin, angelica, ginger, ginseng), in a base of *acidophilus*. Caution: Individuals with diabetes, hypertension, glaucoma, thyroid disease, or pregnant/lactating women should consult their physician or health-care professional prior to using this product.
PHILLIPS NUTRITIONALS, 27071 Cabot Road #122, Laguna Hills, CA 92653; tel: 800-514-5115 or 702-898-8141.

Mega-Stress Complex: Tablets. Replaces the water-soluble vitamins lost during stress; also contains valerian root and chamomile.
NATURE'S PLUS, 548 Broadhollow Road, Melville, NY 11747-3708; tel: 800-645-9500 or 516-293-0030.

Mood Balance: Tablets. Helps deal with daily anxiety, stress, and irritability; contains standardized St. John's wort and valerian extracts; calming compounds such as lemon balm, kava-kava root extract, taurine, and GABA (gamma-aminobutyric acid); also contains amino acids that are used to synthesize neurotransmitters (chemical messengers) that support mental acuity and memory.
SOURCE NATURALS, THRESHOLD ENTERPRISES, 23 Janis Way, Scotts Valley, CA 95066; tel: 800-777-5677 or 831-438-1144.

Mood Support: Liquid. Contains St. John's wort, skullcap, oatseed, nettle, milk thistle, kava-kava, gotu kola, passionflower, schisandra, reishi, Siberian ginseng, and orange and lime oils.

NATURE'S APOTHECARY, P.O. Box 17970, Boulder, CO 80308; tel: 800-999-7422 or 303-664-1600.

Nine Ginsengs by Jade: Liquid or tablets. Chinese herbal tonic to boost vitality, promote alertness and tranquillity, and help circulate and balance energy.

EAST EARTH HERB, INC., P.O. Box 2802, Eugene, OR 97402; tel: 800-827-HERB (4372) or 541-687-0155.

Panax Ginseng: Liquid or tea bags. Made from six-year-old ginseng roots that have been preserved using steam and heat; ginseng is considered an adaptogen for replenishing vital energy.

PRINCE OF PEACE ENTERPRISES, INC., 3450 Third Street #3G, San Francisco, CA 94124; tel: 800-PEACE2U (732-2328).

Pfaffia Paniculata (Suma): Powder. Known in Brazil as "Para Tudo" (for everything), suma has become accepted worldwide as an adaptogen and used to treat chronic diseases characterized by fatigue; provides relief from stress and boosts the immune system; it is a rich source of germanium, allantoin (for wound healing), vitamins, minerals, amino acids, beta ecdysone (to increase oxygen to the cells), sitosterol and stigmasterol (to increase blood circulation), and pfaffosides (found only in *Pfaffia paniculata*) to help inhibit tumor cell growth.

SEDNA, P.O. Box 1453, Andrews, NC 28901; tel: 800-223-0858 or 828-321-2240.

Pregnenolone: Capsules. Pregnenolone is a hormone precursor that the body normally manufactures using cholesterol and can be converted into other hormones, including DHEA, estrogen, testosterone, and progesterone; many people report a sense of enhanced well-being and increased energy after taking it and many physicians and scientists believe that replacement of pregnenolone to youthful levels is an important step in dealing with the symptoms of aging.

LIFEENHANCEMENT PRODUCTS INC., P.O. Box 751390, Petaluma, CA 94975-1390; tel: 800-543-3873 or 707-762-6144.

Pregnenolone: Tablets. Supplementation with pregnenolone has been associated with maintaining positive sleep patterns in humans and improved memory and cognitive thinking in animals; users report improved mood and well-being.

SCHIFF, WEIDER NUTRITION GROUP, 2002 South 5070 West, Salt Lake City, UT 84104; tel: 800-439-8042 or 801-975-5000.

Premium North America Ginseng Men's Formula: Capsules. Assists the body's ability to adapt to stress and fatigue, provides nutritional support for healthy prostate function, and acts as an overall tonifier; contains saw palmetto, smilax, North American ginseng *(Panax quinquefolius)*, oatstraw, horsetail, stinging nettle, pumpkin seed, Siberian ginseng, pygeum, and an enzyme blend.

CHAINATA CORP., 5965 205 A Street, Langley, British Columbia, Canada V3A8C4; tel: 800-406-7668 or 604-533-8883.

Premium North American Ginseng Pure Powdered Root: Capsules. Contains pure North American ginseng known for its ability to help the body maintain its homeostasis when under stress.

CHAINATA CORP., 5965 205 A Street, Langley, British Columbia, Canada V3A8C4; tel: 800-406-7668 or 604-533-8883.

Premium North American Ginseng Ultra Concentrate: Liquid. Ginseng concentrate in an alcohol base that assists the body in adapting to stress, increasing energy and endurance, improving mental alertness, and enhancing physical and mental performance.

CHAINATA CORP., 5965 205 A Street, Langley, British Columbia, Canada V3A8C4; tel: 800-406-7668 or 604-533-8883.

Reishi Mushroom Supreme: Tablets. *Fu Zheng* herbs are used to protect against stress, strengthen resistance, and restore the normal functioning of the body; contains concentrated mature reishi extract, reishi and shiitake mushrooms, astragalus, schisandra, grifola, and poria cocos.

PLANETARY FORMULAS, 23 Janis Way, Scotts Valley, CA 95066; tel: 800-606-6226.

Relax: Caplets or liquid. Herbal blend containing valerian and California poppy that promotes relaxation and ease of mind during the day without inducing drowsiness.

RAINBOW LIGHT, P.O. Box 600, Santa Cruz, CA 95061; tel: 800-635-1233 or 408-429-9089.

Relax Caps. Herbal nutrients to help restore and soothe the body physically and mentally.

CRYSTAL STAR HERBAL NUTRITION, 4069 Wedgeway Court, Earth City, MO 63045; tel: 800-736-6015 or 314-739-7551.

Relax and Sleep: Capsules. Herbal extract of valerian root, catnip, hops, and passionflower for relief of occasional sleeplessness and fatigue due to nervous tension, stress, and exhaustion.

PHILLIPS NUTRITIONALS, 27071 Cabot Road #122, Laguna Hills, CA 92653; tel: 800-514-5115 or 702-898-8141.

RollaDream: Lotion. Ayurvedic aromatherapy formula containing mild, herbal aromatics to encourage rest and relaxation for the body and mind.

VEDA HEALTH INC., P.O. Box 1535, Soquel, CA 95073; tel: 888-856-8334 or 408-465-9084.

Sedalia: Homeopathic tablets. For temporary relief of nervousness, irritability, and hypersensitivity due to stress.

BOIRON, 6 Campus Boulevard, Building A, Newtown Square, PA 19073; tel: 800-264-7661 or 610-325-7464.

Sensi-Stress: Capsules. Formula that replaces water-soluble vitamins lost during stress.

NATURE'S PLUS, 548 Broadhollow Road, Melville, NY 11747-3708; tel: 800-645-9500 or 516-293-0030.

Stabilium (Garum armoricum): Softgels. *Garum armoricum*, a fish and salt preparation discovered by the ancient Celts, has been used traditionally for its high nutritive value. An adaptogen and antidepressant, garum helps balance mood, correct sleep disturbances, and increase energy and stamina.

ALLERGY RESEARCH GROUP/NUTRICOLOGY, P.O. Box 55907, Hayward, CA 94544; tel: 800-545-9960 or 510-487-8526.

St. John's Positive Thoughts: Tablets. Contains St. John's wort, valerian, kava-kava, and lemon balm, with key amino acids, vitamins, and minerals; designed to soothe and uplift one's mood.

SOURCE NATURALS, THRESHOLD ENTERPRISES, 23 Janis Way, Scotts Valley, CA 95066; tel: 800-777-5677 or 831-438-1144.

St. John's Solution Plus: Capsules, softgels, or tablets. Nutritional support for mood balance; contains St. John's wort, passionflower, and lemon balm.

QUANTUM INC., 754 Washington Street, Eugene, OR 97401; tel: 800-448-1448 or 541-345-5556.

St. John's Special Formula: Capsules. Contains St. John's wort extract with a potency of 0.3% hypericin, as well as kava-kava, L-tyrosine, DL-phenylalanine, and ginkgo.

SOLARAY, NUTRACEUTICAL CORP., P.O. Box 681869, Park City, UT 84068; tel: 800-669-8877.

St. John's Wort Formula: Capsules. Contains St. John's wort and herbal energy tonics, adaptogens, and nervines to support the body's effort to overcome chronic fatigue, stress, and weak immunity, as well as tyrosine, magnesium, malic acid, and vitamin B6 to support neurotransmitter function and energy levels.

ZAND HERBAL FORMULAS, 1722 14th Street #230, Boulder, CO 80302; tel: 800-800-0405 or 303-786-8558.

St. John's Wort • Kava Compound: Liquid. Mild relaxing sedative, antispasmodic, and muscle relaxant; indicated in depression and despondency, and associated anxiety, nervous agitation, stress, restlessness, and sleeplessness; ingredients include St. John's wort flower and bud, kava-kava root, skullcap flowering herb, and prickly ash bark.

HERB PHARM, 20260 Williams Highway, Williams, OR 97544; tel: 800-348-4372 or 541-846-6262.

St. John's Wort-Kava Compound: Tablets. Blend of Chinese and Western herbs to promote mental well-being.

PLANETARY FORMULAS, 23 Janis Way, Scotts Valley, CA 95066; tel: 800-606-6226.

St. John's Wort • Melissa SuperComplex: Liquid. Herbal blend containing St. John's wort, lemon balm, and wild indigo.

RAINBOW LIGHT, P.O. Box 600, Santa Cruz, CA 95061; tel: 800-635-1233 or 408-429-9089.

Stress: Capsules. Combination of adaptogenic herbs, coenzyme Q10, vitamins, and plant enzymes, which have been shown to support the body's adrenal glands, help reduce stress, increase energy, overcome exhaustion, and nourish the body.

ALTERNATIVE THERAPY, INC., 1664 Fairlawn Avenue, San Jose, CA 95125; tel: 800-311-7922.

Stress B-Complex: Tablets. Provides a balanced ratio of B-complex vitamins (which are actively involved in the breakdown and metabolism of carbohydrates, proteins, and fats for energy production), with vitamin C and raw stomach, duodenum, and liver concentrates in a yeast-free formula.

ETHICAL NUTRIENTS, 971 Calle Negocio, San Clemente, CA 92673; tel: 800-668-8743 or 949-366-0818.

Stress B-Complex: Capsules. Ingredients include vitamins B1, B2, B6, B12, and C, niacinamide, pantothenic acid (d-calcium pantothenate), biotin, PABA (para-aminobenzoic acid), folic acid, choline bitartrate, and inositol.

TWIN LABS, 150 Motor Parkway, Hauppauge, NY 11788; tel: 800-645-5626.

Stress Bee '60' Sustained Release: Tablets. B complex with 500 mg of vitamin C for people under stress.

NATURE'S PLUS, 548 Broadhollow Road, Melville, NY 11747-3708; tel: 800-645-9500 or 516-293-0030.

Stress-D: Capsules. Herbal formula to help calm the central nervous system during times of stress and fatigue; contains nutrients known to support the adrenal glands and central nervous system, including Siberian ginseng, American ginseng, magnesium, vitamin C, kava-kava root, passionflower, chamomile, and vitamins B1, B2, B3, B5, B6, and B12.

BIODYNAMAX, 6525 Gunpark Drive #150-507, Boulder, CO 80301; tel: 800-926-7525 or 303-530-4665.

Stress Defense: Tablets. Herbal relaxant that contains valerian, passionflower, calcium, vitamins B3 and B6, magnesium, and hops.

NUTRITION NOW, 501 Southeast Columbia Shore Boulevard #350, Vancouver, WA 98661; tel: 800-929-0418 or 360-737-6800.

Stress Ease: Capsules. Contains vitamin and mineral complex, gotu kola, wood betony, guarana, garlic, dandelion root, alfalfa, rose hips, ginseng, and valerian.

WGI, 35008 Emerald Coast Parkway, 5th Floor, Destin, FL 32541; tel: 800-854-8353 or 850-654-4744.

Stress Free: Tablets. Herbal formula for coping with stress; contains valerian root, skullcap, chamomile, wood betony, hops, American ginseng, Siberian ginseng (*Eleutherococcus senticosus*), Chinese zizyphus, and hawthorn berry.

PLANETARY FORMULAS, 23 Janis Way, Scotts Valley, CA 95066; tel: 800-606-6226.

Stress Release: Capsules. Combination of vitamins and herbs to help replenish nutrients lost during stressful conditions such as illness, injury, physical overwork, dieting, or lack of sleep. Caution: May cause drowsiness.

NATURE'S HERBS, 600 East Quality Drive, American Fork, UT 84003; tel: 800-437-2257 or 801-763-0700.

Stress Support: Tablets. Contains GTF (glucose tolerance factor) chromium, antioxidants vitamin C and zinc, and the herbal extracts of hops and melissa.

NEW CHAPTER, 22 High Street, Brattleboro, VT 05301; tel: 800-543-7279 or 802-257-9345.

Student's Formula: Homeopathic lozenges. For relief of tension, anxiety, and restlessness caused by stressful situations.

SUPHERB LTD., P.O. Box 1135, Nahariya 22100, Israel; tel: 800-409-HERB (4372).

Super Vitamin B Complex: Capsules. Formula prepared from the least allergenic B vitamins and related factors.

ALLERGY RESEARCH GROUP/NUTRICOLOGY, P.O. Box 55907, Hayward, CA 94544; tel: 800-545-9960 or 510-487-8526.

TranQaCalm: Tablets. Contains herbs for support of nervous system and a balance of minerals and digestive enzymes.

BIO NATIVUS, P.O. Box 3281, Ogden, UT 84401; tel: 888-628-4887 or 801-732-1294.

Tranquil Spirit: Liquid or tablets. Useful for relieving restlessness, excessive worry, anxiety, or irritability.

FLORA INC., 805 East Badger Road, Lynden, WA 98264; tel: 800-446-2110 or 360-354-2110.

Tranquillity Balance: Tablets. Helps relax and calm the body.

VEDA HEALTH INC., P.O. Box 1535, Soquel, CA 95073; tel: 888-856-8334 or 408-465-9084.

Ultra Stress With Iron: Tablets. Replaces the water-soluble vitamins that are lost during extreme physical stress.

NATURE'S PLUS, 548 Broadhollow Road, Melville, NY 11747-3708; tel: 800-645-9500 or 516-293-0030.

Valerian Combination: Capsules. Contains valerian root, hops, wood betony, skullcap, black cohosh root, passionflower, and cayenne. Caution: May cause drowsiness.

NATURE'S HERBS, 600 East Quality Drive, American Fork, UT 84003; tel: 800-437-2257 or 801-763-0700.

Valerian • Passionflower Compound: Liquid. Gentle, non-narcotic sedative, which is indicated in nervous excitement and hysteria, mental depression due to worry or imagined wrongs, nervous headache, insomnia, and in nervousness associated with menopause.

HERB PHARM, 20260 Williams Highway, Williams, OR 97544; tel: 800-348-4372 or 541-846-6262.

Viva-Lift: Tablets. Pharmaceutical-grade, isolated amino acid formula containing L-tyrosine and pyridoxal-5-phosphate (the active form of vitamin B6) to aid moodiness due to stress or PMS.

THURSDAY PLANTATION INC., NATURE'S PLUS, 548 Broadhollow Road, Melville, NY 11747-3708; tel: 800-645-9500 or 516-293-0030.

Surgery is used by conventional doctors for a wide variety of ailments from eye disorders and cancer to heart disease and dental problems. However necessary (or routine) these procedures may be, surgery sends the body into physical and emotional shock. An incision into the skin removes the body's first defense against disease-causing agents and, in turn, sends the immune system into "emergency" mode. In addition, the feelings of anxiety, fear, and dread that many people experience prior to surgery heighten the impending assault on the body and may impede recovery following the procedure. Typically, recuperation from even minor surgery can take weeks and includes pain, immobility, and weakened immunity (due to prescribed antibiotics and pain medication).

Nutritional and Herbal Support for Surgery

There are specific nutritional and herbal supplements that help in preparation for and recovery from surgery. A review of the medical literature shows that people who prepare for an operation in this way experience less pain and fewer complications and recover more rapidly than those who did no preparation.[193]

For information about the book *Prepare for Surgery, Heal Faster* and the accompanying tape *Relaxation Healing*, call 800-726-4173 or visit the website www.healfaster.com.

Before Surgery

We recommend reading Peggy Huddleston's book *Prepare for Surgery, Heal Faster* (Angel River Press, 1996), which advises how to overcome the fear of surgery and to facilitate the mind/body's healing potential after surgery.

■ Two weeks before surgery, start building up the immune and body defense systems by taking a daily high-potency multivitamin/mineral complex, additional vitamin C, bioflavonoids, the herb echinacea, and antioxidants such as pycnogenol (pine bark or grape seed extract). Eat a diet high in vegetable proteins. Do not attempt any detoxification or cleansing program (except under special circumstances).

■ Forty-eight hours before surgery, take anti-inflammatory nutrients such as protease or bromelain (pineapple enzymes), which will reduce the swelling, inflammation, and pain of surgery. Continue taking liquid ionic trace minerals until the post-surgical healing is complete. Many vital body processes depend on the movement of ions (ionic minerals) across the cell membranes. Minerals in the liquid ionic form can be readily absorbed by the body, providing key nutrients to those areas most in need of repair after surgery.

After Surgery

Severe trauma to the body, such as surgery, suppresses immune function. Supplementation with vitamins A and C following surgery has been shown to boost immunity. Vitamin C also aids in the healing of surgical incisions, as does the amino acid arginine.[194] It is also important to support the adrenal glands in handling the stress of surgery; take adaptogenic herbs such as ginseng or adaptogenic formulas.

To reduce the inflammation caused by surgery, continue to take protease or bromelain; omega-3 essential fatty acids (fish and flaxseed oils) are also anti-inflammatory. An excellent homeopathic remedy for inflammation is *Arnica montana*, in oral and topical form (do not apply the cream or gel directly onto the incision, but only on the skin near it).

If antibiotic therapy is used before or after surgery, take *acidophilus* or a probiotic (beneficial intestinal bacteria) combination during and after the course of antibiotics. This recolonizes these good bacteria killed by the antibiotics and helps prevents an overgrowth of harmful microorganisms normally kept in check by the beneficial flora.

After surgery people are usually on a restricted diet, but this is the time their nutritional needs are greatest. We often recommend a product called One Step, a "predigested" powdered protein and nutrient drink. Free-form amino acids can also provide the body with "predigested" proteins, which stabilize blood sugar levels and aid in wound healing.

To help prevent the constipation that occurs as a result of the metabolism-slowing effects of pain medications and anesthesia, take aloe vera juice and be sure to eat sufficient dietary fiber.

Products for Surgery

ACES Gold: Tablets. Antioxidant formula that contains coenzyme Q10, vitamins A, C, and E, plus glutathione peroxidase support (selenium, glutathione, and N-acetyl-cysteine), superoxide dismutase support (zinc, copper, and manganese), alpha-lipoic acid, citrus bioflavonoids (including quercetin), and odorless garlic (*Allium sativum*).

J.R. Carlson Labs Inc., 15 College Drive, Arlington Heights, IL 60004-1985; tel: 800-323-4141 or 708-255-1600.

Advance Multi-Vitamin and Minerals: Capsules. Contains naturally derived vitamins, organic mineral citrates and pure plant enzymes (helps the body break down and absorb nutrients from the diet); also available in an iron-free formula.

PreVail Corp., 2204-8 Northwest Birdsdale, Gresham, OR 97030; tel: 800-248-0885 or 503-667-5527.

Advanced Stress System: Tablets. Contains phyto-nutrients, B-complex vitamins, botanical extracts, and antioxidants to support the body's response to stress.

Rainbow Light, P.O. Box 600, Santa Cruz, CA 95061; tel: 800-635-1233 or 408-429-9089.

Arnica Montana: Homeopathic remedy. Helpful in dental surgery, shock from trauma, bruises, falls, blows, black eyes, sore muscles, tendon injury, and shin splints.

Standard Homeopathic Co., 201 West 131st, Los Angeles, CA 90061; tel: 800-624-9659 or 310-768-0700.

Body Mend: Homeopathic liquid. For treatment of minor injuries and as an aid in the recovery from surgical procedures.

BioEnergetics, Inc., P.O. Box 127, Sandy, OR 97055; tel: 800-334-4043 or 503-668-7478.

Cat's Claw: Capsules. Contains cat's claw (*Uncaria tomentosa*), which is grown in the Peruvian rainforest and has been used for centuries by native Peruvians; studies have found that cat's claw enhances the activity of white blood cells during phagocytosis (engulfing potentially harmful microorganisms), inhibits platelet aggregation (abnormal blood clotting) and thrombosis, and is effective in the treatment of allergies.

Nature's Pride, Nature's Products, 1301 Sawgrass Corporate Parkway, Sunrise, FL 33323-2813; tel: 800-752-7873 or 954-233-4600.

Concentrated Mineral Drop Complex: Liquid. Helps conduct and generate the body's electrical system; contains complete, soluble, liquid ionic minerals and trace minerals.

BIO NATIVUS, P.O. Box 3281, Ogden, UT 84401; tel: 888-628-4887 or 801-732-1294.

Essential Fatty Acid Complex: Softgels. Contains evening primrose and flaxseed oils, vitamin E, and plant antioxidants from rosemary and sage; helps control a variety of body functions including pain, inflammation, blood pressure, and skin softness.

SCHIFF, WEIDER NUTRITION GROUP, 2002 South 5070 West, Salt Lake City, UT 84104; tel: 800-439-8042 or 801-975-5000.

Essiac: Tea. Nontoxic herbal remedy containing inulin, a starch occurring in certain plants. Inulin acts as an endocrine hormone, enhancing the growth factor of cells; it also helps the immune system, liver, spleen, and pancreas; contains burdock root, slippery elm, sheep sorrel, and Indian rhubarb, which together help normalize body systems by purifying the blood and promoting cell repair.

ESSIAC INTERNATIONAL, 164 Richmond Road, Ottowa, Ontario, Canada K1Z 6W1; tel: 613-729-9111.

Ester C Plus: Capsules. Antioxidant with antihistamine, anti-inflammatory, and immune-enhancing properties; assists healing, strengthens blood vessels, and normalizes high cholesterol. Ester C (a non-acidic form of vitamin C) is absorbed better, excreted significantly slower, and is more biologically active than regular vitamin C; also contains bioflavonoids as cofactors for vitamin C activity in all tissues (especially the circulatory system).

PHILLIPS NUTRITIONALS, 27071 Cabot Road #122, Laguna Hills, CA 92653; tel: 800-514-5115 or 702-898-8141.

Formula VM-2000: Tablets. Multi-nutrient system with a complete balance of vitamins and minerals in a whole food and herbal base; contains high levels of antioxidants, essential vitamins, and multi-chelated blend of minerals in their citrate, aspartate, amino acid, and picolinate forms; specific ingredients include buffered vitamin C, B complex, beta carotene, and nine essential amino acids.

SOLGAR VITAMIN & HERB COMPANY INC., 500 Willow Tree Road, Leonia, NJ 07605; tel: 800-645-2246 or 201-944-2311.

Herbal Aloe Force: Juice or topical gel. Processed aloe vera juice containing vitamins, minerals, enzymes, amino acids, essential fatty acids, growth factors, glycoproteins, sterols, bioflavonoids, and polysaccharides (complex sugars), plus ionized colloidal silver and herbal extracts

(cat's claw, chamomile, burdock root, hawthorn berry, astragalus root, sheep sorrell, pau d'arco bark, slippery elm bark, and rhubarb root).
HERBAL ANSWERS INC., P.O. Box 1110, Saratoga Springs, NY 12866; tel: 888-256-3367 or 518-581-1968.

Hypericum: Homeopathic remedy. Helpful in eye, nerve, and tailbone injury, dental surgery, puncture wounds, splinters, bites, cuts, burns, and post-operative pain.
STANDARD HOMEOPATHIC CO., 201 West 131st Street, Los Angeles, CA 90061; tel: 800-624-9659 or 310-768-0700.

Katsu Kelp Root Tablets. Contains extract and powder of kelp root, a source of iodine, potassium, calcium, amino acids, and plant fiber; supports proper thyroid function.
KENSHIN TRADING, CORP., 1815 West 213th Street #180, Torrance, CA 90501; tel: 800-766-1313.

Kyo-Green: Liquid. Green drink made of a blend of organic barley grass and wheat grass, chlorella, brown rice, green algae, and Pacific kelp; a good source of minerals, especially iodine and potent antioxidant enzymes; a potent blood alkalizer and energizer.
WAKUNAGA OF AMERICA, 23501 Madero, Mission Viejo, CA 92691; tel: 800-421-2998 or 949-855-2776.

One Step: Powder. Body cleansing formula; beverage mix contains predigested soy protein concentrate, vitamins, minerals, antioxidants and anti-aging nutrients, and other nutrients to support immunity, detoxification, and intestinal health.
PROGRESSIVE LABORATORIES INC., 1701 West Walnut Hill Lane, Irving, TX 75038; tel: 800-527-9512 or 972-518-9660.

PB 8 Pro-Biotic Acidophilus: Capsules. Contains the highest potency of *acidophilus* available, 14 billion friendly bacteria per capsule at the time of manufacture.
NUTRITION NOW, 501 Southeast Columbia Shore Boulevard #350, Vancouver, WA 98661; tel: 800-929-0418 or 360-737-6800.

Premier Anti-Oxidant: Capsules. Enhances the supplementation of vitamins A, C, and E, and bioflavonoids; contains the antioxidants glutathione, taurine, ALA (alpha-lipoic acid), the glutathione precursor NAC (N-acetyl-cysteine), and supporting nutrients.

BIO-NUTRITIONAL FORMULAS, 106 East Jericho Turnpike, Mineola, NY 11501; tel: 800-950-8484.

Pycnogenol & Citrus Bioflavonoids: Capsules. Contains pycnogenol from pine bark, a powerful antioxidant that crosses the blood-brain barrier helping to protect the body and the central nervous system from the damaging effects of free radicals.

AMERICAN HEALTH, 4320 Veterans Memorial Highway, Holbrook, NY 11741; tel: 800-445-7137.

Squalene: Capsules or softgels. Squalene, an extract from the liver of the Aizame shark, increases new tissue growth called granulation, which covers wounds; it also supports the activity of the liver, acts as an adaptogen similar to ginseng and antioxidants, stimulates the defensive forces of the body, and enhances resistance to immune system disorders.

OPTIMAL NUTRIENTS, 1163 Chess Drive #F, Foster City, CA 94404; tel: 800-966-8874 or 415-525-0112.

Thyroid Conditions

The thyroid gland affects the operation of all body processes and organs. It controls body temperature, oxygen utilization, the rate at which organs function, and the speed with which the body uses food. Subclinical thyroid hormonal imbalances are quite common in American adults. Due to the fact that thyroid hormone is converted into its active form in the liver, thyroid function is often diminished in times of increased liver stress or liver toxicity. The pituitary gland, parathyroid glands, and sex glands all work together and are influenced by the thyroid. A malfunctioning or imbalanced thyroid gland can be the underlying cause of many chronic illnesses.

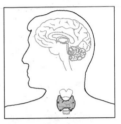

The thyroid gland is the body's metabolic thermostat, controlling body temperature, energy use, and, for children, the body's growth rate.

Types and Causes of Thyroid Conditions

Hyperthyroidism—An overactive thyroid (hyperthyroidism) occurs when the thyroid gland produces too many hormones, speeding up metabolism. Symptoms include nervousness, irritability, increased sweating, insomnia, fatigue, weakness, hair thinning or loss, weight loss, hand tremors, heat intolerance, and bulging eyes. Hyperthyroidism may be associated with and often is called Graves' disease, which is characterized by an enlarged thyroid and the symptom of bulging eyes.

Hypothyroidism—The underproduction of thyroid hormones (hypothyroidism) produces symptoms of fatigue, loss of appetite, weight gain, muscle weakness, dry and scaly skin, loss of eyebrows, constipation, recurrent infections, depression, slow speech, and drooping eyelids. Hypothyroidism can be a hidden factor in a range of health conditions from chronic fatigue syndrome to infertility. Causes of hypothyroidism include accumulated radiation, environmental toxins, overuse of diet pills and other pharmaceuticals, and deficiencies in iodine (the primary mineral nutrient of the thyroid gland), zinc, vitamin A, or vitamin E.[195]

Nutrients and Herbs for Thyroid Conditions

Hypothyroidism is more easily treated through natural therapies than hyperthyroidism.

■ **For hyperthyroidism:** Alan Gaby, M.D., and Jonathan Wright, M.D., have developed a natural protocol for treating the side effects of hyperthyroidism. Daily doses of Super Saturated Potassium Iodine (SSKI) solution, lithium carbonate, and vitamin B12 or Meyer's Cocktail (SEE QUICK DEFINITION) help protect the body from the harmful effects of excess thyroid hormones associated with hyperthyroidism. This protocol is only available under direct medical supervision and can not reverse the condition.[196]

■ **For hypothyroidism:** an organic thyroid glandular extract, given under the supervision of a doctor, can help restore normal thyroid function. We also recommend kelp, which is one of the best natural sources of iodine. Helping the liver to detoxify toxins and excess hormones in turn promotes thyroid hormonal balance. A good product we have found for supporting liver function and detoxification is called LiverGuard. Milk thistle (silymarin), lipoic acid, and B-complex vitamins are also helpful.

Products for Thyroid Conditions

Amino Acids: Capsules, powder, or tablets. Contains only the natural (L) form of the amino acids naturally occurring in plants and animals.

NOW, 550 Mitchell Road, Glendale Heights, IL 60139; tel: 800-283-3500 or 630-545-9098.

AminoHealth: Capsules. Complex of 18 isolated L-crystalline amino acids for times of intense mental and physical stress; also helpful for those exposed to environmental pollution, smokers, or drinkers.

NUTRI-SOURCE, 3290 Cessna Drive, Cameron Park, CA 95682; tel: 800-293-1683 or 530-676-8838.

For information on **testing hormone levels**, see Appendix: Great Smokies Diagnostic Laboratory, pp. 484-485.

Coenzymate B Complex: Tablets. Contains the full spectrum of coenzymated vitamins B1, B2, B3, B6, and B12, and folic acid, biotin, flush-free niacin (it doesn't produce the tingling flush that occurs shortly after taking niacin), pantothenic acid, inositol, and coenzyme Q10.

SOURCE NATURALS, THRESHOLD-ENTERPRISES, 23 Janis Way, Scotts Valley, CA 95066; tel: 800-777-5677 or 831-438-1144.

Concentrated Mineral Drop Complex: Liquid. Helps conduct and generate the body's electrical system; contains complete, soluble, liquid ionic minerals and trace minerals.

BIO NATIVUS, P.O. Box 3281, Ogden, UT 84401; tel: 888-628-4887 or 801-732-1294.

Katsu Kelp Root Tablets. Contains extract and powder of kelp root, a source of iodine, potassium, calcium, amino acids, and plant fiber; supports proper thyroid function.

KENSHIN TRADING CORP., 1815 West 213th Street #180, Torrance, CA 90501; tel: 800-766-1313.

Liver Guard: Tablets. Contains dandelion root and extract, turmeric, silymarin (from milk thistle seed extract), N-acetyl-cysteine, vitamins, minerals, and coenzyme Q10.

SOURCE NATURALS, THRESHOLD ENTERPRISES, 23 Janis Way, Scotts Valley, CA 95066; tel: 800-777-5677 or 831-438-1144.

OptiZinc: Tablets. Contains zinc combined with the essential amino acid methionine. Zinc is necessary for over 100 different enzyme systems, the health of the thymus gland and skin, wound-healing, and carbohydrate metabolism.

SOURCE NATURALS, THRESHOLD ENTERPRISES, 23 Janis Way, Scotts Valley, CA 95066; tel: 800-777-5677 or 831-438-1144.

Thyro-Max Support: Vegitabs. For the health of the thyroid gland; contains a combination of L-tyrosine and L-aspartic acid.

COUNTRY LIFE, 101 Corporate Drive, Hauppauge, NY 11788; tel: 800-645-5768 or 516-231-1031.

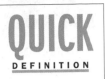

DEFINITION

The **Meyer's Cocktail** is an intravenous vitamin and mineral protocol developed by John Meyers, M.D., a physician at Johns Hopkins University in Baltimore, Maryland, in the 1970s. It contains magnesium chloride hexahydrate (5 cc given), calcium gluconate (2.5 cc), vitamin B2 (1,000 mcg/cc; 1 cc given), vitamin B5 (100 mg/cc; 1 cc given), vitamin B6 (250 mg/cc; 1 cc given), the entire vitamin B complex (100 mg/cc; 1 cc given), and vitamin C (222 mg/oo; 6 oo given). The solution is slowly injected over a 5-15 minute period.

For more about **liver detoxification**, see Liver Disorders, pp. 257-262, and Detoxification in Part III, pp. 446-461.

Urinary Tract Infections

The urinary tract is involved in formation, concentration, and excretion (elimination) of urine from the body. It includes the bladder, urethra (the tube from the bladder to outside the body), kidneys, and ureters (tubes connecting the bladder to the kidneys). Normal urination is four to six times per day, usually in the daytime rather than at night. Infection can occur anywhere along the urinary tract, but is most frequent in the urethra and bladder.

Symptoms and Causes of Urinary Tract Infections

Bladder infection (cystitis) is one kind of urinary tract infection (UTI), usually caused by a bacterial infection ascending the urethra into the bladder. (Infection of the urethra is called urethritis and produces a burning sensation upon urination.) Symptoms of a bladder infection include burning pain with urination, false sensation of needing to urinate urgently and frequently, tenderness in the bladder area, and increased nighttime urination. Cystitis is more common in women because of their much shorter urethra, which makes it easier for bacteria to travel up into the bladder, and due to the proximity of the vagina and anus (potential sources of bacteria) to the urethra's opening. *E. coli*, a bacteria from the intestines, is the source of approximately 85% of UTIs.[197]

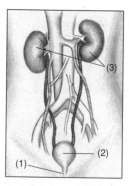

An infection can develop anywhere in the urinary tract. In most cases, the problem starts in the urethra (1) and moves up the system to the bladder (2) and, in severe cases, to the kidneys (3).

Bladder infections generally are not serious if treated quickly. For chronic, recurring bladder infections, it may be necessary to use antibiotics. If a UTI is left untreated, it can ascend to the kidneys, requiring immediate medical care. A descending UTI (moving from the kidneys or bladder down the urethra) is a more serious health condition.

Painful urination and other UTI symptoms may not be the result of a bacterial infection, but can be caused by an acidic urinary pH (SEE QUICK DEFINITION), food allergies, or viral infection, in which case antibiotics are useless.

Treatment of Urinary Tract Infections

If you have a UTI, avoid foods and beverages that cause the body to become acidic and increase your intake of alkalizing foods (see sidebar, p. 396). Aloe vera and green foods, such as chlorella, barley grass, wheat grass, chlorophyll, parsley, and alfalfa, also raise alkalinity. Reduce carbohydrates, sugars, and artificial sweeteners, and eliminate soft drinks. Drink six to eight 8-ounce glasses of pure, filtered water daily; a portion of this fluid intake can be unsweetened cranberry and/or blueberry juice. Juice and extract of these berries are effective in preventing and treating urinary tract infections (even though cranberries are an acid-forming food) due to their property of inhibiting bacteria from adhering to the walls of the urinary tract.[198]

If natural therapies for bladder infections do not appear to be effective within the first 24 to 36 hours, or if a fever or back pain develops along with the bladder symptoms, we recommend you consider conventional antibiotic therapy. As much as we try to avoid using them, antibiotics in this instance will prevent the possible spread of infection into the kidneys, which can be life-threatening.

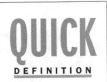

DEFINITION

The term **pH**, which means "potential hydrogen," represents a scale for the relative acidity or alkalinity of a solution. Acidity is measured as a pH of 0.1 to 6.9, alkalinity is 7.1 to 14, and neutral pH is 7.0. Normally, blood is slightly alkaline, at 7.35 to 7.45; urine pH can range from 4.8 to 8.0, but is usually somewhat acidic, with a normal reading between 5.0 and 6.0.

Ask your doctor to culture your urine to see if abnormal bacteria are present and, if so, to perform an antibiotic sensitivity test to determine which antibiotic medication works best for your specific strain of bacterial infection.

While treating a bladder infection, especially if you are taking antibiotics, we recommend using *acidophilus* to decrease the possibility of an overgrowth of *Candida albicans* (yeast-like fungus) or other pathogenic organisms.

Nutrients and Herbs for Urinary Tract Infections

See also **Allergies**, pp. 66-74, and **Viral Infections**, pp. 401-411.

Cantharis and *Apis mellifica* (at potency 6X or 30X) are two homeopathic remedies we have found effective in treating urinary tract and bladder infections.

Among herbs, uva ursi and horsetail have diuretic (urine-increasing) and astringent properties helpful for bladder infections. Echinacea, which is an immune stimulant, has demonstrated effectiveness for UTIs.[199] Goldenseal, colloidal silver, and garlic are natural antibiotics, known to destroy bacteria, fungi, and viruses.[200] Other recommended nutrients for UTIs include vitamin A, aloe vera juice, buchu, juniper berry, parsley, lobelia, ginger, plantain leaf, dandelion leaf, and marshmallow root. As mentioned previously, cranberry and blueberry extracts and/or juice can relieve and prevent recurrence.

As with any infection, strengthening the immune system to release its innate healing abilities is advisable (see Immune Support in Part III).

Products for Urinary Tract Infections

AquaActin: Capsules. Dietary supplement designed to nutritionally support the body's normal water balance; contains green tea, uva ursi, goldenseal, and vitamin B6.

NATURE'S PLUS, 548 Broadhollow Road, Melville, NY 11747-3708; tel: 800-645-9500 or 516-293-0030.

BioBoost: Capsules. Dietary supplement that combines herbs such as echinacea and goldenseal with antioxidant vitamins and minerals to support the body's own defenses.

BIODYNAMAX, 6525 Gunpark Drive #150-507, Boulder, CO 80301; tel: 800-926-7525 or 303-530-4665.

Bladderex by Earth's Bounty: Tablets. Herbal bladder formula that contains *Desmodium* *stracifolium*, corn silk, arbus leaf, herba pyrrosiae, and poria.

MATRIX HEALTH PRODUCTS, 8400 Magnolia Avenue, Suite N, Santee, CA 92071; tel: 800-736-5609 or 619-448-7550.

Chloraid: Capsules. Source of premium chlorophyll, which helps reduce offensive body odors originating in the digestive and urinary tracts.

NATURE'S HERBS, 600 East Quality Drive, American Fork, UT 84003; tel: 800-437-2257 or 801-763-0700.

Colloidal Silver: Liquid. Combination of minute, electrically charged particles of silver and pure water, which work as an antibiotic and immune system enhancer; useful internally for common colds and flu, and externally for cuts and abrasions.

NUPRO, 735-L Park Street, Castle Rock, CO 80104; tel: 800-704-8910 or 303-660-0562.

Cranberry Concentrate: Softgels. Contains concentrated cranberries with the nutritive value equivalent to one ounce of cranberry juice cocktail.

J.R. CARLSON LABS, INC., 15 College Drive, Arlington Heights, IL 60004-1985; tel: 800-323-4141 or 708-255-1600.

Cranberry Defense—Cranberry-Uva Ursi Compound: Tablets. Contains cranberry extract with the botanicals uva ursi and echinacea to support a healthy genitourinary system.

PLANETARY FORMULAS, 23 Janis Way, Scotts Valley, CA 95066; tel: 800-606-6226.

Cranberry Fruit: Capsules. Cranberry fruit helps maintain a healthy urinary tract by preventing the adhesion of bacteria (*E. coli*) to the bladder.

NATURE'S SOURCE, 15451 San Fernando Mission Boulevard, Mission Hills, CA 91345; tel: 800-423-2405 or 818-837-3633.

Cranberry Renal Flush Rx '1500' Complex: Softgels. Nutritional system to help maintain a healthy renal (kidney) system, which combines cranberry juice concentrate, vitamins B6 and C, herbal extracts, and orange and grapefruit concentrate.

PHYTO-THERAPY INC., OPTIMUM HEALTH, 483 West Middle Turnpike, Manchester, CT 06040; tel: 800-228-1507.

Cran-Caplets. For women and men who suffer from poor urinary tract health; contains extract from fresh cranberries.

PHILLIPS NUTRITIONALS, 27071 Cabot Road #122, Laguna Hills, CA 92653; tel: 800-514-5115 or 702-898-8141.

CranGuard: Capsules. Helps maintain healthy urinary function in the female body; contains bee propolis, astragalus, and uva ursi.

NATURAL MAX, NUTRACEUTICAL CORP., P.O. Box 681869, Park City, UT 84068; tel: 800-669-8877.

Echatin Forte: Capsules. Blends extracts of herbs and mushrooms in an echinacea formula; like echinacea, the Chinese herb astragalus contains potent polysaccharides, as do reishi and shiitake mushrooms.

NF FORMULAS INC., 9755 Southwest Commerce Circle, C-5, Wilsonville, OR 97070; tel: 800-547-4891 or 503-682-9755.

Echinacea & Golden Seal Herbal Blend: Capsules. Contains concentrated organically grown echinacea (*E. angustifolia, purpurea,* and *pallida*) with goldenseal and supporting herbs; helps combat infections and boost immunity.

CHAINATA CORP., 5965 205 A Street, Langley, British Columbia, Canada V3A8C4; tel: 800-406-7668 or 604-533-8883.

E.H.B.: Capsules. Blend of three species of echinacea (*E. purpurea, angustifolia,* and *pallida*), goldenseal, and berberis with herbs and vitamins, including licorice, garlic, ginger, bioflavonoids, vitamin C, beta carotene, and zinc.

NF FORMULAS INC., 9755 Southwest Commerce Circle, C-5, Wilsonville, OR 97070; tel: 800-547-4891 or 503-682-9755.

Herbal Aloe Force: Juice or topical gel. Processed aloe vera juice containing vitamins, minerals, enzymes, amino acids, essential fatty acids, growth factors, glycoproteins, sterols, bioflavonoids, and polysaccharides (complex sugars), plus ionized colloidal silver and herbal extracts (cat's claw, chamomile, burdock root, hawthorn berry, *Astragalus membranaceus* root, sheep sorrel, pau d'arco bark, slippery elm bark, and rhubarb root).

HERBAL ANSWERS INC., P.O. Box 1110, Saratoga Springs, NY 12866; tel: 888-256-3367 or 518-581-1968.

Hyland's Bladder Irritation: Sublingual tablets. For relief of symptoms of burning and painful urination associated with bladder irritation.

P & S LABS, 210 West 131st Street, Los Angeles, CA 90061; tel: 800-624-9659 or 310-768-0700.

Katsu Herbal Garlic Complex: Tablets. Concentrated extract of garlic, coix, and rice bran with shark cartilage and vitamin C; garlic is well-known for its ability to inhibit bacteria, fungi, yeast (including *Candida*), and parasites (protozoa and worms), promote immune function, lower cholesterol, reduce platelet aggregation, and aid digestion.
KENSHIN TRADING CORP., P.O. Box 7511, Torrance, CA 90504; tel: 800-766-1313 or 310-212-3199.

KB-Kidney/Bladder: Tablets. Assists in eliminating toxic buildup in the kidneys and bladder, thereby supporting their healthy functioning; contains elecampane root, juniper, parsley, uva ursi, corn silk, cranberry, dandelion, and seaweed.
NATURAL ENERGY PRODUCTS, 21101 Welch Road, Snohomish, WA 98296; tel: 425-486-5956.

KB Formula: Capsules. Ingredients include juniper berries, parsley, ginger root, uva ursi leaves, marshmallow root, cramp bark (*Viburnum opulus*), and goldenseal root, which help provide balance and support for bodily functions.
NATURE'S WAY PRODUCTS, INC., 10 Mountain Springs Parkway, Springville, UT 84663; tel: 800-962-8873 or 801-489-1500.

Kidney Aid: Capsules. Improves circulation to the kidneys, helping them to eliminate accumulated debris; ingredients include cleavers, goldenrod tops, horsetail, hydrangea root, plantain leaf, and kidney glandular substance.
RIDGECREST HERBALS, 1151 South Redwood Road #106, Salt Lake City, UT 84104 3729; tel: 800-242-4649 or 801-978-9633.

Kidney Glandular Plus: Tablets. Blend of nutrients and herbs designed to nutritionally support healthy kidney function and urination.
ETHICAL NUTRIENTS, 971 Calle Negocio, San Clemente, CA 92673; tel: 800-668-8743 or 949-366-0818.

Kyo-Dophilus: Capsules or tablets. Tablets contain one strain of the beneficial bacteria *L. acidophilus*; capsules contain three strains of beneficial bacteria (*L. acidophilus*, *B. bifidum*, and *B. longum*) to help to normalize the intestinal flora.

WAKUNAGA OF AMERICA, 23501 Madero, Mission Viejo, CA 92691; tel: 800-421-2998 or 949-855-2776.

Nephrochel: Capsules. Contains magnesium and potassium citrates, lipoic acid, glutamic acid, vitamin K, the botanicals uva ursi and aloe vera, and glycosaminoglycans that help keep the interior lining of the urinary tract smooth, slippery, elastic, and flexible.

ECOLOGICAL FORMULAS, 1061-B Shary Circle, Concord, CA 94518; tel: 800-888-4585 or 925-827-2636.

Viral Infections

Viruses attach themselves to the cells of their host in order to multiply, taking over these cells to varying degrees, depending on the kind of viruses; some viruses kill the cells they occupy. The viral microorganism has a protective protein shell which renders many drugs ineffective against it because they cannot penetrate the shell. Viruses cannot be killed by antibiotics, for example.

Several hundred viruses cause a wide range of diseases, many of which produce only low-grade, subclinical symptoms. Among the more well-known of the multitude of viruses are influenza, mumps, herpes, hepatitis, Epstein-Barr, and Coxsackie viruses (a group of viruses that particularly affect infants and children).

As is true of bacterial and fungal infections, viruses only gain a hold in the body when immunity is compromised by stress, toxic overload, chronic allergies, or the many other factors which suppress immune function.

Symptoms of Viral Infections

Normally systemic rather than localized (as with many bacterial infections), viral infections are characterized by fever, chills, generalized aches and pains, sensitivity to cold, lowered white-blood-cell count, fatigue, and general weakness.

Nutrients and Herbs for Viral Infections

Given that viruses thrive when the immune system is weak, an important part of treatment is strengthening the immune system. We recommend avoiding sugar and limiting your consumption of fats (these do not include essential fatty acids); research has demonstrated that dietary sugars decrease immunity and a low-fat diet can increase resistance to infection.[201] Further, deficiencies in vitamin A or the B vitamins (particularly B5, B6, and folic acid) impair immunity and increase susceptibility to infection. Vitamin A, as well as vitamin E and essential fatty acids, enhance immune response.

The following supplements and herbs are also useful in working against a viral infection:

■ **Vitamin C and zinc:** vitamin C reduces the severity and duration of viral infections, including the common cold; zinc has the same effects on a cold.[202]

■ **Astragalus:** strengthens the body's ability to resist infection and reduces the frequency and length of colds and other viral conditions.

■ **Garlic:** helps in fighting infectious agents, including viruses.

■ **Grapefruit seed extract:** antibiotic for viral infections; can be used topically or internally.

■ **Olive leaf extract:** antibacterial and antiviral; effective against numerous viruses, including herpes, influenza, and Coxsackie virus.[203]

■ **Quercetin:** antiviral bioflavonoid (antioxidant plant pigment) that appears to inhibit both the ability of viruses to infect and to replicate.[204]

■ **Tea tree oil:** antiseptic; assists in fighting a broad range of infectious agents, including viruses.

Products for Viral Infections

ACES Gold: Tablets. Antioxidant formula that contains coenzyme Q10, vitamins A, C, and E, and glutathione peroxidase support (selenium, glutathione, and N-acetyl-cysteine), superoxide dismutase support (zinc, copper, and manganese), alpha-lipoic acid, citrus bioflavonoids, quercetin bioflavonoid, and odorless garlic (*Allium sativum*).

J.R. CARLSON LABS, INC., 15 College Drive, Arlington Heights, IL 60004-1985; tel: 800-323-4141 or 708-255-1600.

Advance Multi-Vitamin and Minerals: Capsules. Contains naturally derived vitamins, organic mineral citrates, pure plant enzymes (helps the body break down and absorb nutrients from the diet), and other ingredients for maximum absorption and activity in the body; also available in iron-free formula.

PREVAIL CORP., 2204-8 Northwest Birdsdale, Gresham, OR 97030; tel: 800-248-0885 or 503-667-5527.

AminoMune: Capsules. Formula rich in the amino acid L-lysine and 18 pharmaceutical-grade, isolated L-crystalline amino acids; helpful for viral infections, such as cold sores and fever blisters.

NUTRI-SOURCE, 3290 Cessna Drive, Cameron Park, CA 95682; tel: 800-293-1683 or 530-676-8838.

Anti-Bio Caps: Capsules or liquid. Herbal formula that has antiviral, antibacterial, and antiseptic properties; ingredients include echinacea, goldenseal, capsicum, marshmallow, black walnut hulls, elecampane, propolis, myrrh gum, turmeric, and potassium chloride.

CRYSTAL STAR HERBAL NUTRITION, 4069 Wedgeway Court, Earth City, MO 63045; tel: 800-736-6015 or 314-739-7551.

Astragalus Formula: Liquid and tablets. Provides support for immune deficiency and chronic viral infections and is a lung tonic for people with a history of chronic respiratory problems; increases recovery and energy after colds, flu, and illness; part of an herbal rotational program that also includes Insure Herbal, an echincea and goldenseal formula.

ZAND HERBAL FORMULAS, 1722 14th Street #230, Boulder, CO 80302; tel: 800-800-0405 or 303-786-8558.

Begone: Liquid. Herbal remedy for viral, yeast, fungal, and bacterial control; contains concentrated glycerine extract of echinacea, lovage root, and myrrh gum with herbal dilution and flower essences.

OLYMPIC BOTANICALS, 231 Otto Street, Port Townsend, WA 98368; tel: 800-558-7372 or 360-385-9468.

BioBoost: Capsules. Dietary supplement that combines herbs such as echinacea and goldenseal with antioxidant vitamins and minerals to support the body's own defenses.

BIODYNAMAX, 6525 Gunpark Drive #150-507, Boulder, CO 80301; tel: 800-926-7525 or 303-530-4665.

BioPro Thymic Protein A: Sublingual powder. Activates T4 cells (white blood cells vital for immunity), increases the number of properly functioning T4 cells, and allows the body to fight off infections ranging from flu to herpes; useful in chronic fatigue syndrome and any illness involving weakened immunity; contains purified, intact thymus protein.

KLABIN MARKETING, 2067 Broadway #700, New York, NY 10023; tel: 800-933-9440 or 212-877-3632.

Buffered Vitamin C Powder or Beet Source "Buffered Vitamin C": Capsules or powder. Contains ascorbic acid, derived from a hypoallergenic, non-corn source, and buffered with the carbonates of potassium, calcium, and magnesium; some severely ill, allergic, or hypersensitive people are able to tolerate this product if unable to tolerate other vitamin C products.

ALLERGY RESEARCH GROUP/NUTRICOLOGY, P.O. Box 55907, Hayward, CA 94544; tel: 800-545-9960 or 510-487-8526.

Cat's Claw Defense Complex: Tablets. Combines cat's claw with reishi mushroom, the herbs pau d'arco, aloe vera, St. John's wort, astragalus, and two categories of antioxidants.

SOURCE NATURALS, THRESHOLD ENTERPRISES, 23 Janis Way, Scotts Valley, CA 95066; tel: 800-777-5677 or 831-438-1144.

Cat's Claw Plus Ezseac Tea: Liquid. Contains cat's claw concentrated tea combined with a formula of distilled water, burdock root, sheep sorrel, slippery elm bark, water cress, and turkey rhubarb root.

PERUVIAN RAINFOREST BOTANICALS, NUTRAMEDIX, 212 North U.S. Highway 1 #17, Tequesta, FL 33469; tel: 800-730-3130.

Colloidal Silver: Liquid. Combination of minute, electrically charged particles of silver and pure water, which work as an antibiotic and immune-system enhancer; useful internally for common colds and flu and externally for cuts and abrasions.

NUPRO, 735-L Park Street, Castle Rock, CO 80104; tel: 800-704-8910 or 303-660-0562.

Deep Defense: Caplets or liquid. Contains Chinese herbs known as *qi* (also referred to as *chi*, vital life energy) tonics traditionally used to support the body after long-term weakness or chronic deficiency; also includes the healing mushrooms reishi and shiitake plus astragalus.

RAINBOW LIGHT, P.O. Box 600, Santa Cruz, CA 95061; tel: 800-635-1233 or or 408-429-9089.

Echatin Forte: Capsules. Blends extracts of herbs and mushrooms in an echinacea formula; like echinacea, the Chinese herb astragalus contains potent polysaccharides, as do reishi and shiitake mushrooms.

NF FORMULAS, INC. 9755 Southwest Commerce Circle, C-5, Wilsonville, OR 97070; tel: 800-547-4891 or 503-682-9755.

Echinacea Astragalus: Capsules or liquid. Enhances natural resistance.

FRONTIER COOPERATIVE HERBS, 3021 78th Street, Norway, IA 52318; tel: 800-669-3275 or 319-227-7996.

Echinacea/Astragalus/Reishi: Capsules. Helpful during the winter season; ingredients include certified organically grown *Echinacea pur-*

purea, astragalus root, and reishi (*Ganoderma lucidum*) mushroom.
NATURE'S WAY PRODUCTS, INC., 10 Mountain Springs Parkway, Springville, UT 84663; tel: 800-962-8873 or 801-489-1500 .

Echinacea Glycerites: Liquid. Sweet glycerin alternative to traditional liquid extract supplements, which often have a bitter, pungent taste that is difficult for many people, especially children, to ingest.
PLANETARY FORMULAS, 23 Janis Way, Scotts Valley, CA 95066; tel: 800-606-6226.

Echinacea Goldenseal: Capsules or liquid. Provides resistance during cold and flu season.
FRONTIER COOPERATIVE HERBS, 3021 78th Street, Norway, IA 52318; tel: 800-669-3275 or 319-227-7996.

Echinacea-Goldenseal Combination: Capsules. Herbal dietary supplement providing the benefits of echinacea and other herbs.
NATURE'S HERBS, 600 East Quality Drive, American Fork, UT 84003; tel: 800-437-2257 or 801-763-0700.

Echinacea • Goldenseal Compound: Liquid. Remedy for colds and flu accompanied by nasal congestion and other respiratory symptoms; can also be used as a strengthening, preventative tonic for those susceptible to colds and flu; ingredients include echinacea root, goldenseal rhizome and roots, osha root, spilanthes flowering herb and root, yerba santa leaf, horseradish root, elder flower, yarrow flower, watercress herb, and wild indigo root.
HERB PHARM, 20260 Williams Highway, Williams, OR 97544; tel: 800-348-4372 or 541-846-6262.

Echinashield: Chewable tablets or liquid. Ingredients include echinacea, the antioxidant vitamins A, B6, and C, plus zinc; available in assorted flavors.
NF FORMULAS INC., 9755 Southwest Commerce Circle, C-5, Wilsonville, OR 97070; tel: 800-547-4891 or 503-682-9755.

E.H.B.: Capsules. Blend of echinacea, goldenseal, and berberis (which have been standardized to ensure potency of active ingredients) with herbs and vitamins, including vitamin C, beta carotene, and zinc.
NF FORMULAS INC., 9755 Southwest Commerce Circle, C-5, Wilsonville, OR 97070; tel: 800-547-4891 or 503-682-9755.

E-mergen-C: Powder. Replenishes electrolytes and minerals, and fights off free-radical damage; contains vitamin C mineral ascorbates, vitamins B1, B2, B6, and B12, potassium, magnesium, manganese, calcium, zinc, and chromium.

ALACER CORP., 19631 Pauling, Foothill Ranch, CA 92610; tel: 800-854-0249 or 949-454-3900.

Essiac: Tea. Nontoxic herbal remedy, which contains inulin, starch occurring in certain plants. Inulin is an immune system modulator that attaches to white blood cells (T cells) and makes them work better; ingredients include burdock root, slippery elm, sheep sorrel, and Indian rhubarb, which together help normalize body systems by purifying the blood, promoting cell repair, and aiding effective assimilation and elimination.

ESSIAC INTERNATIONAL, 164 Richmond Road, Ottowa, Ontario, Canada K1Z 6W1; tel: 613-729-9111.

Ester-C: Vegitabs. Ester C, a special form of vitamin C, is bound to calcium to create a calcium ascorbate complex; non-acidic (pH neutral); also contains naturally occuring metabolites of vitamin C and active bioflavonoids.

COUNTRY LIFE, 101 Corporate Drive, Hauppauge, NY 11788; tel: 800-645-5768 or 516-231-1031.

Ester C Plus: Capsules. Non-acidic form of vitamin C, which possesses healing, antioxidant, antihistamine, anti-inflammatory, and immune-enhancing properties; strengthens blood vessels; and normalizes high cholesterol.

PHILLIPS NUTRITIONALS, 27071 Cabot Road #122, Laguna Hills, CA 92653; tel: 800-514-5115 or 702-898-8141.

Esterol With Ester-C: Capsules. Contains ester C, water-soluble antioxidant bioflavonoids (quercetin, rutin, and proanthocyanidins from grape seed), and calcium; highly absorbable and non-acidic, making it minimally irritating to the intestines for those with sensitive digestive systems.

ALLERGY RESEARCH GROUP/NUTRICOLOGY, P.O. Box 55907, Hayward, CA 94544; tel: 800-545-9960 or 510-487-8526.

Garlic, Echinacea, Goldenseal Plus: Tablets. Contains echinacea extract and an echinacea herbal blend, plus goldenseal and garlic for overall immune support.

FUTUREBIOTICS, 145 Ricefield Lane, Hauppauge, NY 11788; tel: 800-FOR-LIFE (367-5433) or 516-273-6300.

Garlic-Power: Tablets. Concentrated garlic extract from a Chinese formula of red and white garlic equivalent to 1,200 mg of fresh garlic; contains higher allicin potential (minimum 3 mg of total allicin potential calculated as allicin content and relative allinase enzyme activity per tablet) than any other garlic supplement; odor-controlled.

NATURE'S HERBS, 600 East Quality Drive, American Fork, UT 84003; tel: 800-437-2257 or 801-763-0700.

Garlic Power Rx: Softgels. Contains organic garlic that is five times more potent than fresh garlic, plus vitamin E, hawthorn berry, and parsley.

PHYTO-THERAPY, INC., OPTIMUM HEALTH, 483 West Middle Turnpike, Manchester, CT 06040; tel: 800-228-1507.

Garlinase 4000: Tablets. Daily supplement that contains beneficial allicin (the active component of garlic) while promising odor-free breath.

ENZYMATIC THERAPY, 825 Challenger Drive, Green Bay, WI 54311-8328; tel: 800-558-7372 or 920-469-1313.

GSE Liquid Concentrate (Grapefruit Seed Extract): Capsules, liquid, or tablets. Use internally as a dental, nasal, ear, and vaginal rinse, and throat gargle or externally as a facial cleanser, skin rinse, nail and scalp treatment, and all-purpose cleaner (for toothbrushes, vegetables, fruits, meats, dishes, utensils, and cutting boards).

NUTRIBIOTIC, NUTRITION RESOURCES INC., P.O. Box 238, Lakeport, CA 95453; tel: 800-225-4345 or 707-263-0411.

Health-Gard With Echinacea: Capsules. Helps strengthen the body's natural defenses; contains beta carotene, vitamins C and E, zinc, selenium, blended with echinacea, white willow, odorless garlic, astragalus, reishi and shiitake mushrooms, pau d'arco, goldenseal root, broccoli, selenium, and the amino acid L-methionine.

NATURE'S HERBS, 600 East Quality Drive, American Fork, UT 84003; tel: 800-437-2257 or 801-763-0700.

Herbal Aloe Force: Juice or topical gel. Processed aloe vera juice containing vitamins, minerals, enzymes, amino acids, essential fatty acids, growth factors, glycoproteins, sterols, bioflavonoids, and polysaccharides (complex sugars), plus ionized colloidal silver and herbal extracts (cat's claw, chamomile, burdock root, hawthorn berry, astragalus root, sheep sorrell, pau d'arco bark, slippery elm bark, and rhubarb root).

HERBAL ANSWERS INC., P.O. Box 1110, Saratoga Springs, NY 12866; tel: 888-256-3367 or 518-581-1968.

Herbal Defense: Liquid. Contains extracts of echinacea, Siberian ginseng, and astragalus; also contains the support herbs burdock, dandelion, angelica, ginger, rosemary, peppermint, sage, goldenseal, chamomile, licorice, and reishi and shiitake mushrooms in a base of purified water, brown rice syrup, honey natural flavor, natural color, and 20% USP alcohol.

NATURE'S APOTHECARY, P.O. Box 17970, Boulder, CO 80308; tel: 800-999-7422 or 303-664-1600.

Immune-Action: Capsules. Ingredients include astragalus root, lingustrum berries, schisandra fruit, shiitake mushroom, echinacea root, young barley leaves, and pau d'arco bark.

NATURE' S PLUS, 548 Broadhollow Road, Melville, NY 11747-3708; tel: 800-645-9500 or 516-293-0030.

Immune Formula: Tablets. Contains carotenoids, vitamins A, C, and E, selenium, echinacea, zinc, and ginseng, which help to maintain strong, healthy immune function.

NATURE'S LIFE, 7180 Lampson Avenue, Garden Grove, CA 92841-3914; tel: 800-854-6837 or 714-379-6500.

Immune-Neem by Farmacopia: Capsules or tea. Contains neem leaf (a mainstay of the Ayurvedic health system of India; laboratory studies have shown its antibacterial, antifungal, and antiviral activities), ginger, stevia, peppermint, lemon grass, cinnamon, licorice, and natural flavors.

BOTANICAL PRODUCTS INTERNATIONAL, P.O. Box 174, Hakalau, HI 96710; tel: 808-963-6771.

Katsu Herbal Garlic Complex: Tablets. Concentrated extract of garlic, coix, and rice bran, with shark cartilage and vitamin C; garlic is well-known for its ability to inhibit bacteria, fungi, yeast (including *Candida*), and parasites (protozoa and worms), promote immune functions, lower cholesterol, reduce platelet aggregation (abnormal blood clotting), and aid digestion.

KENSHIN TRADING CORP., P.O. Box 7511, Torrance, CA 90504; tel: 800-766-1313 or 310-212-3199.

Monolauren: Capsules. Monolaurin (lauricidin) is a patented ester of lauric acid, a fatty acid found naturally in coconut milk, which can dissolve the lipid envelope of a virus making it difficult for the virus to replicate.

ECOLOGICAL FORMULAS, 1061-B Shary Circle, Concord, CA 94518; tel: 800-888-4585 or 925-827-2636.

Multi Mushroom Complex: Capsules. Contains Kombucha (a cultured tea), shiitake, maitake, and reishi mushrooms; helpful for cardiovascular, immune, and endocrine systems.

SCHIFF, WEIDER NUTRITION GROUP, 2002 South 5070 West, Salt Lake City, UT 84104; tel: 800-439-8042 or 801-975-5000.

#1 Garlic Plus Ester-C and FOS: Capsules. Contains garlic, an important herb for the immune and cardiovascular systems, ester C, vitamin C, and FOS (fructo-oligosacchrides, which support the friendly intestinal bacteria).

NUTRITION NOW, 501 Southeast Columbia Shore Boulevard #350, Vancouver, WA 98661; tel: 800-929-0418 or 360-737-6800.

Olive Leaf Extract: Capsules. Contains 250 mg of extract guaranteed to contain a minimum of 17% (42.5 mg) of the active compound, oleuropein.

SOLARAY, NUTRACEUTICAL CORP., P.O. Box 681869, Park City, UT 84068; tel: 800-669-8877.

Oxy-Caps by Earth's Bounty. Releases molecular oxygen once it comes in contact with the stomach's hydrochloric acid; increased levels of oxygen can help the body work more efficiently and boost the immune system; research has reported that stabilized oxygen is an effective disinfectant against some viruses, bacteria, and fungi.

MATRIX HEALTH PRODUCTS, 8400 Magnolia Avenue, Suite N, Santee, CA 92071; tel: 800-736-5609 or 619-448-7550.

OxyEssence: Liquid. Stabilized oxygen plus homeopathic trace elements, flowers, and botanical essences, which help kill viruses, yeasts, fungi, and anaerobic bacteria, including *Streptococcus* and *Cryptosporidium.*

OLYMPIC BOTANICALS, 231 Otto Street, Port Townsend, WA 98368; tel: 800-310-6924 or 360-385-9468.

Oxy-Max by Earth's Bounty: Liquid. High potency, stabilized oxygen supplement that provides electrolytes of stabilized oxygen, a form readily utilized by the body. A shortage of oxygen in the body leaves it susceptible to bacterial, fungal, and viral infections, as well as a loss of mental acuity.

MATRIX HEALTH PRODUCTS, 8400 Magnolia Avenue, Suite N, Santee, CA 92071; tel: 800-736-5609 or 619-448-7550.

Oxystat: Capsules. Contains major antioxidants, NAC (N-acetyl-cysteine), standardized green tea (50% catechins), standardized silymarin, choline, methionine, amino acids, glutathione, chlorophyll, coenzyme Q10, calcium D-glucarate, and other nutritional cofactors.

NF FORMULAS INC., 9755 Southwest Commerce Circle, C-5, Wilsonville, OR 97070; tel: 800-547-4891 or 503-682-9755.

Reishi Mushroom Supreme: Tablets. *Fu Zheng* herbs, also known as adaptogens, are used to strengthen resistance, restore the normal functioning of the body, and protect against stress; contains concentrated mature reishi extract, reishi mycelia (the vegetative part of the mushroom), shiitake mushroom, astragalus, schisandra, grifola, and poria cocos.

PLANETARY FORMULAS, 23 Janis Way, Scotts Valley, CA 95066; tel: 800-606-6226.

Royal Scandinavian Colloidal Silver 500 ppm: Liquid. Highest-quality silver with a fine particle size to ensure maximum permeability through body tissues; can be used internally or as a sinus flush; *acidophilus* should be used after administration.

BIO-NUTRITIONAL FORMULAS, 106 East Jericho Turnpike, Mineola, NY 11501; tel: 800-950-8484.

Silver: Liquid. Electro-processsed and chemical-free; ingredients include de-ionized water and colloidal silver, which is tasteless, non-toxic, and contains no artificial ingredients, preservatives, or additives.

FUTUREBIOTICS, 145 Ricefield Lane, Hauppauge, NY 11788; tel: 800-FOR-LIFE (367-5433) or 516-273-6300.

SP-21 Echinacea-Goldenseal Blend: Capsules. Ingredients include *Echinacea purpurea* root, goldenseal root, myrrh gum, garlic, licorice root, vervain, butternut bark, and kelp with a homeopathically prepared mineral formula.

SOLARAY, NUTRACEUTICAL CORP., P.O. Box 681869, Park City, UT 84068; tel: 800-669-8877.

Squalene: Softgels. Squalene is an extract from the liver of the Aizame shark; increases new tissue growth (granulation which covers wounds), supports the activity of the liver, acts as an adaptogen similar to ginseng and antioxidants, stimulates the defensive forces of the body, and enhances the resistance to immune system disorders.

OPTIMAL NUTRIENTS, 1163 Chess Drive #F, Foster City, CA 94404; tel: 800-966-8874 or 650-525-0112.

Wellness Formula: Tablets. Contains large doses of vitamin C, antioxidants, herbs, and other vitamins and ingredients to provide nutritional protection during the winter months and throughout the year.

SOURCE NATURALS, THRESHOLD ENTERPRISES, 23 Janis Way, Scotts Valley, CA 95066; tel: 800-777-5677 or 831-438-1144.

Weight, Excess

Weight loss is a national obsession in the United States. At any given time, 40% of women and 24% of men are trying to lose weight through diets, exercise, behavior modification, drugs, and other weight-loss methods. Behind this obsession is a physical reality—one-quarter to one-third of Americans are overweight, and obesity has been linked to numerous health conditions, including heart disease, high blood pressure, diabetes, gallbladder disease, respiratory conditions, complications of pregnancy, and even certain cancers.[205]

There are many factors that contribute to an inability to lose weight and keep it off, including underlying organic dysfunction such as a hormonal imbalance in thyroid, insulin (which enables the body to utilize sugar and carbohydrates), or other hormones.

See **Diabetes**, pp. 160-163, **Thyroid Conditions**, pp. 391-393, **Gastrointestinal Disorders**, pp. 198-217, and **Detoxification** in Part III, pp. 446-461.

Metabolism (conversion of food into energy) and the utilization of fats also affect weight. People who are trying to lose unwanted pounds need to be conscious of their fat intake in relation to their individual metabolic rate. Fat is not easily or fully burned and utilized; if the metabolism is sluggish (which can be due to a thyroid problem) or if certain nutrients (such as the enzyme lipase) aren't available to properly digest and utilize fat, the body stores it as a source for future energy.

Poor digestion and elimination can also contribute to excess weight. An overload of toxins in the colon and/or liver can make it difficult for a person to break down fat and lose weight; most adults have between five and 40 pounds of toxic residues amassed on their intestinal walls. Dietary practices obviously have an integral role in the health of digestion and the buildup of toxins in the colon. Other lifestyle components, such as exercise and psychological and emotional issues, involved in weight gain are also important to consider.

With these factors in mind, we recommend the following: a diet containing as few processed foods as possible and no animal fats; six to eight 8-ounce glasses of pure, filtered water daily; regular, significant exercise; thyroid glandular extracts and other nutritional support for a sluggish thyroid, if needed; and counseling, stress reduction, or other approaches to help address underlying emotional causes of weight gain.

Nutrients and Herbs for Excess Weight

Appetite Suppressants—By providing assimilable proteins that balance and stabilize blood sugar, free-form amino acids and spirulina and other blue-green algae help suppress the appetite; blue-green algae is rich in other nutrients as well. Ephedra *(ma huang)* is also an appetite suppressant; its primary function in weight loss, however, seems to be in increasing the metabolic rate of fat tissue.[206]

General Weight Loss Nutrients

■ **Fiber:** fiber products (such as psyllium or guar gum) mixed with water or juice produce a gelatinous mass that, when taken before a meal, creates a feeling of fullness and thus reduces appetite. This mixture also assists in controlling blood sugar, decreasing the number of calories absorbed, and cleaning out the intestinal tract.[207] Colon cleansing is an important part of any weight-loss program. Supplementing with fiber compared to only reducing calories can result in 50% to 100% more weight loss.[208] (Note: The absorption of nutritional supplements or other medications into the body may be decreased by fiber, so they should be taken at least an hour before or after fiber intake.)

■ **Essential fatty acids:** supplementing with essential fatty acids (EFAs) assists the body in breaking down dietary fats, cholesterol, triglycerides (neutral fats, see below), and stored body fats. Gamma-linolenic acid (GLA), the EFA in evening primrose, borage, and black currant seed oils, has been shown to help control the appetite.[209]

■ **Medium-chain triglycerides (MCTs):** saturated fats found in milk fat and palm kernel and coconut oils, MCTs are easily absorbed and quickly metabolized, so they are not stored as fat in tissues. They can help reverse fat malabsorption problems.[210] Unlike other saturated fats, MCTs do not appear to cause weight gain and actually increase the rate at which calories are burned.

■ **Chromium picolinate:** assists in weight loss by promoting lean (muscle) body mass, seemingly by increasing the body's sensitivity to insulin, which results in improved sugar and carbohydrate metabolism.[211]

■ **Coenzyme Q10:** deficiencies may be a factor in some cases of obesity since coQ10 is integral to the manufacture of energy.[212]

Pregnant women or people with high blood pressure or heart disease should not use ephedra.

■ **Kelp:** rich in minerals and iodine, which support the thyroid and enhance fat-burning during exercise.[213]

■ **Lipase enzymes:** aid in weight loss by breaking down dietary fats for proper utilization by the body and thereby improving digestion as well.

■ **Malabar tamarind** (*Garcinia*): its active ingredient, hydroxycitric acid (HCA), is proving effective for weight management by curbing appetite and inhibiting fat formation; HCA is found in a number of natural diet products.[214]

■ **Wild yam:** contains DHEA (SEE QUICK DEFINITION), low levels of DHEA have been linked to obesity.[215]

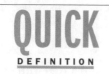

DEFINITION

DHEA (dehydroepiandrosterone) is naturally produced by the human adrenal glands and gonads, with optimal levels occurring around age 20 for women and age 25 for men. After those ages, DHEA levels gradually decline so that a person 80 years old produces only a fraction of the DHEA they did when they were 20. As an antioxidant, hormone regulator, and the building block from which estrogen and testosterone are produced, DHEA is vital to health. Test subjects using supplemental DHEA reported improved sleeping patterns, better memory, an improved ability to cope with stress, decreased joint pain, increases in lean muscle, and decreases in body fat. No serious side effects have been reported to date, although acne, oily skin, facial hair growth on women, deepening of the voice, irritability, insomnia, and fatigue have been reported with high DHEA doses.

Products for Excess Weight

Aqua-Trim: Capsules. Gentle diuretic with potassium for relief of the bloating, puffiness, and fatigue associated with periods; ingredients include uva ursi, natural caffeine, potassium, and the extracts of buchu leaf, juniper berry, and horse chestnut seed.

NATURE'S HERBS, 600 East Quality Drive, American Fork, UT 84003; tel: 800-437-2257 or 801-763-0700.

Basic #3: Tablets. Contains essential nutritional support and nutrients that help control food urges; contains chromium polynicotinate.

ATKINS NUTRITIONALS, INC., 185 Oser Avenue, Hauppauge, NY 11788; tel: 800-628-5467 or 516-951-7171; or CANADIAN AMERICAN RESOURCES, 327 West Fayette Street, Suite 211, Syracuse, NY 13202; tel: 315-476-4944.

Calorie Burners: Caplets. Boosts metabolism, increases caloric expenditure without ephedra or caffeine; provides green orange extract and *Panax ginseng* extract for metabolic stimulation, red pepper and cinnamon powder as thermogenic (promoting heat production in the body to burn fat rather than store it) and digestive aids, and parsley as an herbal diuretic.

SYNERGY PLUS, IVC, 500 Halls Mill Road, Freehold, NJ 07728; tel: 800-666-8482.

Celium: Powder. Daily supplement of soluble fiber to aid regularity; celium contains 98% pure psyllium husks for maximum bulking (contains 2% seed particles).

SIERRA HEALTH PRODUCTS, INC., 7949 Woodley Avenue, Van Nuys, CA 91406; tel: 818-375-5029.

Cellu-Stop: Capsules. Controls formation of cellulite (subcutaneous fatty deposits) and reduces existing deposits; contains herbs that break down cellulite and help flush it from the system.

NATURE'S PRIDE, NATURE'S PRODUCTS, 1301 Sawgrass Corporation Parkway, Sunrise, FL 33323-2813; tel: 800-752-7873 or 954-233-4600.

Chitosan: Capsules. Dietary fiber derived from chitin, an aminopolysaccharide found in the shells of various shellfish.

SOURCE NATURALS, THRESHOLD ENTERPRISES, 23 Janis Way, Scotts Valley, CA 95066; tel: 800-777-5677 or 831-438-1144.

Chromium Power-Herb: Capsules. Glycemic-edge formula providing chromium and nutrients blended with *Gymnema sylvestre* extract.

NATURE'S HERBS, 600 East Quality Drive, American Fork, UT 84003; tel: 800-437-2257 or 801-763-0700.

CitriMax: Capsules. Derived from the dried rind (pericarp) of tamarind (*Garcinia cambogia*), a natural appetite suppressant.

SPORTS ONE INC., 47 Capital Drive, Wallingford, CT 06492; tel: 800-624-8787 or 203-294-6370.

Citrimax-Power: Capsules. Combines *Garcinia cambogia* extract (standardized to 50% hydroxycitric acid), a fat-metabolizing component of *Garcinia* with chromium picolinate.

NATURE'S HERBS, 600 East Quality Drive, American Fork, UT 84003; tel: 800-437-2257 or 801-763-0700.

Day Time Body Management: Caplets. Combination of thermogenic (helps increase fat-burning) herbs, minerals, and amino acids, which help manage weight, energy, mental clarity, appetite, and blood-sugar regulation; contains ephedra (*ma huang*), white willow, kola nut, ginger, bladderwrack, *Ginkgo biloba*, gotu kola, saw palmetto (*Serenoa repens*), ginseng, L-carnitine, chromium picolinate, choline, boron citrate, and zinc proteinate.

NUPRO, 735-L Park Street, Castle Rock, CO 80104; tel: 800-704-8910 or 303-660-0562.

Diet by Jade: Tablets. Helps increase metabolic rate, suppress appetite, and decrease water retention; also aids digestion and increases energy. Caution: not recommended for pregnant or nursing mothers.

EAST EARTH HERB, INC., P.O. Box 2802, Eugene, OR 97402; tel: 800-827-HERB (4372) or 541-687-0155.

Diet-Phen: Tablets. Herbal dieting aid that contains St. John's wort, phenylalanine (an essential amino acid that is converted by the body into tyrosine), chromium, and low levels of ephedra.

SOURCE NATURALS, THRESHOLD ENTERPRISES, 23 Janis Way, Scotts Valley, CA 95066; tel: 800-777-5677 or 831-438-1144.

Diet Power: Vegitabs. Contains nutritional thermogenics and herbs to curb appetite and activate metabolism without stimulants.

COUNTRY LIFE, 101 Corporate Drive, Hauppauge, NY 11788; tel: 800-645-5768 or 516-231-1031.

Diet Pro: Capsules. Aids endurance during strenuous workouts by promoting glucogenesis, the formation of glucose from glycogen (the form in which sugars are stored in the body) to use in energy production, and by increasing energy levels; also contains fat burners and appetite suppressants, such as citrilene (an extract from papaya that is known to burn fat as energy) and carnitine.

UNIVERSAL, 3 Terminal Road, New Brunswick, NJ 08901; tel: 800-872-0101 or 732-545-3130.

Dieter's Advantage: Tablets. Nutritional formula that helps the body's ability to use food for energy and repair instead of storing it as body fat.

ATKINS NUTRITIONALS INC., 185 Oser Avenue, Hauppauge, NY 11788; tel: 800-628-5467 or 516-951-7171; or CANADIAN AMERICAN RESOURCES, 327 West Fayette Street, Suite 211, Syracuse, NY 13202; tel: 315-476-4944.

Dieter's Multiple: Tablets. Contains vitamins and minerals for dietary support.

NATURE'S PRIDE, NATURE'S PRODUCTS, 1301 Sawgrass Corporation Parkway, Sunrise, FL 33323-2813; tel: 800-752-7873 or 954-233-4600.

Diet Support: Tablets. Helps promote lean muscle mass, inhibit fat storage, reduce sugar cravings, and increase energy; ingredients include citrimax (*Garcinia cambogia*), plant cellulose, *Commiphora mukul*, shave grass, *Gymnema sylvestre*, zinc, and chromium.

NUTRITION NOW, 501 Southeast Columbia Shore Boulevard #350, Vancouver, WA 98661; tel: 800-929-0418 or 360-737-6800.

Endurox Excel: Caplets. Contains standardized extract of the herb ciwujia plus the antioxidant vitamin E to help build endurance, raise the lactate threshold, speed workout recovery, and increase cardiac efficiency by lowering heart rate.

PACIFIC HEALTH LABS, INC., 1480 Route 9 North #204, Woodbridge, NJ 07095; tel: 800-39P-ROVE (7-7683).

EnerTrim: Capsules. Supports a healthy weight without stimulants such as ephedra (*ma huang*) or kola nut. HCA (hydroxycitric acid) and Peptide FM (a combination of hydrolyzed bovine globin protein, wheat gluten, and casin) help the body burn rather than store fat, L-carnitine helps transport fatty acids into the body's cells where they can be burned for energy, and chromium supports healthy blood sugar levels.

BIODYNAMAX, 6525 Gunpark Drive #150-507, Boulder, CO 80301; tel: 800-926-7525 or 303-530-4665.

Enzyme & Herbal Formula #2: Capsules. For people who are having trouble losing weight (however, other digestive problems must also be addressed, such as sugar and protein intolerance); contains the enzymes protease, amylase, and lipase, plus the herbs bilberry extract, fenugreek seeds, *Ginkgo biloba* leaf, and dandelion root.

21ST CENTURY NUTRITION, 6421 Enterprise Lane, Madison, WI 53719; tel: 800-662-2630 or 608 273 8100.

Enzyme & Herbal Formula #5: Capsules. Helps decrease a big appetite; contains the digestive enzymes protease, amylase, lipase, and disaccharidases, plus nettle leaf, prickly ash bark, marshmallow root, and rose hips.

21ST CENTURY NUTRITION, 6421 Enterprise Lane, Madison, WI 53719; tel: 800-662-2630 or 608-273-8100.

EverSlender: Capsules. Blend of vegetable, citrus, and herbal fiber that provides a feeling of fullness; also contains uva ursi, shave grass, corn silk, and watermelon seed.

NATURE'S HERBS, 600 East Quality Drive, American Fork, UT 84003; tel: 800-437-2257 or 801-763-0700.

Fat Absorber: Capsules. Combination of soluble and insoluble fiber, which binds to dietary fat and flushes it out of the body; contains psyllium seed husk mucilage.

NATURE'S PRIDE, NATURE'S PRODUCTS, 1301 Sawgrass Corporation Parkway, Sunrise, FL 33323-2813; tel: 800-752-7873 or 954-233-4600.

Fat Burners and Super Fat Burners: Tablets. Blend of lipotropics (substances that metabolize cholesterol and fat), L-carnitine (an amino acid that helps convert body matter into energy), and chromium picolinate (a trace mineral that may help restore the body's sensitivity to insulin and therefore make better use of glucose).

HEALTH PLUS, 13837 Magnolia Avenue, Chino, CA 91710; tel: 800-822-6225 or 909-627-9393.

Fat Enzyme Formula: Capsules. High-lipase digestive supplement that contains pure plant enzymes to help the body digest fats, proteins, carbohydrates, and fiber.

PREVAIL CORP., 2204-8 Northwest Birdsdale, Gresham, OR 97030; tel: 800-248-0885 or 503-667-5527.

5-HTP SeroTonic: Capsules. Scientists have discovered that conditions of depression, carbohydrate cravings (with resultant weight gain), anxiety, sleeplessness, obsessions, and compulsions are all connected to reduced levels of serotonin in the brain—furthermore, if serotonin levels are restored, these conditions often disappear. The amino acid 5-HTP is a metabolic precursor of serotonin, which increases its production and availability; 5-HTP SeroTonic contains 50 mg of 5-HTP per capsule with St. John's wort (10 mg) and 5-pyridoxal phosphate (15 mg), plus cofactors magnesium hydroxide, inositol hexanicotinate, and calcium citrate.

LIFEENHANCEMENT PRODUCTS INC., P.O. Box 751390, Petaluma, CA 94975-1390; tel: 800-543-3873 or 707-762-6144.

FMF # 24: Tablets. Contains L-carnitine, lecithin, bromelain, choline, and inositol, which help with weight loss.

ATKINS NUTRITIONALS, INC., 185 Oser Avenue, Hauppauge, NY 11788; tel: 800-628-5467 or 516-951-7171; or CANADIAN AMERICAN

RESOURCES, 327 West Fayette Street, Suite 211, Syracuse, NY 13202; tel: 315-476-4944.

Grapeseed Oil. A source of medium-chain triglycerides (MCTs), which are saturated fats helpful for weight loss. Diabetics and those with liver disorders should avoid MCTs entirely or use them only under a doctor's supervision.

SPECTRUM NATURALS, 133 Copeland Street, Petaluma, CA 94952; tel: 707-778-8900.

Green Diet Eaze: Vegitabs. Contains chlorella with dahlulin, a complex carbohydrate derived from the root of the dahlia plant, which helps fight hunger and the desire to overeat, as well as providing energy and nourishment while dieting.

COUNTRY LIFE, 101 Corporate Drive, Hauppauge, NY 11788; tel: 800-645-5768 or 516-231-1031.

Heat Wave: Powder and tablets. Two-part thermogenic formula for weight management. Thermo-Lift Powder contains potassium and magnesium phosphates to activate muscle thermogenesis, which supports the body's calorie and fat burning mechanisms; Thermo-Plex Tablets contain a stimulant-free combination of spice extracts traditionally considered thermogenic, balanced with the cooling extract of mint.

RAINBOW LIGHT, P.O. Box 600, Santa Cruz, CA 95061; tel: 800-635-1233 or or 408-429-9089.

Herb Trim: Capsules. Dietary supplement that contains guarana extract, *ma huang* extract, white willow extract, and cayenne.

NATURE'S HERBS, 600 East Quality Drive, American Fork, UT 84003; tel: 800 437 2257 or 801-763-0700.

Lean Body Factors: Tablets. Supplies more than 20 whole food nutrients known for their ability to help the body with weight management.

NEW CHAPTER, 22 High Street, Brattleboro, VT 05301; tel: 800-543-7279 or 802-257-9345.

Lipolysia: Powder. Meal replacement drink that limits the amount of carbohydrates and adds essential fats and proteins derived from whey isolates and glutamine peptides; for dieters and body builders who want to gain lean mass.

ATKINS NUTRITIONALS, INC., 185 Oser Avenue, Hauppauge, NY 11788; tel: 800-628-5467 or 516-951-7171; or CANADIAN AMERICAN RESOURCES, 327 West Fayette Street, Suite 211, Syracuse, NY 13202; tel: 315-476-4944.

Maxi-Lean: Caplets. Diet aid that helps curb appetite; contains standardized extracts of *ma huang* and cholinate, chromium picolinate, vitamin C, potassium, vegetable and fruit concentrates, magnesium aspartate, white willow, and cayenne; useful in a total weight management program (a low-fat diet, exercise, and rest at night). Note: Individuals with diabetes, hypertension, glaucoma, thyroid disease or pregnant/lactating women should consult their physician or health professional prior to using this product.

PHILLIPS NUTRITIONALS, 27071 Cabot Road #122, Laguna Hills, CA 92653; tel: 800-514-5115 or 702-898-8141.

Maxi-Lean Fat Toner With Chromium Picolinate: Caplets. Herbal/vitamin combination that contains fat-burning chromium picolinate and maxi-choline complex, which helps maintain muscle activity and cellular strength.

PHILLIPS NUTRITIONALS, 27071 Cabot Road #122, Laguna Hills, CA 92653; tel: 800-514-5115 or 702-898-8141.

Max Omega: Oil. Contains black currant seed oil, which is the most complete source of essential fatty acids (EFAs); also contains linoleic acid (an omega-6 EFA) and, unlike primrose or borage oil, alpha linolenic acid (ALA, an omega-3 EFA). Also, unlike flaxseed, black currant seed oil contains 18% gamma-linolenic acid (GLA), twice the amount in primrose oil.

BIO-NUTRITIONAL FORMULAS, 106 East Jericho Turnpike, Mineola, NY 11501; tel: 800 950-8484.

MCT Oil. Contains medium-chain triglycerides (MCTs), which, unlike other types of fat, tend to be rapidly burned up rather than stored as fat. Diabetics and those with liver disorders should avoid MCTs entirely or use them only under a doctor's supervision.

SOUND NUTRITION, P.O. Box 555, Dover, ID 83825; tel: 800-844-6645 or 208-263-6183.

More Than A Diet: Tablets. Contains dietary elements for maintaining a lean and healthy body and important daily nutrients, including chromium, lipoactives, amino acid and herbal thermogenic factors, fiber, enzymes, EFAs and appetite and fluid factors.

AMERICAN HEALTH, 4320 Veterans Memorial Highway, Holbrook, NY 11741; tel: 800-445-7137.

Multi-Fiber Complex: Capsules. Contains fiber from five sources plus the herbs licorice root and slippery elm bark; useful as a part of a weight-loss program or as an everyday fiber supplement to help maintain regularity.

NATROL, INC., 21411 Prairie Street, Chatsworth, CA 91311; tel: 818-739-6000.

Nature Cleanse Fiber Diet: Capsules. Contains 77% dietary fiber, which provides a filling effect to reduce appetite.

NATURE'S PLUS, 548 Broadhollow Road, Melville, NY 11747-3708; tel: 800-645-9500 or 516-293-0030.

Night Time Body Manager: Caplets. Combination of 14 amino acids, vitamins, minerals, and herbs to nourish the body while promoting sleep and rest; helps manage stress, fat, and body tone by increasing basal metabolic rate, which is a weight-regulating mechanism.

NUPRO, 735-L Park Street, Castle Rock, CO 80104; tel: 303-660-0562 or 800-704-8910.

Phencal: Tablets. For maintaining a healthy diet by warding off cravings and binge impulses; contains no diuretics or stimulants.

SCHIFF, WEIDER NUTRITION GROUP, 2002 South 5070 West, Salt Lake City, UT 84104; tel: 800-439-8042 or 801-975-5000.

PhosGold: Powder. Creatine-enhanced high-protein powder that provides a formulation of seven protein sources, which assist the building of solid muscle while promoting fat loss.

SPORTS ONE INC., 47 Capital Drive, Wallingford, CT 06492; tel: 800-624-8787 or 203-294-6370.

ProZone: Powder. Fat-reducing drink mix containing 30% protein, 30% fat, and 40% carbohydrate.

NUTRIBIOTIC, NUTRITION RESOURCES, INC., P.O. Box 238, Lakeport, CA 95453; tel: 800-225-4345.

Quick Trim Weight Loss Shakes. Weight-loss formula that contains soy protein and whey protein concentrate, which is vitamin-enriched and contains chromium picolinate, citrimax, and selenium.

CYBERGENICS AMERICA, LLC., 417 Fifth Avenue, New York, NY 10016; tel: 800-635-8970 or 212-252-7782.

Skinny (SK) Formula: Capsules. Herbal dietary fiber supplement to help increase daily fiber consumption and aid in weight loss when used in conjunction with a doctor's diet program and exercise; contains chickweed, vegetable fiber, licorice root, saffron flowers, gotu kola, Norwegian kelp, echinacea root, black walnut hulls, fennel seed, parthenium root, dandelion root, hawthorn berries, and papaya leaves.

NATURE'S HERBS, 600 East Quality Drive, American Fork, UT 84003; tel: 800-437-2257 or 801-763-0700.

Slim and Tone Shake: Powder. Contains vitamins, minerals, and proteins, fortified with ten essential amino acids, extra calcium, magnesium, L-carnitine, and dietary fiber.

SPORTS ONE INC., 47 Capital Drive, Wallingford, CT 06492; tel: 800-624-8787 or 203-294-6370.

Spirulina Herbal Diet: Tablets. A 100% pure green-food formula designed to support weight loss and a balanced metabolism.

RAINBOW LIGHT, P.O. Box 600, Santa Cruz, CA 95061; tel: 800-635-1233 or or 408-429-9089.

SoyDiet Program: Caplets. Weight-loss program to reduce the appetite and increase energy; ingredients include dehydrated, sprouted mungbeans and oatbran, which provide essential nutrients without calories.

SCANDINAVIAN NATURAL HEALTH & BEAUTY PRODUCTS INC., 13 North 7th Street, Perkasie, PA 18944; tel: 800-688-2276.

Sugar Control: Capsules. Contains chromium polynicotinate, amino acids, and herbs designed as a nutritional aid for people concerned about curbing sugar cravings.

NATURE'S PLUS, 548 Broadhollow Road, Melville, NY 11747-3708; tel: 800-645-9500 or 516-293-0030.

Super DietMax: Capsules. Contains thermogenic and support herbs and lipotropics (substances that metabolize cholesterol and fat).

NATURAL MAX, NUTRACEUTICAL CORP., P.O. Box 681869, Park City, UT 84068; tel: 800-669-8877.

Super Fat Control: Caplets. Contains chitosan (a form of fiber derived from shellfish) with citrimax *(Garcinia cambogia)*, L-carnitine, and chromium picolinate to provide nutritive support for normal metabolism of fat.

NATURAL MAX, NUTRACEUTICAL CORP., P.O. Box 681869, Park City, UT 84068; tel: 800-669-8877.

T-Lite: Capsules. Blend of 14 herbs, vitamin B complex, and chromium picolinate, which works by suppressing the appetite, increasing the metabolism, and burning fat; does not contain *ma huang* or any forms of ephedra and is safe for diabetics and patients with high blood pressure and heart problems.

WGI, 35008 Emerald Coast Parkway, 5th Floor, Destin, FL 32541; tel: 800-854-8353 or 850-654-4744.

T-Lite Energy: Capsules. Blend of 12 ingredients (without ephedrine or *ma huang*) helps with losing weight and boosting energy; ingredients include kola nut, ginger root, ginkgo, and gotu kola.

WGI, 35008 Emerald Coast Parkway, 5th Floor, Destin, FL 32541; tel: 800-854-8353 or 850-654-4744.

Trim Pak: Caplets. Helps with weight loss, improved body tone, energy, stress control, rest, and fat control.

NUPRO, 735-L Park Street, Castle Rock, CO 80104; tel: 800-704-8910 or 303-660-0562.

Triphala Herbal Diet Program: Tablets. Contains supplement nutrients and cleansing herbs to promote overall health.

PLANETARY FORMULAS, 23 Janis Way, Scotts Valley, CA 95066; tel: 800-606-6226.

Veg-Omega Organic Borage Oil. Source of essential fatty acids necessary for health, maintaining cell structure, and producing energy; also a source of phytosterols, beta-sistosterin, and phospholipids, which aid in the digestion of fats; contains twice the omega-3 of fish oil.

SPECTRUM NATURALS, 133 Copeland Street, Petaluma, CA 94952; tel: 800-995-2705 or 707-778-8900.

Weight Loss Formulae: Homeopathic liquid. Helps reduce weight that was gained because of depression, eating disorders, and hypertension (high blood pressure).

LIDDELL LABORATORIES, 1036 Country Club Drive, Moraga, CA 94556; tel: 800-460-7733 or 925-377-3000.

Zinc Pico Plus: Tablets. Contains zinc picolinate; picolinic acid absorption is normally produced in the pancreas and forms a complex with zinc, which helps facilitate its absorption through the gastrointestinal wall and into the circulation.

ETHICAL NUTRIENTS, 971 Calle Negocio, San Clemente, CA 92673; tel: 800-668-8743 or 949-366-0818.

Many health conditions
are a result of detrimental lifestyle,
faulty dietary practices,
and the aging process.
While the functioning of the brain,
organs, and circulatory, digestive,
and immune systems tends
to decline over time, healthy habits
and nutritional supplements
can support brain power,
detoxify the body, and help
prevent degenerative diseases
from developing.

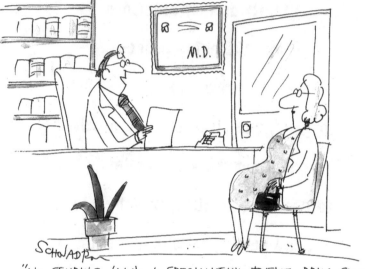

"I'M SENDING YOU TO A SPECIALIST WHO TREATS DRUG SIDE EFFECTS FROM DRUG SIDE EFFECTS."

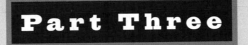

Part Three

Supplements as Preventive Medicine

Brain Power and Longevity

Aging is a fact of life, but many of the health conditions typically associated with aging are more a function of detrimental lifestyle and dietary practices than of aging itself. While the functioning of the brain, organs, and circulatory, digestive, and immune systems does tend to decline with age, healthy habits and nutritional supplements can support brain power, strengthen the body, and help prevent degenerative diseases from developing.

Any chronic burden on the body contributes to an acceleration of the natural aging process, as well as degenerative disorders. Lifestyle factors such as chronic stress, high alcohol consumption, or long-term cigarette smoking are implicated. A high-fat, low-fiber, or high-caloric diet, or excessive sugar or salt intake, are dietary influences on aging. Poor digestion and elimination allow toxins to accumulate in the colon and eventually enter the bloodstream, creating the need for continual immune activation. A buildup in the body of toxins such as environmental chemicals depletes the kidneys and liver, the organs responsible for processing toxins. Finally, the increased presence of free radicals (SEE QUICK DEFINITION) has been linked to both aging and degenerative diseases. This makes it vital to raise your antioxidant (SEE QUICK DEFINITION) intake as you get older.

Nutrients and Herbs for Brain Power and Longevity

To Reduce Free-Radical Damage—The following antioxidant nutrients are helpful: vitamin A, beta carotene, vitamin C, vitamin E, bioflavonoids, pycnogenol, the amino acid cysteine, NADH (coenzyme of vitamin B3), selenium, and zinc; copper, a cofactor for antioxidants, and manganese, an important nutrient in the formation of manganese superoxide dismutase; and the enzymes catalase, glutathione, and superoxide dismutase (SOD).

To Improve Brain Power—Phosphatidyl choline, found in lecithin, is the nutrient precursor to acetylcholine, an important brain chemical involved in both memory and thought. DMAE (dimethylamine ethanol) also promotes the production of acetylcholine and has been shown to increase memory.[1]

Phosphatidyl serine (PS) supports and revitalizes nerve cells and has been shown in numerous studies to slow or reverse cognitive losses attributed to aging.

To Reduce the Effects of Aging—Deficiency of the B vitamins can result in numerous conditions related to the brain and nervous system, including memory loss or impairment, disorientation or confusion, irritability or emotional (mood) swings, fatigue, or depression.[2]

It is estimated that at least 30% of elderly Americans who have been institutionalized are deficient in niacin (vitamin B3).[3] Niacin helps support the healthy functioning of the nervous system (brain and nerves) and the digestive system by lowering cholesterol levels and improving the circulation of blood and oxygen throughout the body.[4]

Numerous observational studies have found insufficient levels of vitamin B6 (pyridoxine) in many elderly Americans. Pyridoxine supports the digestive, immune, and nervous systems, and normal brain function.

Vitamin B12 (cyanocobalamin) supports the formation and maintenance of the covering of the nerves (myelin sheath) throughout the body. It is involved in the formation of the neurotransmitter acetylcholine, which supports cognitive functions such as the ability to learn new concepts and remember them.

Most effective when combined with vitamins C and B12, folic acid is important during the aging process because it provides nourishment for the brain. Folic-acid supports the production of energy in the body, and the production of red and white (immune) blood cells. Supplementing with folic acid is important for preventing or treating folic-acid anemia and it may also help in the treatment of depression.

Fats and oils found in foods are made up of fatty acids. Essential fatty acids (EFAs) are the

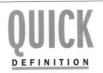

QUICK

DEFINITION

A **free radical** is an unstable, toxic molecule of oxygen with an unpaired electron that steals an electron from another molecule and produces harmful effects. Free radicals are formed when molecules within cells react with oxygen (oxidize) as part of normal metabolic processes. Free radicals then begin to break down cells, especially the cell membranes, often in a matter of minutes to an hour. A single free radical can destroy a cell. While free radicals are normal products of metabolism, uncontrolled free-radical production plays a major role in the development of degenerative disease, including cancer and heart disease.

An **antioxidant** (meaning "against oxidation") is a natural biochemical substance that protects living cells against damage from harmful free radicals. Antioxidants work against the process of oxidation—the robbing of electrons from substances.

Aging is a fact of life, but many of the health conditions typically associated with aging are more a function of detrimental lifestyle and dietary practices than of aging itself.

"healthy" fats required for the proper maintenance of numerous body systems. Our bodies cannot make essential fatty acids; they can only be obtained through dietary sources or nutritional supplements. There are two main types of EFAs: omega-3, which is found in fresh, deep-water fish and in some vegetable oils such as canola or flaxseed; and omega-6, which is found in beans (legumes), nuts, seeds, and unsaturated vegetable oils such as borage and evening primrose. Over 60 different health conditions and disease states can be helped by supplementing the diet with essential fatty acids.[5]

Coenzyme Q10 is a potent antioxidant nutrient found in every cell of the body. It assists the cells (including brain cells) with energy production and has been shown to be very beneficial for treating cardiovascular disease. Coenzyme Q10 is non-toxic and has no side effects if used properly.[6]

The amino acids (building-blocks of protein) responsible for brain and nervous system functions include arginine, glutamine, methionine, phenylalanine, and tryptophan (now available by prescription only). We recommend, unless under the direct supervision of a qualified nutritionist or doctor, that people take free-form, USP, pharmaceutical-grade amino acid formulas containing balanced ratios of individual amino acids.[7]

Ionic minerals (in liquid form) are easily absorbed into the blood through the small intestine. Each ionic mineral (there can be up to 70 in a formula) has either a negative or positive charge and distinguishable properties that allow them to participate as biochemical cofactors in cellular communication, nerve transmission, and/or in the ionic transport of minerals and nutrients across the cell wall. Ionic minerals have the ability to protect the body from the effects of other, toxic minerals which may be absorbed or ingested.[8]

Ginkgo biloba helps to improve the circulation of blood and oxygen to the entire body and the brain. Standardized extracts of ginkgo have been shown in numerous double-blind studies to be able to greatly improve the supply of blood and oxygen to the brain and improve brain function in cases of cerebral dysfunction (dementia related to depression or insufficient blood supply, but not to Alzheimer's disease).[9]

The ginseng root is a potent adaptogenic herb, which assists the body in adapting to both physical and mental stress and protecting against stress-related health conditions. Ginseng also has the ability to improve mental function and stamina as well as physical endurance. Siberian ginseng is most often recommended to improve mental function.[10]

"Green" powder drinks and supplements are called superfoods because they provide a variety of food-based micronutrients. These products usually contain live food concentrates, such as organically grown, freeze-dried barley, wheat, and oat grasses; live plants and organisms, such as chlorella, blue-green algae, and kelp, which are known to be nutritionally high in chlorophyll and an excellent source of minerals (especially iodine) and antioxidant enzymes. Vitamins, minerals, amino acids, adaptogenic herbs, antioxidant nutrients, and other ingredients are also added to green powder drinks.

Green tea, taken as a tea or in a capsule, is a potent natural antioxidant. Numerous studies have shown the antitumor and anticancer properties of green tea. It is a good source of bioflavonoids, which help prevent strokes. Some people report that the small amount of

Alzheimer's Disease

A mental disease of the aged, Alzheimer's disease involves progressive deterioration of intellectual function and memory, disturbances in gait and speech, disorientation, and aggressive behavior.

Causes of Alzheimer's Disease—Both pernicious anemia (a severe form of this blood disease) and cerebral vascular insufficiency (lack of blood supply to the brain due to constricted arteries) can produce a type of senile dementia that is often misdiagnosed as Alzheimer's. Drug reactions, nutritional deficiencies, and systemic overgrowth of Candida albicans are other sources of mental deterioration.[11]

While the causes of Alzheimer's have not been definitively identified, environmental factors—heavy metals, paints, and industrial pollutants—may contribute to mental deterioration. Problematic substances found in foods may have similar effects. These substances include herbicide and pesticide residues, artificial additives, hormones, antibiotics, preservatives, and synthetic or genetically altered ingredients.

Certain food additives called excitotoxins (used to enhance the flavor of food) can cause damage or even kill brain cells through over-stimulation. Experimental studies suggest that long-term consumption of excitotoxins may be associated with Alzheimer's disease, amyotrophic lateral sclerosis (ALS), Huntington's disease, Parkinson's disease, and other neurodegenerative diseases. Examples of excitotoxins found in many food products include aspartame (Nutrasweet®), aspartic acid, hydrolyzed protein, and monosodium glutamate (MSG).[12]

caffeine in green tea improves their ability to think more clearly.[13]

Pycnogenol, an extract derived from grape seeds or pine bark, provides antioxidant protection to the brain and central nervous system. It strengthens blood vessel and capillary walls and improves circulation. Increased blood flow helps prevent ischemia (lack of oxygen due to poor blood flow) in brain tissue and, in turn, reduce mental deterioration.[14]

Other nutrients and herbs known to support brain function and longevity include: *acidophilus*, adequate filtered water, lecithin, acetyl-L-carnitine, germanium, mucopolysaccharides, digestive enzymes, *ashwagandha* (Ayurvedic), bilberry, capsicum, fiber (to promote a clear colon), *fo-ti tieng* (Chinese), garlic, gotu kola, peppermint leaf, rosemary, sarsaparilla, skullcap, and wood betony.

Products for Brain Power and Longevity

ACES Gold: Tablets. Antioxidant formula that contains coenzyme Q10, vitamins A, C, and E, and glutathione peroxidase support (selenium, glutathione, and N-acetyl-cysteine), superoxide dismutase support (zinc, copper, and manganese), alpha-lipoic acid, citrus bioflavonoids, quercetin, and odorless garlic.

J.R. CARLSON LABS INC., 15 College Drive, Arlington Heights, IL 60004-1985; tel: 800-323-4141 or 708-255-1600.

Advanced Antioxidant Formula: Vegicaps. Contains vitamins, minerals, and plant-based antioxidants plus SOD (superoxide dismutase) inducers in a food and herbal base.

SOLGAR VITAMIN & HERB COMPANY INC., 500 Willow Tree Road, Leonia, NJ 07605; tel: 800-645-2246 or 201-944-2311.

Advanced Mature Gold: Tablets. Multivitamin and mineral product for people ages 50 and older; contains higher levels of the most important antioxidants, vitamins, and minerals.

BRONSON LABORATORIES INC., 600 East Quality Drive, American Fork, UT 84003; tel: 800-235-3200 or 801-756-5670.

Advanced Multi-Vitamin and Minerals: Capsules. Contains naturally derived vitamins, organic mineral citrates, pure plant enzymes (helps the body break down and absorb nutrients from the diet), and other ingredients for maximum absorption and activity in the body; also available in an iron-free formula.

PREVAIL CORP., 2204-8 Northwest Birdsdale, Gresham, OR 97030; tel: 800-248-0885 or 503-667-5527.

Antioxidant Formula: Capsules. Contains the beneficial properties of vitamin E and beta carotene (natural, mixed carotenoid complex derived primarily from the sea algae *Dunaliella salina*) in a base of antioxidant-supportive food concentrates, nutrients, and herbs to reduce free-radical formation; other sources of carotenoids include alpha carotene, zeazanthin, cryptoxanthin, and lutein, and whole-food sources of beta carotene such as broccoli, carrot, and blue-green algae; also contains concentrated powdered extracts of grape seed, green tea, and pine bark, which are all proven antioxidants.

ZAND HERBAL FORMULAS, 1722 14th Street #230, Boulder, CO 80302; tel: 800-800-0405 or 303-786-8558.

Amino-Mag 200: Tablets. Contains elemental magnesium as an amino acid chelate (magnesium glycinate/lysinate combination), which can be absorbed intact without gastrointestinal side effects.

AMNI, 2247 National Avenue, Hayward, CA 94540-5012; tel: 800-437-8888 or 510-783-6969.

AminoTrate: Capsules. Complex of 14 isolated L-crystalline amino acids to support mental activities; contains a high concentration of L-glutamine (sometimes called the "thinker's amino") and other amino acids considered to excite brain function.

THURSDAY PLANTATION INC., NATURE'S PLUS, 548 Broadhollow Road, Melville, NY 11747-3708; tel: 800-645-9500 or 516-293-0030.

Baby Boomer Mind: Tablets. Supports brain activity with ginkgo (which has been shown to increase blood flow to the brain and enhance concentration and memory), the hormone pregnenolone, *Panax ginseng*, and phosphatidyl serine (all have been linked to healthy brain function).

AMERIFIT, 166 Highland Park Drive, Bloomfield, CT 06002; tel: 800-990-FIRM (3476) or 860-242-3476.

Balanced B-100: Tablets. Contains B vitamins that work together to convert food into energy and are necessary for the nervous system.

NATURE MADE LLC, NATURE'S RESOURCE, P.O. Box 9606 Mission Hills, CA 91346-9606; tel: 800-314-HERB (4372).

BioEnhance: Capsules. Contains 42 antioxidants, vitamins, minerals, amino acids, and other nutrients determined to be helpful for longevity and cognitive enhancement.

LifeEnhancement Products Inc., P.O. Box 751390, Petaluma, CA 94975-1390; tel: 800-543-3873 or 707-762-6144.

Brain Care: Tablets. Contains the neuronutrients vitamin E, phosphatidyl serine (which helps membrane flexibility), phosphatidyl choline, coenzyme Q10, ginkgo, alpha-linolenic acid, and the marine lipids DHA (docosahexaenoic acid) and EPA (eicosapentaenoic acid) that are rich in omega-3 fatty acids.

Quantum Inc., 754 Washington Street, Eugene, OR 97401; tel: 800-448-1448 or 541-345-5556.

Brain Fuel: Tablets. Nutritional support for the brain; contains neurotransmitter (substances that transmit nerve impulses to the brain) precursors; ingredients include ginkgo, guarana, gotu kola, American and Korean ginseng, licorice extract, tyrosine, glutathione, phosphatidyl choline, vitamins B5, B6, B12, C, and E, folic acid, potassium, bromelain, betaine HCl, L-methionine, RNA (ribonucleic acid), and PABA (para-aminobenzoic acid).

Futurebiotics, 145 Ricefield Lane, Hauppauge, NY 11788; tel: 800-FOR-LIFE (367-5433) or 516-273-6300.

Brain Modulators: Tablets. Supports brain functioning, neurotransmission, cerebral blood flow, and membrane fluidity (which permits neurons to communicate more efficiently); contains phosphatidyl choline, acetyl-L-carnitine, vitamin B12 (cyanocobalamin), folic acid, phosphatidyl serine, DHA (docosahexaenoic acid, an omega-3 oil), and ginkgo.

Solgar Vitamin & Herb Company Inc., 500 Willow Tree Road, Leonia, NJ 07605; tel: 800-645-2246 or 201-944-2311.

Brain Power: Vegitabs. Combination of neural-enhancing nutrients and specific amino acids for an increased level of mental activity.

Country Life, 101 Corporate Drive, Hauppauge, NY 11788; tel: 800-645-5768 or 516-231-1031.

Brain-Vita With Ginkgo Biloba: Tablets. Combination of vitamins, amino acids, minerals, and herbs to stimulate the brain.

Health Plus, 13837 Magnolia Avenue, Chino, CA 91710; tel: 800-822-6225 or 909-627-9393.

Bronson Memory Formula: Tablets. Blend of nutrients and herbs to supplement the body's ability to enhance mental function and memory.

BRONSON LABORATORIES INC., 600 East Quality Drive, American Fork, UT 84003; tel: 800-235-3200 or 801-756-5670.

Calms: Tablets. Contains four botanicals (passionflower, hops, wild oats, and chamomile) long used in homeopathy to soothe and quiet irritated nerves without sedatives or tranquilizers.

For **products related to depression**, See Depression in Part II, pp. 155-159.

P & S LABS, 210 West 131st Street, Los Angeles, CA 90061; tel: 800-624-9659 or 310-768-0700.

Clear Mind: Tablets. Contains ginkgo and gotu kola for greater mental energy and awareness.

PLANETARY FORMULAS, 23 Janis Way, Scotts Valley, CA 95066; tel: 800-606-6226.

Coenzyme Q-10 Rx (Q-Gel): Softgels. Powerful cellular energizer that research has shown to be the only hydrosoluble coenzyme Q10 product; has up to four times more bio-availability than other delivery systems.

PHYTO-THERAPY INC., OPTIMUM HEALTH, 483 West Middle Turnpike, Manchester, CT 06040; tel: 800-228-1507.

CoQ10 (Coenzyme Q10): Capsules. Assists the antioxidant vitamins C and E; helps provide oxygen to cells and strengthen the heart muscle.

TWIN LABS, 150 Motor Parkway, Hauppauge, NY 11788; tel: 800-645-5626.

Elan Vital: Tablets. Multiple antioxidant that also supports structural integrity, energy generation, neurotransmitter production, and liver health; contains the antioxidants N-acetyl-cysteine, vitamins C and E, beta carotene, and selenium, plus niacin, biotin, chromium, coenzyme Q10, ginkgo, DMAE (an amino-acid complex originating from soy beans), silymarin, bilberry, N-acetyl-glucosamine, quercetin, N-acetyl L-tyrosine, lipoic and succinic acids.

SOURCE NATURALS, THRESHOLD ENTERPRISES, 23 Janis Way, Scotts Valley, CA 95066; tel: 800-777-5677 or 831-438-1144.

Enada NADH: Tablets. NADH (coenzyme vitamin B3) is involved in production of cellular energy and is required for synthesis of neurotransmitters, which may explain its effects on maintaining healthy mood and mental functions; users report improved feelings of well-being and energy.

SCHIFF, WEIDER NUTRITION GROUP, 2002 South 5070 West, Salt Lake City, UT 84104; tel: 800-439-8042 or 801-975-5000.

Ester C Plus: Capsules. Strong antioxidant with antihistamine, anti-inflammatory, and immune-enhancing properties; assists healing, strengthens blood vessels, and normalizes high cholesterol. Ester C (a non-acidic form of vitamin C) is absorbed better and is more biologically active then regular vitamin C; also contains bioflavonoids, including quercetin and bromelain, as cofactors for their activity in all tissues (especially the circulatory system).

PHILLIPS NUTRITIONALS, 27071 Cabot Road #122, Laguna Hills, CA 92653; tel: 800-514-5115 or 702-898-8141.

Formula 3/6/9: Softgels. Natural source of essential fatty acids (EFAs); ingredients include borage oil, fish oil, flaxseed oil, gamma-linolenic acid, omega-3 fatty acids, and linoleic acids.

PHILLIPS NUTRITIONALS, 27071 Cabot Road #122, Laguna Hills, CA 92653; tel: 800-514-5115 or 702-898-8141.

4 Thought: Vegitabs. Nutritional complex that energizes and nourishes the brain.

COUNTRY LIFE, 101 Corporate Drive, Hauppauge, NY 11788; tel: 800-645-5768 or 516-231-1031.

Functional Greens: Powder or tablets. Superfood concentrate with 42 bioactive ingredients and plant nutrients.

ETHICAL NUTRIENTS, 971 Calle Negocio, San Clemente, CA 92673; tel: 800-668-8743 or 949-366-0818.

Garlic Power Rx: Softgels. Contains organic garlic that is five times more potent than fresh garlic, vitamin E, hawthorn berry, and parsley.

PHYTO-THERAPY INC., OPTIMUM HEALTH, 483 West Middle Turnpike, Manchester, CT 06040; tel: 800-228-1507.

Garlinase 4000: Tablets. Daily supplement that contains beneficial allicin while promising odor-free breath.

ENZYMATIC THERAPY, 825 Challenger Drive, Green Bay, WI 54311-8328; tel: 800-558-7372 or 920-469-1313.

Ginkgo Biloba Forte With Maxicholine: Caplets. Each active ingredient is helpful for mental nutrition; maxicholine is a proprietary combination of phosphatidyl choline and choline complex.

PHILLIPS NUTRITIONALS, 27071 Cabot Road #122, Laguna Hills, CA 92653; tel: 800-514-5115 or 702-898-8141.

Ginkgo Biloba Leaf Extract: Capsules. Helps increase peripheral circulation and improve oxygenation of the blood, thereby enhancing blood flow to the brain.

NATURE'S SOURCE, 15451 San Fernando Mission Boulevard, Mission Hills, CA 91345; tel: 800-423-2405 or 818-837-3633.

Ginkgo Biloba Plus L-Glutamine: Softgels. Standardized extracts to help brain functioning and memory.

J.R. CARLSON LABS INC., 15 College Drive, Arlington Heights, IL 60004-1985; tel: 800-323-4141 or 708-255-1600.

Ginkgo-Go!: Caplets. Daily formula containing 120 mg of ginkgo extract (120 mg of a 50:1 extract) per caplet.

WAKUNAGA OF AMERICA, 23501 Madero, Mission Viejo, CA 92691; tel: 800-421-2998 or 949-855-2776.

Ginkgo Gotu Kola: Capsules or liquid. Support for healthy memory function; contains ginkgo for its oxygen-enhancing benefits, gotu kola for its stimulating effects on thinking, Siberian ginseng for its ability to enhance performance, peppermint and astragalus for support and tone, and rosemary for enhancing memory.

FRONTIER COOPERATIVE HERBS, 3021 78th Street, Norway, IA 52318; tel: 800-669-3275 or 319-227-7996.

Ginkgo Phytosome Plus Choline: Softgels. Helps increase blood circulation to the brain; contains herbal extracts, soybean phospholipids (lecithin), choline, and the antioxidant vitamin E.

NATURE'S HERBS, 600 East Quality Drive, American Fork, UT 84003; tel: 800-437-2257 or 801-763-0700.

Ginkoba: Tablets. Clinical evidence shows that the standardized extract of ginkgo leaf in this formula increases the flow of oxygen to the brain, which can help improve memory and concentration, enhance mental focus.

BOEHRINGER INGELHEIM PHARMACEUTICALS INC., 900 Ridgebury Road, Ridgefield, CT 06877; tel: 800-243-0127.

Ginseng Ginkgo: Capsules or liquid. Contains the herbs *Ginkgo biloba*,

Siberian ginseng, and Korean ginseng, which promote mental alertness and physical endurance.

FRONTIER COOPERATIVE HERBS, 3021 78th Street, Norway, IA 52318; tel: 800-669-3275 or 319-227-7996.

Golden Years: Tablets. Multivitamin for mature adults with higher potencies of calcium, magnesium, betaine HCl, phosphatidyl choline, RNA (ribonucleic acid), DNA (deoxyribonucleic acid), and additional antioxidant protectors.

NATURE'S PLUS, 548 Broadhollow Road, Melville, NY 11747-3708; tel: 800-645-9500 or 516-293-0030.

Gotu Kola • Ginkgo Compound: Liquid. Indicated for mental fatigue from studying and other memory work, failing memory of old age, and Alzheimer's disease and other dementias; can aid recovery from strokes and enhance meditation or mental work; contains gotu kola herb and root, ginkgo leaf, passionflower flowering tips, skullcap flowering herb, calamus rhizome, and rosemary flowering branches.

HERB PHARM, 20260 Williams Highway, Williams, OR 97544; tel: 800-348-4372 or 541-846-6262.

Green Tea Extract: Tablets. Contains one of green tea's active components, epigallocatechin gallate (EGCg), a powerful antioxidant that test results suggest is 200 times more powerful than vitamin E.

SOURCE NATURALS, THRESHOLD ENTERPRISES, 23 Janis Way, Scotts Valley, CA 95066; tel: 800-777-5677 or 831-438-1144.

Hypericalm: Capsules. Contains St. John's wort extract for healthy mental and nervous system function.

ENZYMATIC THERAPY, 825 Challenger Drive, Green Bay, WI 54311-8328; tel: 800-558-7372 or 920-469-1313.

KYOLIC Formula 105: Tablets. Contains 200 mg of Aged Garlic Extract (a Wakunaga of America product), vitamins A, C, and E, selenium, and green tea, all of which are known for their antioxidant properties; dairy-free.

WAKUNAGA OF AMERICA, 23501 Madero, Mission Viejo, CA 92691; tel: 800-421-2998 or 949-855-2776.

L-5-HTP: Capsules. Contains natural L-5-HTP, vitamins B6 and C, and bioflavonoids. Clinical studies indicate that L-5-HTP enhances synthesis of serotonin in the brain.

SOLARAY, NUTRACEUTICAL CORP., P.O. Box 681869, Park City, UT 84068; tel: 800-669-8877.

Life Maintenance Formula: Packets. Contains antioxidants to optimize neurological, cardiovascular, and immune system nutrition while combating the effects of stress, tension, and pollution.
NATURE'S PRIDE, NATURE'S PRODUCTS, 1301 Sawgrass Corporate Parkway, Sunrise, FL 33323-2813; tel: 800-752-7873.

LifeSpan 2000: Vegitabs. Helps compensate for the natural aging process; contains DMAE (an amino-acid complex originating from soybeans), choline, phosphatidyl choline, NAC (N-acetyl-cysteine), ester C, vanadyl sulfide, ginkgo, grape seed extract, bilberry, vitamins A and E, and beta carotene.
COUNTRY LIFE, 101 Corporate Drive, Hauppauge, NY 11788; tel: 800-645-5768 or 516-231-1031.

Maxicholine: Caplets. Contains a high concentration of free choline, currently being studied in age-related diseases and disorders concerning loss of smell, taste, and movement.
PHILLIPS NUTRITIONALS, 27071 Cabot Road #122, Laguna Hills, CA 92653; tel: 800-514-5115 or 702-898-8141.

MC-Memory/Circulation: Tablets. Oral chelator, which aids in the breakdown of plaque attached to the veins and arteries, thereby increasing circulation throughout the body and improving memory functions; contains lecithin, gotu kola, RNA (ribonucleic acid) powder, capsicum, seaweed, and barberry.
NATURAL ENERGY PRODUCTS, 21101 Welch Road, Snohomish, WA 98296; tel: 425-486-5956.

MemorActin: Capsules. Supports brain functions; contains standardized ginkgo leaf, phosphatidyl choline, phosphatidyl serine, and other botanicals and nutrients.
NATURE'S PLUS, 548 Broadhollow Road, Melville, NY 11747-3708; tel: 800-645-9500 or 516-293-0030.

Mental Edge: Tablets. Contains vitamins, minerals, and herbal extracts that nourish and protect the brain by providing essential building blocks for neurotransmitters and the production of energy; also includes nutrients and herbal antioxidants to protect the brain from oxidative damage; helps enhance and sharpen mental acuity.

SOURCE NATURALS, THRESHOLD ENTERPRISES, 23 Janis Way, Scotts Valley, CA 95066; tel: 800-777-5677 or 831-438-1144.

Mental Support Formula With Ginkgo Biloba: Capsules. Research has shown that ginkgo increases peripheral blood flow, thereby enhancing oxygen flow to the brain; it helps fortify brain-body health for complex mental tasks; also contains gotu kola, Siberian ginseng root, reishi mycelium, and ginger root.

NATROL INC., 21411 Prairie Street, Chatsworth, CA 91311; tel: 818-739-6000.

Mind Peak by Jade: Liquid or tablets. Chinese herbal clear-thinking formula to help sustain high-level mental energy and enhance mental clarity.

EAST EARTH HERB INC., P.O. Box 2802 Eugene, OR 97402; tel: 800-827-HERB or 541-687-0155.

Mood Balance: Tablets. Helps deal with daily anxiety, stress, and irritability; contains standardized St. John's wort and valerian extracts; calming compounds such as lemon balm, kava-kava root extract, taurine, and GABA (gamma-aminobutyric acid); also contains amino acids that are used to synthesize neurotransmitters (chemical messengers) that support mental acuity and memory.

SOURCE NATURALS, THRESHOLD ENTERPRISES, 23 Janis Way, Scotts Valley, CA 95066; tel: 800-777-5677 or 831-438-1144.

Mood Swing Support: Capsules. Contains St. John's wort (*Hypericum perforatum*), which provides support for depressed moods and mild anxiety.

NUTRITION NOW, 501 Southeast Columbia Shore Boulevard #350, Vancouver, WA 98661; tel: 800-929-0418 or 360-737-6800.

Natural Vitamin E + (With Selenium & Chromium): Capsules. Contains a dry (non-oil) form of vitamin E, selenium, and chromium; vitamin E is an active antioxidant, enhances vitamin A activity, and acts as a vasodilator and an anticoagulant; selenium boosts vitamin E activity; chromium aids fat/carbohydrate metabolism and promotes a leaner, stronger physique. Both selenium and chromium are common deficiencies in Americans.

INFINITY HEALTH, 1519 Contra Costa Boulevard, Pleasant Hill, CA 94523; tel: 800-733-9293 or 925-676-8982.

Ocean Nutrition of Canada Brain Nutrition: Capsules. Contains DHA (docosahexaenoic acid, an essential fatty acid), the most abundant fatty acid in the gray matter of the brain.

OCEAN NUTRITION CANADA LTD., 757 Bedford Highway, Bedford, Nova Scotia, Canada B2A3Z7; tel: 888-980-8889 or 902-457-2399.

OptiZinc: Tablets. OptiZinc (a patented combination of zinc and the essential amino acid methionine) for the health of the thymus gland, which is important for skin health, wound-healing, carbohydrate metabolism, and enzyme systems.

SOURCE NATURALS, THRESHOLD ENTERPRISES, 23 Janis Way, Scotts Valley, CA 95066; tel: 800-777-5677 or 831-438-1144.

Oral Chelation and Age-Less Formulas: Liquid. Oral chelation and vitamin, mineral, and nutrient replenishment formula; Oral Chelation I Formula contains nutrients that can cross the blood-brain barrier to bind with and flush mercury and heavy metals out of the body; ingredients include EDTA (an amino acid), alginate, garlic, activated attapulgite clay, chlorella, methionine, cysteine, lipoic acid, vitamin C, and lipotropics; Age-Less II Formula replenishes the nutrients that are removed by chelation and helps support and detoxify the liver; contains minerals, vitamins, phytonutrients, antioxidants, amino acids, and lipotropics; both formulas contain plant-based bromelain, lipase, and catalase enzymes for optimal digestion, assimilation, and utilization of nutrients.

EXTREME HEALTH INC., 50 Oak Court, Suite 212, Danville, CA 94526; tel: 800-800-1285 or 925-855-1262.

Original AntiOx: Capsules. Contains key nutrients in combination with the minerals necessary for the antioxidant enzymes as well as the B vitamins that act as cofactors to help support and recharge the antioxidant defenses.

ALLERGY RESEARCH GROUP/NUTRICOLOGY, P.O. Box 55907, Hayward, CA 94544; tel: 800-545-9960 or 510-487-8526.

Phosphatidyl Serine Complex: Capsules. Peer-reviewed studies suggest that phosphatidyl serine (PS), a phospholipid, is vital to brain cell structure and function and helps maintain or improve cognitive functions such as memory and learning in adults over age 50; PS also plays important roles in neurotransmitter (chemical messengers in the brain) systems, metabolism levels, and maintaining nerve connections in the brain.

OPTIMAL NUTRIENTS, 1163 Chess Drive #F, Foster City, CA 94404; tel: 800-966-8874 or 650-525-0112.

Pregnenolone: Capsules. Many physicians and scientists believe that supplementing with pregnenolone (a hormone precursor manufactured by the body, which can be converted into other hormones including DHEA, estrogen, testosterone, and progesterone) is an important step in dealing with the symptoms of aging; many people report enhanced memory, well-being, and energy after taking pregnenolone.

LIFEENHANCEMENT PRODUCTS INC., P.O. Box 751390, Petaluma, CA 94975-1390; tel: 800-543-3873 or 707-762-6144.

Pregnenolone: Tablets. Supplementation with pregnenolone, which has been called a brain neurosteroid (since there are high levels of it in the brain tissues) is linked with improved sleep and brain function.

SCHIFF, WEIDER NUTRITION GROUP, 2002 South 5070 West, Salt Lake City, UT 84104; tel: 800-439-8042 or 801-975-5000.

Premier Anti-Oxidant: Capsules. Formula designed to enhance the supplementation of vitamins A, C, and E, and bioflavonoids; contains the antioxidants glutathione, taurine, ALA (alpha-lipoic acid), and the glutathione precursor NAC (N-acetyl-cysteine).

BIO-NUTRITIONAL FORMULAS, 106 East Jericho Turnpike, Mineola, NY 11501; tel: 800-950-8484.

Premium North American Ginseng Chewable With Vitamin C: Tablets. Contains 50 mg of fresh pure powdered North American ginseng (*Panax quinquefolius*) blended with vitamins A, B6, and C, zinc, and beta carotene in a base containing sorbitol, fructose, vegetable stearin, and flavored with natural licorice.

CHAINATA CORP., 5965 205 A Street, Langley, British Columbia, Canada V3A8C4; tel: 800-406-7668 or 604-533-8883.

Premium North American Ginseng Sarsaparilla: Liquid. Antioxidant formula to help defend the body against free radicals caused by our environment; contains extracts of American ginseng roots combined with vitamin C and other vitamins and minerals; nonalcoholic.

CHAINATA CORP., 5965 205 A Street, Langley, British Columbia, Canada V3A8C4; tel: 800-406-7668 or 604-533-8883.

Premium North American Ginseng Ultra Concentrate: Liquid. Contains the essence of North American ginseng (*Panax quinquefolius*) roots, which assist the body in adapting to stress, increasing energy and endurance, improving mental alertness, and enhancing physical and mental performance; concentrated for instant absorption.

CHAINATA CORP., 5965 205 A Street, Langley, British Columbia, Canada V3A8C4; tel: 800-406-7668 or 604-533-8883.

Pycnogenol & Citrus Bioflavonoids: Capsules. Contains pycnogenol, from pine bark, a powerful antioxidant that crosses the blood-brain barrier helping to protect the body and the central nervous system from the damaging effects of free radicals.

AMERICAN HEALTH, 4320 Veterans Memorial Highway, Holbrook, NY 11741; tel: 800-445-7137.

Quintessence Garlic Plus Ginkgo: Capsules. Contains garlic (odorless) combined with ginkgo (24% ginkgo flavonoid glycosides).

PURE-GAR, 21411 Prairie Street, Chatsworth, CA 91311; tel: 800-537-7695 or 818-739-6046.

Respond: Tablets. Contains the nutrients niacinamide, vitamins B6 and C, L-glutamine, ginkgo, and zinc, which are all involved in healthy brain function.

J.R. CARLSON LABS INC., 15 College Drive, Arlington Heights, IL 60004-1985; tel: 800-323-4141 or 708-255-1600.

Sphingolin-MS: Capsules. Contains prepared extract of bovine myelin sheath (insulation around nerve bundles), a rich source of naturally occuring sphingomyelin; the formula's delicate enzymes are protected by lyophilization (a type of freeze-drying process).

ECOLOGICAL FORMULAS, 1061-B Shary Circle, Concord, CA 94518; tel: 800-888-4585 or 925-827-2636.

Stay Sharp: Capsules. Provides nourishment for heightened mental energy and alertness; ingredients include alfalfa juice concentrate, chlorella, spirulina, kola nut extract, pantothenic acid, American ginseng, gotu kola, *Panax ginseng* extract, niacin, and ginkgo extract.

BIODYNAMAX, 6525 Gunpark Drive #150-507, Boulder, CO 80301; tel: 800-926-7525 or 303-530-4665.

Super Defense Antioxidant Formula: Capsules. Antioxidant formula containing high levels of beta carotene, vitamins C and E, and the mineral selenium.

BRONSON LABORATORIES INC., 600 East Quality Drive, American Fork, UT 84003; tel: 800-235-3200 or 801-756-5670.

Super Minerals: Liquid. Highly charged, bio-stable mineral supplement that contains minerals and trace minerals in a blend of non-ionic colloidal minerals and polyelectrolytes (two forms of minerals that work well together).

R GARDEN, 3881 Enzyme Lane, Kettle Falls, WA 99141; tel: 800-700-7767 or 425-271-0539.

Super 10 Antioxidant: Vegitabs. Contains potent antioxidants such as polyphenols found in red wine extract, polyphenols and similar antioxidants found in green tea extract, and bromelain, an enzyme from pineapples that enhances the absorption of quercetin and other bioflavonoids.

COUNTRY LIFE, 101 Corporate Drive, Hauppauge, NY 11788; tel: 800-645-5768 or 516-231-1031.

The Mind System: Tablets. Blend of antioxidant nutrients, amino acids, superfoods, and herbal extracts (such as ginkgo and gotu kola) to help support mental functioning.

RAINBOW LIGHT, P.O. Box 600, Santa Cruz, CA 95061; tel: 800-635-1233 or 408-429-9089.

Think of It: Tablets. Contains high levels of neuronutrients and co-factors for brain health, including Maxicholine, which has been added for higher uptake of choline, plus herbs and vitamins.

PHILLIPS NUTRITIONALS, 27071 Cabot Road #122, Laguna Hills, CA 92653; tel: 800-514-5115 or 702-898-8141.

Triple Action Antioxidant +: Capsules. Combination of proanthocyanidins (proven stronger than pycnogenol), citrus bioflavonoids, and vitamin C to nourish the body, enhance joint flexibility, provide protection from free radicals, and promote healthy blood vessels and pliable, youthful skin.

NUPRO, 735-L Park Street, Castle Rock, CO 80104; tel: 303-660-0562 or 800-704-8910.

Ultra Antioxidants: Tablets. Contains 21 antioxidants including selenium, zinc, grape seed extract, green tea, garlic, and others.

BioDynamax, 6525 Gunpark Drive #150-507, Boulder, CO 80301; tel: 800-926-7525 or 303-530-4665.

Ultra Antioxidant Plus: Softgels. Contains pycnogenol, coenzyme Q10, SOD (superoxide dismutase), glutathione, zinc, beta carotene, vitamins C and E, and selenium to neutralize free radical production. Clinical data has shown the damaging effects of free radicals and single oxygen on cells and body systems.

Phillips Nutritionals, 27071 Cabot Road #122, Laguna Hills, CA 92653; tel: 800-514-5115 or 702-898-8141.

Ultra Oils: Softgels. Contains the oils of flaxseed, pumpkin seed, borage, black currant, vitamin E, and rosemary; provides the ideal ratios of omega-3, -6, and -9 essential fatty acids that have proven healing and balancing properties.

Country Life, 101 Corporate Drive, Hauppauge, NY 11788; tel: 800-645-5768 or 516-231-1031.

Ultra-One: Tablets. Multivitamin and mineral that contains 100 mg of all the B vitamins plus other vitamins and amino acid–chelated minerals.

Nature's Plus, 548 Broadhollow Road, Melville, NY 11747-3708; tel: 800-645-9500 or 516-293-0030.

Ultra-Two: Tablets. Multivitamin and mineral formula that contains high potencies of essential vitamins and minerals and a complete combination of trace minerals.

Nature's Plus, 548 Broadhollow Road, Melville, NY 11747-3708; tel: 800-645-9500 or 516-293-0030.

Detoxification

The body's five organs of elimination and detoxification are the colon (large intestine), kidneys, liver, lungs, and skin. When the body is healthy, these organs are able to fulfill their function of processing and removing toxins and unwanted substances. When these systems break down or become overloaded, however, toxins build up in the body. If the accumulation is unchecked by detoxification protocols, health begins to decline and degenerative diseases can develop.

Symptoms and Causes of Toxic Overload

Common symptoms associated with toxins accumulating in the colon and tissues of the body include general aches and pains, chronic tiredness, headaches, and skin reactions. Toxic buildup can be the predisposing factor in a wide range of illnesses including chronic fatigue syndrome, environmental illness (SEE QUICK DEFINITION), and cancer. When combined with other stresses on the body, toxic overload can be the proverbial last straw in the development of disease.

For many Americans, at least three of their five organs of detoxification are likely to be overburdened, due to chronic exposure to human-made chemicals and heavy metals in the environment, cigarette smoking, extensive use of drugs (prescription or recreational), and overconsumption of frozen, canned, cooked, and processed foods, alcohol, coffee, sugar, and fat.

Cellular, intestinal, and liver detoxification can help rid the body of its toxic burden, an important step in disease prevention.

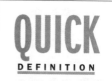

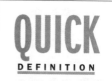

DEFINITION

Environmental illness is a multiple-symptom, debilitating, chronic disorder involving prolonged, heightened, and often incapacitating allergies or sensitivities to numerous common substances found in one's environment. Symptoms may include headaches, fatigue, muscle pain and/or weakness, coughing or wheezing, asthma, weight loss, infections, and emotional fluctuations, depression, and/or irritability.

Cellular Detoxification

Cellular detoxification involves identifying and eliminating toxins that have been absorbed, ingested, or inhaled over a lifetime. This is body-wide detoxification to pull toxins from tissue cells where they are stored.

Nutrients for Cellular Detoxification—Vitamin A, vitamin B complex (especially B2, B3, B6, and B12), vitamin C with bioflavonoids, choline, coenzyme Q10, copper, folic acid, free-form amino acids (especially cysteine, glutathione, glycine, methionine, and taurine), magnesium, N-acetyl-cysteine (NAC), protease enzymes, spirulina, superoxide dismutase (SOD), and zinc.

Herbs for Cellular Detoxification—Alfalfa, barley grass, burdock root, cayenne (capsaicin), chaparral, chlorophyll, devil's claw, garlic, ginger root, ginkgo, gotu kola, horsetail, lemon grass, Oregon grape root, parsley leaf, pau d'arco bark, red clover blossom, rose hips, turmeric (curcumin), and yellowdock.

Intestinal Detoxification

A diet devoid or lacking in live enzymes (such as overly cooked, canned, or processed food) or a diet consisting of allergy-triggering foods (such as sugar, dairy, wheat, or corn) can cause an over-secretion of mucus in the intestinal tract. Even toxic by-products of pathologic intestinal flora (bacteria, viruses, yeast, or mold) or intestinal parasites can trigger the secretion of this mucus. Also called mucoid plaque, the mucus layer acts as a protective barrier to prevent the absorption of toxic substances; it is a natural self-defense mechanism that probably evolved to handle the occasional ingestion of rotten food or other toxins. Once the danger had passed, the body would strip away the mucoid lining it had created. Unfortunately, the standard American diet consists largely of mucus-promoting foods that put a constant stress on the gastrointestinal tract.[15]

Under such stress, the normal lymphatic drainage system becomes overloaded as it attempts to absorb the constant supply of mucus, pathogenic organisms, and other toxins present in an unhealthy intestinal system. The mucoid plaque that can not be absorbed by the lymphatic system remains in the intestinal tract creating a false lining along the intestinal wall. The space between this false mucoid lining and the actual intestinal wall is a breeding ground for microbial organisms such as bacteria, viruses, yeast, and parasites. Toxic by-products from the microbial organisms burden the liver (where many toxins are neutralized) and eventually the immune system. The mucoid lining has also been linked to colon and gastric cancer.[16]

Intestinal detoxification drains the stored mucus and

See **Gastrointestinal Disorders** in Part II, pp. 198-217.

other toxins from the lymphatic system. The false mucoid lining in the intestines is also broken apart and removed in order to restore healthy intestinal function and improve peristaltic action (muscle contraction that moves matter along the digestive tract). Most detoxification protocols focus on the colon as that is where the majority of the buildup occurs.

If a colon cleanse is aggressive or a high level of toxicity is present, some people will feel worse while this process is under way. Common symptoms include fatigue, headaches, general body aches, and foul-smelling urine and feces. It is extremely important to proceed with a cleanse at a pace your body can tolerate. If the colon cleanse is performed too quickly, these symptoms may become more serious, with abdominal cramping, diarrhea, or low-grade fever, prompting some people to terminate the cleansing process before it is complete.

There are a number of oral supplement programs for cleansing the colon. We recommend that people (especially those who are sensitive) start with a smaller dose of the colon-cleansing product and gradually work up to the recommended dose. Most manufacturers of these products address individual needs with instructions on how to move ahead or slow down to get the desired results. During a colon cleanse, we recommend increasing your intake of pure water and mainly eating organic vegetables, fruits, and grains.

As an adjunct to colon cleansing, taking protease enzymes on an empty stomach aids the body in getting rid of the toxins loosened by the cleanse. The toxins circulate in the body until they are processed and eliminated. With a large toxic load, this can be a big job for the detoxification systems. Protease enzymes assist by entering the bloodstream and lymphatic system where they act as scavengers, "eating" the circulating toxins. The sooner you can get the toxins out of your body, the less symptoms and discomfort you will have.

Nutrients and Herbs for Colon Cleansing

■ **Lipex and Everyday Fiber:** we often advise our patients to use these products to improve regularity and cleanse the colon; both are non-irritating and work well for people who travel a lot or who do not want to use the powdered colon-cleansing drinks.

■ **Arise & Shine Cleanse Thyself™ Program:** we recommend this comprehensive oral supplement cleansing package for people who want to do a more extensive intestinal cleanse.

■ **Bentonite clay:** by binding with heavy metals, bentonite assists in their elimination from the body.

■ *Acidophilus*, **magnesium, and fiber:** a low population of beneficial *acidophilus* bacteria in the intestines, low dietary fiber, and magnesium deficiency can contribute to constipation and toxic buildup in the intestines. We do not usually recommend psyllium fiber products for people with sensitive bodies; however, vegetable or apple/pear pectin fiber can be used instead.

■ **Aloe vera juice:** it promotes intestinal health and helps loosen stools.

■ **Cascara sagrada or senna:** these are strong herbs that work as well as laxatives, but should not be used continuously for long periods of time because the body can become dependent on them.

Additional Supplements for Intestinal Detoxification—Vitamins A, B complex, E, and C, beta carotene, bioflavonoids, chlorophyll, flaxseed, fructo-oligosaccharides (FOS, "food" for beneficial intestinal flora), garlic, glutathione, guar gum, molybdenum, oat bran, plant enzymes (amylase, lipase, trypsin, chymotrypsin), quercetin, selenium, superoxide dismutase (SOD), vanadium, and zinc.

Additional Herbs for Intestinal Detoxification—Barberry bark, black walnut hulls, buckthorn, cayenne (capsicum), dandelion root, echinacea, fennel seed, goldenseal, licorice root, Oregon grape root, rhubarb root, sarsaparilla root, and yellowdock.

Liver Detoxification

The symptoms of a toxic or overworked liver are often diffuse and can involve nearly every organ or system in the body. Some specific symptoms and signs include headaches, skin conditions (acne, psoriasis, rashes, dry and itchy skin), candidiasis (an overgrowth of yeast in the body), fatigue, food allergies, chemical sensitivities, premenstrual syndrome, depression, poor digestion (bad breath, bloating, constipation, gallbladder problems), achy joints and muscles, sore or burning feet, or deficiencies in fat-soluble vitamins (vitamins A, D, E, and K) and essential fatty acids.[17] A unique feature of the liver is its ability to heal itself and regenerate cells, especially when supported by nutritional supplementation and herbs.

Nutrients and Herbs for Liver Detoxification

■ **Artichoke:** it protects the liver from toxic substances, and acts in the regeneration of liver cells; also used for treating liver disease and lowering cholesterol levels.[18]

See **Liver Disorders** in Part II, pp. 257-262.

■ **Catechin:** an antioxidant flavonoid, used in cases of hepatitis or chemical, drug, or alcohol damage to the liver.

■ **Lipoic acid:** a powerful antioxidant, lipoic acid detoxifies the body of substances such as mercury, arsenic, lead, and other heavy metals; it is used in cases of alcohol-related liver disease, hepatitis, drug coma, and mushroom poisoning.

■ **Milk thistle (silymarin):** the active component of milk thistle is silymarin, a potent antioxidant, that promotes liver function and prevents liver degeneration and destruction.

■ **N-acetyl-cysteine (NAC):** a sulfur-containing amino acid that supports the immune system; used to treat liver toxicity caused by prolonged and excessive use of acetaminophen (such as Tylenol[R]).

■ **Vitamin C:** an antioxidant that is used in large doses (via intravenous drip or oral dosages to bowel tolerance) to treat chemical sensitivities or food and airborne allergies.[19]

Additional Supplements for Liver Detoxification—Antioxidants, vitamin B complex (sublingual), catechins (bioflavonoids from green tea), choline, coenzyme Q10, vitamin E, free-form amino acids (sublingual, especially cysteine and methionine), garlic, grape seed extract (pycnogenol), inositol (a B vitamin), multivitamin complex, multimineral complex, and selenium.

Products for Detoxification

FOR CELLULAR DETOXIFICATION

Alpha Lipoic Acid: Tablets. Helps scavenge harmful free radicals in the body and protects cells from damage caused by pollution, stress, and smoking; also features NutriVin, a protective antioxidant complex made from red grape seeds, skin, leaves, and stems.

AMERIFIT, 166 Highland Park Drive, Bloomfield, CT 06002; tel: 800-990- FIRM (3476) or 860-242-3476.

Antioxidant Formula: Capsules. Contains antioxidants and nutrients that enhance the uptake of vitamin C and cellular function; ingredients include vitamins A, C, and E, beta and alpha carotenes, coenzyme forms of vitamins B1, B2, and B6, N-acetyl-L-cysteine, ferulic acid, malic acid, lipoic acid, calcium, copper, manganese, magnesium, selenium, zinc, pycnogenols, and green tea catechins.

HEALTH PRODUCTS DISTRIBUTORS INC., 23847 Peaceful Ridge Road, Smithsburg, MD 21783; tel: 800-228-4265 or 301-416-0500.

Cell Guard: Capsules. Combination of SOD (superoxide dismutase), glutathione peroxidase, and catalase, which acts to promote maximum cellular protection and health.

BIOTEC FOODS, 5152 Borsa Avenue, Suite 101, Huntington Beach, CA 92649; tel: 800-788-1084 or 714-899-3477.

Detox Caps With Goldenseal: Capsules. Stimulates the body to eliminate wastes rapidly; may be accompanied by mild symptoms of a "healing crisis" such as headache, bad breath, slight nausea, body odor, and concentrated urine.

CRYSTAL STAR HERBAL NUTRITION, 4069 Wedgeway Court, Earth City, MO 63045; tel: 800-736-6015 or 314-739-7551.

DetoxCleanse: Capsules. Herbal formula that assists in detoxifying the body and bloodstream by cleansing the liver, improving digestion, binding and excreting toxins within the gastrointestinal tract, and promoting regularity.

BIODYNAMAX, 6525 Gunpark Drive #150-507, Boulder, CO 80301; tel: 800-926-7525 or 303-530-4665.

Detox Enzyme Formula: Capsules. Contains antioxidants, vitamins, minerals, and amino acids that play key roles in the body's detoxification pathways; also contains calcium D-glucarate and plant enzymes to enhance absorption.

PREVAIL CORP., 2204-8 Northwest Birdsdale, Gresham, OR 97030; tel: 800-248-0885 or 503-667-5527.

L-Glutathione: Vegicaps. Modulators assist in the production of L-glutathione, an amino acid, antioxidant, and detoxifier. Glutathione neutralizes cell-damaging free radicals, detoxifies the liver, and binds with heavy metals (such as mercury and cadmium); contains NAC (N-acetyl-cysteine), alpha-lipoic acid, and selenium, which are essential for the synthesis of glutathione; also includes vitamin C, which studies indicate can increase tissue glutathione levels.

SOLGAR VITAMIN & HERB COMPANY, Inc., 500 Willow Tree Road, Leonia, NJ 07605; tel: 800-645-2246 or 201-944-2311.

Heavy Metal Cleanz Caps: Capsules. Contains barley grass to help neutralize and cleanse.

CRYSTAL STAR HERBAL NUTRITION, 4069 Wedgeway Court, Earth City, MO 63045; tel: 800-736-6015 or 314-739-7551.

Herbal Aloe Force: Juice or topical gel. Processed aloe vera juice containing vitamins, minerals, enzymes, amino acids, essential fatty acids, growth factors, glycoproteins, sterols, bioflavonoids, and polysaccharides (complex sugars), plus ionized colloidal silver and herbal extracts (cat's claw, chamomile, burdock root, hawthorn berry, *Astragalus membranaceus* root, sheep sorrell, pau d'arco bark, slippery elm bark, and rhubarb root).

HERBAL ANSWERS, INC., P.O. Box 1110, Saratoga Springs, NY 12866; tel: 888-256-3367 or 518-581-1968.

Liv-Alive Tea. Cleansing herbal blend to re-establish an alkaline environment; contains the roots of dandelion, licorice, Oregon grape, and yellowdock, hyssop, milk thistle seed, pau d'arco bark, parsley, hibiscus flower, watercress leaf, red sage leaf, anise, and white sage oil.

CRYSTAL STAR HERBAL NUTRITION, 4069 Wedgeway Court, Earth City, MO 63045; tel: 800-736-6015 or 314-739-7551.

Magnesium Malate: Tablets. Contains magnesium (45% of the U.S. RDA) and malic acid (found in apples and also produced by the body); malic acid is involved in the manufacture of energy in the cells; it also crosses the blood-brain barrier and has been shown to bind to aluminum and flush it out of the body; by binding to aluminum, malic acid frees receptor sites for magnesium.

SOURCE NATURALS, THRESHOLD ENTERPRISES, 23 Janis Way, Scotts Valley, CA 95066; tel: 800-777-5677 or 831-438-1144.

Oxystat: Capsules. Contains the antioxidants NAC (N-acetyl-cysteine), standardized green tea (50% catechins), standardized silymarin, choline, methionine, amino acids, glutathione, chlorophyll, coenzyme Q10, calcium D-glucarate, and other important nutritional cofactors.

NF FORMULAS INC., 9755 Southwest Commerce Circle, C-5, Wilsonville, OR 97070; tel: 800-547-4891 or 503-682-9755.

Pau d'Arco Burdock: Capsules or liquid. Contains pau d'arco, red clover, burdock, yellowdock, and nettle for general purification and tonification.

FRONTIER COOPERATIVE HERBS, 3021 78th Street, Norway, IA 52318; tel: 800-669-3275 or 319-227-7996.

Phyto-Pro: Liquid. High-protein vegetarian "green" drink for additional nutritional support; ingredients include a blend of organic grasses, such as chlorella and spirulina, with amino acids, adaptogenic nutrients, antioxidants, and superfoods.

NF FORMULAS INC., 9755 Southwest Commerce Circle, C-5, Wilsonville, OR 97070; tel: 800-547-4891 or 503-682-9755.

FOR INTESTINAL DETOXIFICATION

Arise & Shine Cleanse Thyself™ Program. A comprehensive intestinal cleansing kit consisting of nutritional support and detoxifying agents, a shaker bottle for preparation of cleansing drinks, pH paper to test acid-alkaline balance and monitor electrolyte levels, and specific instructions, including the educational book *Cleanse and Purify Thyself* written by Richard Anderson, N.D., N.M.D., developer of the program.

ARISE AND SHINE, P.O. Box 901, Mount Shasta, CA, 96067; tel: 800-688-2444 or 530-926-0891.

Alkalizer: Powder. Concentrated source of organic potassium, sodium, calcium, phosphate, chloride, magnesium, and other alkaline electrolyte minerals for people with low alkaline reserves; not recommended for people who have sugar problems such as hypoglycemia, diabetes, or candidiasis.

ARISE AND SHINE, P.O. Box 1439, Mount Shasta, CA 96067; tel: 800-688-2444 or 530-926-0891.

BWL Tone IBS Caps: Capsules. Contains peppermint and slippery elm to soothe and tone the intestines.

CRYSTAL STAR HERBAL NUTRITION, 4069 Wedgeway Court, Earth City, MO 63045; tel: 800-736-6015 or 314-739-7551.

Cayenne (Capsicum): Capsules. Cayenne, a harmless internal disinfectant, has been found to be an effective nutritional support for migraine and cluster-type headaches; it is one of the highest sources of vitamins A and C, has the complete vitamin B complex, and is rich in organic calcium and potassium.

ARISE AND SHINE, P.O. Box 1439, Mount Shasta, CA 96067; tel: 800-688-2444 or 530-926-0891.

Chomper: Vegicaps. Herbal laxative that thoroughly cleanses the alimentary canal (passage from mouth to anus), liver, deep cell tissues, and other organs.

ARISE AND SHINE, P.O. Box 1439, Mount Shasta, CA 96067; tel: 800-688-2444 or 530-926-0891.

Cleansing Laxative Formula: Tablets. Herbal laxative for occasional constipation and colon-cleansing regimens; contains the herb cascara sagrada, kaolin clay, and other ingredients to support bowel detoxification.

ZAND HERBAL FORMULAS, 1722 14th Street #230, Boulder, CO 80302; tel: 800-800-0405 or 303-786-8558.

Colon Balance: Tablets. Helps support the body's natural balance and a healthy elimination system.

VEDA HEALTH INC., P.O. Box 1535, Soquel, CA 95073; tel: 888-856-8334 or 408-465-9084.

Colon Cleanse: Capsules. Provides psyllium husk fiber (without seeds which can irritate the colon), an essential soluble fiber that expands; psyllium acts as a soft and gentle brush inside the colon and provides lubrication to the lining of the colon helping in the removal of waste matter generated in the body.

HEALTH PLUS, 13837 Magnolia Avenue, Chino, CA 91710; tel: 800-822-6225 or 909-627-9393.

Daytime/Nighttime Daily Cleanse: Tablets. Multiple herbs and fiber supplement program.

AMERICAN HEALTH, 4320 Veterans Memorial Highway, Holbrook, NY 11741; tel: 800-445-7137.

Detox-Zyme: Vegicaps. Blend of enzymes that break down proteins, fats, carbohydrates, and fiber, plus herbs traditionally used to support the cleansing and eliminative functions of the body.

RAINBOW LIGHT, P.O. Box 600, Santa Cruz, CA 95061; tel: 800-635-1233 or 408-429-9089.

Evacu Lax RX: Caplets. Intestinal/colon probiotic and cleansing system that helps promote, cleanse, and re-establish a healthy colon.

PHYTO-THERAPY INC., OPTIMUM HEALTH, 483 West Middle Turnpike, Manchester, CT 06040; tel: 800-228-1507.

Everyday Fiber System: Powder. Fiber supplement for maintaining daily regularity; contains a blend of three soluble fibers plus supporting herbs such as ginger, FOS (fructo-oligosaccharides; a carbohydrate that supports the friendly intestinal bacteria), chlorophyll, and plant-source enzymes.

RAINBOW LIGHT, P.O. Box 600, Santa Cruz, CA 95061; tel: 800-635-1233 or 408-429-9089.

Fiber & Herbs Cleanse Caps: Capsules. Balance of herbal nutrients for complete colon cleansing.

CRYSTAL STAR HERBAL NUTRITION, 4069 Wedgeway Court, Earth City, MO 63045; tel: 800-736-6015 or 314-739-7551.

Flora Grow: Vegicaps. Restores the healthy intestinal bacteria (flora) normally depleted by the use of antibiotics and poor eating habits; beneficial bacteria are essential for a strong immune system, assimilation of vitamins, proteins, fats, carbohydrates, and the manufacture of B vitamins, vitamin K, and various amino acids.

ARISE AND SHINE, P.O. Box 1439, Mount Shasta, CA 96067; tel: 800-688-2444 or 530-926-0891.

Gentle-Cleanse: Capsules. Contains natural plant fiber (psyllium hydrophyllic mucilloid), which the body needs to help eliminate waste, and the extract casanthranol from aged cascara sagrada that gently promotes comfortable relief of occasional irregularity.

NATURE'S HERBS, 600 East Quality Drive, American Fork, UT 84003; tel: 800-437-2257 or 801-763-0700.

Health Cleanse: Powder. Contains highly soluble, sugar-free fibers and herbs that help cleanse and detoxify the colon and intestinal tract.

BIODYNAMAX, 6525 Gunpark Drive #150-507, Boulder, CO 80301; tel: 800-926-7525 or 303-530-4665.

Herbal Aloe Force: (See Cellular Detoxification product listing, above)

Herbal Nutrition: Vegicaps. Helps the body remove the mucoid plaque that lines the walls of the alimentary canal.

ARISE AND SHINE, P.O. Box 1439, Mount Shasta, CA 96067; tel: 800-688-2444 or 530-926-0891.

Intestinal Cleanser: Powder. Contains powdered psyllium seed and husk; helps remove old mucus, feces, and putrefying toxins that can accumulate in pockets of the large intestine (colon).

SONNE'S ORGANIC FOODS INC., P.O. Box 2160, Cottonwood, CA 96022; tel: 800-544-8147 or 530-347-5868.

LB Formula: Capsules or tablets. Vegetable laxative with cascara sagrada bark in a base of goldenseal root, barberry bark, ginger root, red raspberry leaves, rhubarb root, fennel seed, cayenne, and lobelia herb.

NATURE'S HERBS, 600 East Quality Drive, American Fork, UT 84003; tel: 800-437-2257 or 801-763-0700.

Lipex: Powder. Fiber supplement with lecithin, which contains dietary fibers, carrageenan, guar gum, and other nutrients that support metabolism of fat and cholesterol.

AMNI, 2247 National Avenue, Hayward, CA 94540-5012; tel: 800-437-8888 or 510-783-6969.

Liquid Bentonite. Bentonite clay has been used for centuries as an internal and external purification aid; it is known for its highly absorptive properties, drawing out metals, drugs, and toxins for release from the body.

ARISE AND SHINE, P.O. Box 1439, Mount Shasta, CA 96067; tel: 800-688-2444 or 530-926-0891.

LX-Elimination: Tablets. Helps digestion, assimilation, and elimination; contains aloe, buckthorn, bayberry, seaweed, white oak bark, myrrh, ginger, and cider vinegar.

NATURAL ENERGY PRODUCTS, 21101 Welch Road, Snohomish, WA 98296; tel: 425-486-5956.

Nature Cleanse: Tablets. Contains a blend of fiber and herbs with digestive enzymes to maximize the cleansing process.

NATURE'S PLUS, 548 Broadhollow Road, Melville, NY 11747-3708; tel: 800-645-9500 or 516-293-0030.

Oxy-Cleanse by Earth's Bounty: Capsules. Oxygen colon conditioner that works without psyllium or herbs to break down debris into very small pieces that can be easily and gently eliminated.

MATRIX HEALTH PRODUCTS, 8400 Magnolia Avenue, Suite N, Santee, CA 92071; tel: 800-736-5609 or 619-448-7550.

pH Paper. pH Paper (to test acid/alkaline balance) is used to gauge the body's electrolyte levels during the cleansing program.

ARISE AND SHINE, P.O. Box 1439, Mount Shasta, CA 96067; tel: 800-688-2444 or 530-926-0891.

Psyllium Husk Powder. Fibrous bulking agent that gels and thickens when mixed with water or juice and helps detoxify the alimentary canal.

ARISE AND SHINE, P.O. Box 1439, Mount Shasta, CA 96067; tel: 800-688-2444 or 530-926-0891.

Quick Cleanse Program Kit. One-week internal detoxification program that cleanses the colon and aids in the elimination of toxins from the liver and blood; contains Cleansing Fiber capsules, Cleansing Laxative tablets, and Thistle Cleanse capsules; can be customized for individual intake needs.

ZAND HERBAL FORMULAS, 1722 14th Street #230, Boulder, CO 80302; tel: 800-800-0405 or 303-786-8558.

Regucil: Capsules. Formula works with the body to help keep it regular; combines two natural stimulant laxatives, aloe vera and casanthranol (extract of cascara sagrada), in a base of fennel, ginger, raspberry leaves, goldenseal root, barberry bark, and cayenne; for overnight relief of occasional irregularity.

NATURE'S HERBS, 600 East Quality Drive, American Fork, UT 84003; tel: 800-437-2257 or 801-763-0700.

Senna Extract (*Cassia angustifolia*): Capsules. Useful for overnight relief of irregularity; suitable for cases of chronic constipation and for children.

NATURE'S HERBS, 600 East Quality Drive, American Fork, UT 84003; tel: 800-437-2257 or 801-763-0700.

Super Colon Cleanse: Capsules or powder. Formula combines the benefits of pure psyllium, herbs, and *acidophilus*; pure psyllium has bulking and lubricating properties for cleansing the colon; the herbs senna, fennel seed, celery seed, cascara sagrada, Oregon grape root, and buckthorn bark provide laxative action; digestive enzymes from papaya and Oregon grape root help digest food; and rose hips, peppermint, and Oregon grape root soothe and help overcome irritation of the colon.

HEALTH PLUS, 13837 Magnolia Avenue, Chino, CA 91710; tel: 800-822-6225 or 909-627-9393.

Triphala: Tablets. Internal cleanser to invigorate, strengthen, and tone the gastrointestinal system; for long-term preventive maintenance or for a concentrated cleansing program; provides nutritional support for indigestion, carbohydrate intolerance, elevated cholesterol, diabetes, chronic lung disease, hypertension, anemia, yeast infections, eye disease, and skin disorders.

PLANETARY FORMULAS, 23 Janis Way, Scotts Valley, CA 95066; tel: 800-606-6226.

FOR LIVER DETOXIFICATION

Bupleurum Calmative Compound (Xiao Yao Wan): Tablets. In traditional Chinese medicine, the liver is considered to be the organ primarily associated with emotional stability; cleanses and tonifies the liver to restore a sense of peace and well-being to the entire body.

PLANETARY FORMULAS, 23 Janis Way, Scotts Valley, CA 95066; tel: 800-606-6226.

Dandelion Burdock: Capsules or liquid. Helps enhance digestion and support the activity of the liver and gallbladder; includes dandelion and burdock roots, artichoke leaves, and milk thistle seed.

FRONTIER COOPERATIVE HERBS, 3021 78th Street, Norway, IA 52318; tel: 800-669-3275 or 319-227-7996.

Dandelion & Milk Thistle: Capsules. Herbal formula to help protect and detoxify the liver.

NUTRITION NOW, 501 Southeast Columbia Shore Boulevard #350, Vancouver, WA 98661; tel: 800-929-0418 or 360-737-6800.

Dandelion • Milk Thistle Compound: Liquid. Restorative and protective tonic for the liver and cleanser for the liver and gallbladder; can be used as an occasional maintenance tonic, after illness or abuse, as adjunct therapy in chronic constipation, or as post-surgical treatment of cholecystectomy (gallbladder removal); helpful for sluggish bile and gallstones, hepatitis, and jaundice; ingredients include dandelion (root, leaf, and flower), Oregon grape root, mature seed of milk thistle, artichoke leaf, beet leaf, and fennel seed.

HERB PHARM, 20260 Williams Highway, Williams, OR 97544; tel: 800-348-4372 or 541-846-6262.

DetoxCleanse: Capsules. Helps detoxify the body and bloodstream through cleansing the liver, improving digestion, binding and excreting toxins within the gastrointestinal tract, and promoting regularity.

BIODYNAMAX, 6525 Gunpark Drive #150-507, Boulder, CO 80301; tel: 800-926-7525 or 303-530-4665.

Fundamental Sulfur: Tablets. Supplies biologically active sulfur (a mineral element missing from many diets) that supports connective tissues, immune function, and detoxification; the liver also depends on sulfur to detoxify food or airborne compounds that are foreign to the body.

AMNI, 2247 National Avenue, Hayward, CA 94540-5012; tel: 800-437-8888 or 510-783-6969.

Hepa Plus: Capsules. Contains milk thistle extract (standardized to greater than 80% silymarin), dandelion root extract, alpha-lipoic acid, NAC (N-acetyl-cysteine), TTFD (thiamin tetrahydrofurfuryl disulfide), ornithine, alpha-ketoglutarate, glycine, taurine, and the minerals molybdenum and selenium.

HEALTH PRODUCTS DISTRIBUTORS INC., 23847 Peaceful Ridge Road, Smithsburg, MD 21783; tel: 800-228-4265 or 301-416-0500.

Hepato-Pure: Tablets. Facilitates deep internal detoxification while nurturing and strengthening the liver; dredges the system of stored toxins and waste products.

PLANETARY FORMULAS, 23 Janis Way, Scotts Valley, CA 95066; tel: 800-606-6226.

Herbal Aloe Force: (See product listing for Cellular Detoxification, above)

Herbal Liver Complex: Vegicaps. Formula for the support of normal healthy liver function.

SOLGAR VITAMIN & HERB COMPANY, INC., 500 Willow Tree Road, Leonia, NJ 07605; tel: 800-645-2246 or 201-944-2311.

Lipoic Acid: Capsules. Lipoic acid is a powerful antioxidant that protects other antioxidants (vitamins C and E and glutathione) in the body; it also chelates (binds with) heavy metals such as lead, cadmium, mercury, and free iron and copper and eliminates them from the body.

HEALTH PRODUCTS DISTRIBUTORS INC., 23847 Peaceful Ridge Road, Smithsburg, MD 21783; tel: 800-228-4265 or 301-416-0500.

LIV-WELL: Caplets. Contains the flavonoids silymarin, quercetin, cynarin, and capillarisin, which have been shown to improve liver metabolism and promote detoxification of the liver and body in general; aids in the elimination of excess water through the kidneys, and stimulates bile flow (through the gallbladder) and other digestive substances, which improves digestion.

EXTREME HEALTH INC., 50 Oak Court, Suite 212, Danville, CA 94526; tel: 800-800-1285 or 925-855-1262.

LiverClean: Capsules. Nourishes, balances, and detoxifies the liver; ingredients include barberry root bark, blessed thistle, dandelion root, boldo leaves, black radish seed, wild yam root, fennel seed, and cloves.

RIDGECREST HERBALS, 1151 South Redwood Road #106, Salt Lake City, UT 84104-3729; tel: 800-242-4649 or 801-978-9633.

Liver Glandular Plus: Tablets. Contains raw liver concentrate, methyl donors (which help carry oxygen, increase circulation, and metabolize fats), vitamin B6, and herbs designed to support liver function; the bovine glandular concentrate in this product is guaranteed raw (processed below 37° C).

ETHICAL NUTRIENTS, 971 Calle Negocio, San Clemente, CA 92673; tel: 800-668-8743 or 949-366-0818.

Liver Guard: Tablets. Contains 25 of the most important nutrients and related substances identified in scientific studies as either nourishment or protection for the liver.

SOURCE NATURALS, THRESHOLD ENTERPRISES, 23 Janis Way, Scotts Valley, CA 95066; tel: 800-777-5677 or 831-438-1144.

Liver Support With Milk Thistle Extract: Capsules. Contains milk thistle extract (a powerful natural antioxidant, which helps maintain healthy liver functions while it deals with pollutants and other toxins, including alcohol), dandelion root, ginger, burdock root, parsley root, and black radish root.

NATROL INC., 21411 Prairie Street, Chatsworth, CA 91311; tel: 818-739-6000.

Liv-R-Actin: Vegicaps. Contains milk thistle extract and an herbal blend of dandelion, barberry, goldenseal, wild Oregon grape, and celery seed.

NATURE'S PLUS, 548 Broadhollow Road, Melville, NY 11747-3708; tel: 800-645-9500 or 516-293-0030.

Metabolic Liver Formula: Capsules. Combines plant enzymes with fat-processing lipotropic nutrients, herbs, and liver extract; ingredients include choline, methionine, inositol, milk thistle seed, Russian black radish, and beet leaf, all traditionally used for liver support.

PREVAIL CORP., 2204-8 Northwest Birdsdale, Gresham, OR 97030; tel: 800-248-0885 or 503-667-5527.

Milk Thistle: Tablets. Standardized to 80% silymarin, which has antioxidant properties and supports healthy liver function and detoxification.

ETHICAL NUTRIENTS, 971 Calle Negocio, San Clemente, CA 92673; tel: 800-668-8743 or 949-366-0818.

Milk Thistle Extract: Capsules. Through its antioxidant properties, milk thistle extract helps maintain healthy liver function; used by people concerned about cigarette smoke, alcohol, or environmental toxins.

NATURE'S SOURCE, 15451 San Fernando Mission Boulevard, Mission Hills, CA 91345; tel: 800-423-2405 or 818-837-3633.

Milk-Thistle Power: Capsules. Concentrated, standardized extract of milk thistle combined with artichoke and turmeric to support healthy liver function.

NATURE'S HERBS, 600 East Quality Drive, American Fork, UT 84003; tel: 800-437-2257 or 801-763-0700.

Quick Cleanse Program Kit: (See product listing for Intestinal Detoxification, above)

Whole Beet Juice Tablets. Beets, which are high in iron, can help support liver function and detoxification, and also establish a favorable environment in the intestines for support of healthy intestinal flora.

SONNE'S ORGANIC FOODS INC., P.O. Box 2160, Cottonwood, CA 96022; tel: 800-544-8147 or 530-347-5868.

Immune Support

Bacteria, fungi, and viruses are continually present in our bodies, mainly in the skin, eyes, respiratory system, gastrointestinal tract (stomach and intestines), and urinary tract (kidneys, bladder, and urethra). We are also additionally exposed on occasion to highly infectious bacteria, viruses, and parasites. A healthy immune system is generally able to prevent both microorganisms present in the body and outside invaders from producing illness.

The immune "workers" dispatched by the immune system to fight infection are various white blood cells including one trillion lymphocytes and 100 million trillion antibodies produced and secreted by the lymphocytes. Lymphocytes (T and B cells) are found in high numbers in the lymph nodes, bone marrow, spleen, and thymus gland. Lymph nodes are clusters of immune tissue that work as filters or "inspection stations" for detecting foreign and potentially harmful substances in the lymph fluid that flows in the lymphatic vessels throughout the body.

Of all the body's systems, the immune system is the most vulnerable to nutritional deficiencies. Therefore, providing optimal nutrition to keep the immune system strong and able to fulfill its defensive function is an important step in both disease prevention and the maintenance of overall health. As immune system efficiency declines with age—beginning to drop off after 40 and becoming much less effective by 70—nutritional supplementation is particularly recommended for people over 50.

Nutrients and Herbs for Immune Support

Adaptogens—This category of nutrients helps the body adapt to stress. One of the best products we have used is Adaptogem, which contains the adaptogenic herbs Siberian ginseng root, schisandra fruit, echinacea root, wild oats, bladderwrack, and gotu kola.

See also **Stress** in Part II, pp. 369-384. For more about **amino acids**, see An A-Z Nutrient Guide in Part I, pp. 24-62.

Adrenal Glandular Extracts—A primary function of the adrenal glands is to help the body adjust to stressful environments or conditions. Chronic stress depletes these glands which in turn lowers immunity. By supporting the adrenals, glandular extracts improve immunity. Adrenal Glandular Plus is a formula we have used with success.

Antibiotic Nutrients—Garlic, olive leaf extract, goldenseal, and grapefruit seed extract are antimicrobial agents which can aid the immune system in preventing or eliminating infection.

Antioxidants—These vital nutrients protect the body by neutralizing potentially damaging free radicals (SEE QUICK DEFINITION). If left uncontrolled, free radicals can weaken the immune system and lead to illness and degenerative diseases. Supplementation with antioxidants has proven effective in increasing immunity.[20] Antioxidant nutrients include vitamins A, C, and E, beta carotene, selenium, coenzyme Q10, pycnogenol (grape seed extract), L-glutathione, superoxide dismutase (SOD), bioflavonoids, ginkgo, and garlic. When antioxidants are taken in combination, the effect is stronger than when they are used individually.

While many people take antioxidants primarily for immune health, it should be understood that these nutrients are equally important for the cardiovascular, nervous, and, indeed, all body systems.

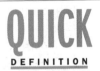

DEFINITION

A **free radical** is an unstable, toxic molecule of oxygen with an unpaired electron that steals an electron from another molecule and produces harmful effects. Free radicals are formed when molecules within cells react with oxygen (oxidize) as part of normal metabolic processes. Free radicals then begin to break down cells, especially the cell membranes, often in a matter of minutes to an hour. A single free radical can destroy a cell. While free radicals are normal products of metabolism, uncontrolled free-radical production plays a major role in the development of degenerative disease, including cancer and heart disease.

Free-Form Amino Acids—Under immune challenge, the body may need three to four times its usual requirement of amino acids, which are essential to immune function. When the immune system has been weakened, however, digestion is often sluggish and heavy meat proteins (a typical source of amino acids) are difficult for the body to process. Amino acid supplements are readily digested and assimilated and do not put stress on the kidneys as heavy proteins often do. AminoHealth is one free-form amino acid product that we take ourselves and often recommend. Pro Support, a powdered drink mix, is another good source, as is Aminomune.

Minerals—Deficiencies in zinc, iron, selenium, and copper have all been shown to impair immune response.[21]

Additional Immune-Enhancing Nutrients—Other nutrients and herbs we often recommend for immune system support are dimethyl glycine (DMG), germanium, aloe vera, pau d'arco, cat's claw, astragalus, echinacea, shiitake and reishi mushrooms, barberry (berberine), *acidophilus*, "green" foods such as blue-green algae, chorella, spirulina, and wheat grass (blood detoxifiers), and sea vegetables such as kelp, nori, and dulse (high in trace minerals).

Products for Immune Support

The number of products for support of immune health is extensive. To make our listing more useful to the reader, we have grouped the products according to the following categories (in the order in which they appear): General Immune Support, Antioxidants, Echinacea and Goldenseal, Garlic, "Green" Food Products, and Minerals.

GENERAL IMMUNE SUPPORT

Adaptogem: Caplets. Contains adaptogenic herbs traditionally used to help the body adapt to physical and emotional change; particularly recommended after stress or overwork.

RAINBOW LIGHT, P.O. Box 600, Santa Cruz, CA 95061; tel: 800-635-1233 or 408-429-9089.

Adrenal Glandular Plus: Tablets. Combines bovine adrenal glandular extract and B vitamins involved in hormone production and regulation; nutritional support for adrenal function.

ETHICAL NUTRIENTS, 971 Calle Negocio, San Clemente, CA 92673; tel: 800-668-8743 or 949-366-0818.

Alkyrol: Capsules. Purified and standardized shark liver oil, which clinical studies have proven to be an immune stimulant; helps prevent colds and other infections, reduce symptoms of asthma and psoriasis, and lessen the side effects of chemotherapy and radiation treatments.

SCANDINAVIAN NATURAL HEALTH & BEAUTY PRODUCTS, INC., 13 North 7th Street, Perkasie, PA 18944; tel: 800-688-2276.

AminoHealth: Capsules. Complex of 18 isolated L-crystalline amino acids for times of mental and physical stress; contains the sulfur-bearing amino acids, which constitute a high percentage of the amino acids found in hair, skin, and nails and also play a role in detoxification.

NUTRI-SOURCE, 3290 Cessna Drive, Cameron Park, CA 95682; tel: 800-293-1683 or 530-676-8838.

AminoMune: Capsules. Contains an arginine-free, balanced complex of 18 isolated L-crystalline amino acids and the amino acid L-lysine;

for viral infections, such as cold sores or underlying viral conditions. NUTRI-SOURCE, 3290 Cessna Drive, Cameron Park, CA 95682; tel: 800-293-1683 or 530-676-8838.

Anti-Bio Caps: Capsules or liquid. Herbal formula that has antiviral, antibacterial, and antiseptic properties; contains echinacea, goldenseal, capsicum, marshmallow, black walnut hulls, elecampane, propolis, myrrh gum, turmeric, and potassium chloride.
CRYSTAL STAR HERBAL NUTRITION, 4069 Wedgeway Court, Earth City, MO 63045; tel: 800-736-6015 or 314-739-7551.

Astragalus Formula: Liquid and tablets. Provides support for immune deficiency, chronic viral infections and is a lung tonic for people with a history of chronic respiratory problems; increases recovery and energy after colds, flu, and illness; part of an herbal rotational program that also includes Insure Herbal, an echinacea and goldenseal formula.
ZAND HERBAL FORMULAS, 1722 14th Street #230, Boulder, CO 80302; tel: 800-800-0405 or 303-786-8558.

BioPectin: Tablets. Contains modified citrus pectin, a complex carbohydrate extracted from the pulp of citrus fruits; citrus pectin is absorbed into the bloodstream where it attaches to undesirable cells and helps the body to eliminate them.
FLORA INC., 805 East Badger Road, Lynden, WA 98264; tel: 800-446-2110 or 360-354-2110.

BioPro Thymic Protein A: Sublingual powder. Contains thymic protein A, which increases the number of functioning key white blood cells and allows the body to fight off infections (from flu to herpes); also useful in cancer therapy, chronic fatigue syndrome, low white blood cell count, and any other illness involving weakened immunity.
KLABIN MARKETING, 2067 Broadway #700, New York, NY 10023; tel: 800-933-9440 or 212-877-3632.

Cat's Claw: Capsules. Contains cat's claw; studies have found that cat's claw enhances the activity of white blood cells during phagocytosis (engulfing potentially harmful microorganisms), inhibits platelet aggregation, and is effective in the treatment of allergies.
NATURE'S PRIDE, NATURE'S PRODUCTS, 1301 Sawgrass Corporate Parkway, Sunrise, FL 33323-2813; tel: 800-752-7873 or 954-233-4600.

Cat's Claw: Liquid, tablets, or tea bags. Liquid contains extract of cat's claw inner bark, 20% pure grain alcohol, and filtered water; tablets contain concentrated cat's claw (three times the active ingredient of an identically weighted dosage); tea bags contain concentrated cat's claw extract with cinnamon, ginger, and cardamom.

PERUVIAN RAINFOREST BOTANICALS, NUTRAMEDIX, 212 North U.S. Highway 1 #17, Tequesta, FL 33469; tel: 800-730-3130.

Cat's Claw and Aloe Vera: Capsules. Combination of cat's claw concentrate plus 100 mg of a 200:1 concentrate of whole-leaf aloe vera.

PERUVIAN RAINFOREST BOTANICALS, NUTRAMEDIX, 212 North U.S. Highway 1 #17, Tequesta, FL 33469; tel: 800-730-3130.

Cat's Claw Defense Complex: Tablets. Combines cat's claw with herbs such as pau d'arco, aloe vera, St. John's wort, reishi mushroom, and astragalus, and two categories of antioxidants.

SOURCE NATURALS, THRESHOLD ENTERPRISES, 23 Janis Way, Scotts Valley, CA 95066; tel: 800-777-5677 or 831-438-1144.

Cat's Claw Plus Ezseac Tea: Liquid. Contains cat's claw concentrated tea combined with a formula of distilled water, burdock root, sheep sorrel, slippery elm bark, water cress, and turkey rhubarb root.

PERUVIAN RAINFOREST BOTANICALS, NUTRAMEDIX, 212 North U.S. Highway 1 #17, Tequesta, FL 33469; tel: 800-730-3130.

Deep Defense: Caplets or liquid. Contains Chinese herbs known as *qi* (also referred to as *chi*, vital life energy) tonics to support the body after long-term weakness or chronic deficiency; ingredients include the healing mushrooms reishi and shiitake, plus astragalus.

RAINBOW LIGHT, P.O. Box 600, Santa Cruz, CA 95061; tel: 800-635-1233 or 408-429-9089.

Defense Formula: Capsules. Protective dietary supplement with a blend of nutrients, herbs (two species of echinacea), and thymus glandular extracts to enhance the body's resistance.

PREVAIL CORP., 2204-8 Northwest Birdsdale, Gresham, OR 97030; tel: 800-248-0885 or 503-667-5527.

East Star Formula: Liquid. Contains pau d'arco, *Pfaffia paniculata*, chaparral, and Chinese astragalus prepared in a 20% ethanol base.

SEDNA, P.O. Box 1453, Andrews, NC 28901; tel: 800-223-0858 or 828-321-2240.

Echatin Forte: Capsules. Contains immune stimulators that can help increase the white blood cell count; ingredients include echinacea, astragalus, and reishi and shiitake mushrooms.

NF FORMULAS INC., 9755 Southwest Commerce Circle, C-5, Wilsonville, OR 97070; tel: 800-547-4891 or 503-682-9755.

Ecogen 851 Soy Liquid. Contains fermented soy, a bioavailable source of whole protein; beneficial properties of fermented soy are more easily assimilated than unfermented soy; good for weak digestive systems and in the treatment of cancer and immune-deficiency states.

KLABIN MARKETING, 2067 Broadway #700, New York, NY 10023; tel: 800-933-9440 or 212-877-3632.

Ecogen Soy Isoflavone: Powder or tablets. Contains a high potency concentrate of soy isoflavones (the main protective elements in soy), including genistein and diadzein.

KLABIN MARKETING, 2067 Broadway #700, New York, NY 10023; tel: 800-933-9440 or 212-877-3632.

ESI-20: Liquid. Contains sheep sorrel, turkey rhubarb, slippery elm, burdock root (*Arctium lappa*), and watercress prepared in a 20% ethanol base.

SEDNA, P.O. Box 1453, Andrews, NC 28901; tel: 800-223-0858 or 828-321-2240.

Essiac Herbal Tea. Herbal remedy that contains inulin, a starch occurring naturally in certain plants that attaches to white blood cells and improves their function; ingredients include burdock root, slippery elm (*Ulmus rubra*), sheep sorrel, and Indian rhubarb, which can help normalize body systems by purifying the blood, promoting cellular repair, and aiding effective assimilation and elimination; nontoxic and herbicide-free.

ESSIAC INTERNATIONAL, 164 Richmond Road, Ottawa, Ontario, Canada K1Z 6W1; tel: 613-729-9111.

Flora • Essence: Liquid. Formula of eight herbs that work together to cleanse, stimulate, and strengthen the body; ingredients include burdock root, sheep sorrel, slippery elm, watercress, Turkish rhubarb, kelp, blessed thistle, and red clover.

FLORA INC., 805 East Badger Road, Lynden, WA 98264; tel: 800-446-2110 or 360-354-2110.

Farmacopia by Immune-Neem: Capsules or tea. Contains neem leaf (a mainstay of the Ayurvedic health system of India; laboratory studies have shown its antifungal, antibacterial, and antiviral activities), ginger, stevia, peppermint, lemon grass, cinnamon, and licorice.

BOTANICAL PRODUCTS INTERNATIONAL, P.O. Box 174, Hakalau, HI 96710; tel: 808-963-6771.

Germanium: Capsules. Contains germanium Ge-132 (bis-carboxyethyl germanium sesquioxide); organic germanium may increase production of interferon (protein released by white blood cells), thereby making it an immune stimulant; animal experiments suggest a role for organic germanium in hypertension and heart disease.

OPTIMAL NUTRIENTS, 1163 Chess Drive #F, Foster City, CA 94404; tel: 800-966-8874 or 650-525-0112.

Health-Gard With Echinacea: Capsules. Helps strengthen the body's natural defenses; contains beta carotene, vitamins C and E, zinc, selenium, echinacea, white willow, odorless garlic, astragalus, reishi and shiitake mushrooms, pau d'arco, goldenseal root, broccoli, natural aromatic oil, selenium, and the amino acid L-methionine.

NATURE'S HERBS, 600 East Quality Drive, American Fork, UT 84003; tel: 800-437-2257 or 801-763-0700.

Herbal Aloe Force: Juice or topical gel. Processed aloe vera juice containing vitamins, minerals, enzymes, amino acids, essential fatty acids, growth factors, glycoproteins, sterols, bioflavonoids, and polysaccharides (complex sugars), plus ionized colloidal silver and herbal extracts (cat's claw, chamomile, burdock root, hawthorn berry, astragalus root, sheep sorrell, pau d'arco bark, slippery elm bark, and rhubarb root).

HERBAL ANSWERS INC., P.O. Box 1110, Saratoga Springs, NY 12866; tel: 888-256-3367 or 518-581-1968.

Herbal Defense: Liquid. Contains extracts of echinacea, Siberian ginseng, *Astragalus membranaceus*, the support herbs burdock, dandelion, angelica, ginger, rosemary, peppermint, sage, goldenseal, chamomile, licorice, and reishi and shiitake mushrooms in a base of purified water, brown rice syrup, honey natural flavor, natural color, and 20% USP alcohol.

NATURE'S APOTHECARY, P.O. Box 17970, Boulder, CO 80308; tel: 800-999-7422 or 303-664-1600.

Herbal Resistance: Liquid. Contains osha root, lomatium, and echinacea, which have been used to nutritionally support good health and strengthen respiratory functions during periods of health imbalance. NOW, 550 Mitchell Road, Glendale Heights, IL 60139; tel: 800-283-3500 or 630-545-9098.

Immune-Action: Capsules. Ingredients include astragalus root, lingustrum berries, schisandra fruit, shiitake mushrooms, echinacea root, young barley leaves, and pau d'arco bark.
NATURE'S PLUS, 548 Broadhollow Road, Melville, NY 11747-3708; tel: 800-645-9500 or 516-293-0030.

ImmuneActin: Capsules or syrup. Capsules contain echinacea, goldenseal, and antioxidants that nutritionally support the body's normal adaptogenic functions; syrup contains elderberry, slippery elm, echinacea, white willow, and goldenseal.
NATURE'S PLUS, 548 Broadhollow Road, Melville, NY 11747-3708; tel: 800-645-9500 or 516-293-0030.

Immune Formula: Tablets. Contains carotenoids, vitamins A, C, and E, selenium, echinacea, zinc, and ginseng, which help to maintain strong, healthy immune function.
NATURE'S LIFE, 7180 Lampson Avenue, Garden Grove, CA 92841-3914; tel: 800-854-6837 or 714-379-6500.

Laktoferrin: Capsules. Contains lactoferrin, a naturally occurring iron-binding protein, derived from New Zealand grain-fed cattle; pathogens involved in the disease process feed off of free-floating iron; lactoferrin supports the immune system by binding with the food source and starving iron-feeding pathogens.
ALLERGY RESEARCH GROUP/NUTRICOLOGY, P.O. Box 55907, Hayward, CA 94544; tel: 800-545-9960 or 510-487-8526.

LDM-100 (Lomatium Dissectum): Liquid. Contains the herb *Lomatium dissectum*, which has antibacterial and antiviral properties; useful for colds, *Streptococcus* and *Staphylococcus* infections, and other infections.
SEDNA, P.O. Box 1453, Andrews, NC 28901; tel: 800-223-0858 or 828-321-2240.

Lysine-Power: Capsules. Contains the amino acid L-lysine, with zinc, vitamin C, quercetin, and extracts of grape skin, green tea, propolis, echinacea, St. John's wort, and licorice root.

NATURE'S HERBS, 600 East Quality Drive, American Fork, UT 84003; tel: 800-437-2257 or 801-763-0700.

Maitake Mushroom Extract D Fraction: Liquid. Researchers have identified maitake's stimulatory effect upon the immune system and have isolated the maitake mushroom's active component, a beta-glucan called D-fraction; contains at least 900 mg of maitake D-fraction.

SHOKO'S NATURAL PRODUCTS, 3402 Edgmont Avenue #373, Brookhaven, PA 19015; tel: 800-654-4394 or 610-876-9850.

Multi Mushroom Complex: Capsules. Contains Kombucha, shiitake, maitake, and reishi mushrooms, which are beneficial to the body's cardiovascular, immune, and endocrine systems.

SCHIFF, WEIDER NUTRITION GROUP, 2002 South 5070 West, Salt Lake City, UT 84104; tel: 800-439-8042 or 801-975-5000.

Mycoceutics 10 Mushroom Extract: Capsules. For improving natural immunity or as an adjunct treatment of cancer and other immuno-deficiency diseases; contains extracts of the Chinese mushrooms *Lentinus* and *Coriolus versicolor*, which studies have found to have immune-stimulating and anticancer properties, plus eight other potent mushroom extracts.

KLABIN MARKETING, 2067 Broadway #700, New York, NY 10023; tel: 800-933-9440 or 212-877-3632.

Natural Defense Balance: Tablets. Helps support a healthy defense system; contains herbal combinations created by Ayurvedic physicians.

VEDA HEALTH INC., P.O. Box 1535, Soquel, CA 95073; tel: 888-856-8334 or 408-465-9084.

Noni Hawaiian Morinda Citrifolia by Earth's Bounty: Capsules. The noni plant grows best in mineral-rich Hawaiian volcanic ash; used for boosting immune system, easing joint pain, and regenerating cells.

MATRIX HEALTH PRODUCTS, 8400 Magnolia Avenue, Suite N, Santee, CA 92071; tel: 800-736-5609 or 619-448-7550.

NSC-24 and NSC-100: Capsules. Beta-glucan immune enhancers; NSC-24 contains 3 mg of beta glucans for the maintenance of a healthy immune system; NSC-100 is for protection of compromised or weakened immune systems such as cancer or severe allergies.

NUTRITIONAL SUPPLY CORP., 2533 North Carson Street #3127, Carson City, NV; tel: 888-24-NSC (672)-24 or 702-888-6900.

Ocean Nutrition Canada Shark Liver Oil. Immune-system booster.
OCEAN NUTRITION CANADA LTD., 757 Bedford Highway, Bedford, Nova Scotia, Canada B2A3Z7; tel: 888-980-8889 or 902-457-2399.

OxyEssence: Liquid. Stabilized oxygen plus homeopathic trace elements, flowers, and botanical essences, which help kill viruses, yeast, fungi, and bacteria, including *Streptococcus* and *Cryptosperidium*.
OLYMPIC BOTANICALS, 231 Otto Street, Port Townsend, WA 98368; tel: 800-310-6924 or 360-385-9468.

PDL-500: Liquid. Ingredients include herbs from North America and the Yucatan rainforest.
SEDNA, P.O. Box 1453, Andrews, NC 28901; tel: 800-223-0858 or 828-321-2240.

Pfaffia Paniculata (Suma): Powder. Known in Brazil as "Para Tudo" (for everything), suma has become accepted worldwide as an adaptogen and has been used to treat chronic diseases characterized by fatigue; provides relief from stress and helps enhance immune system function; it is a rich source of germanium, allantoin (which promotes wound healing), vitamins, minerals, amino acids, beta-ecdysone (which helps increase oxygenation of the cells), sitosterol and stigmasterol (which help increase coronary circulation), and pfaffosides (which are found only in *Pfaffia paniculata* and help inhibit tumor cell growth).
SEDNA, P.O. Box 1453, Andrews, NC 28901; tel: 800-223-0858 or 828-321-2240.

Reishi Mushroom Supreme: Tablets. *Fu Zheng* herbs are used to strengthen resistance, restore the normal functioning of the body, and protect against stress; contains concentrated mature reishi extract, reishi mycelia (the vegetative part of the mushroom), shiitake mushroom, astragalus, schisandra, grifola, and poria cocos.
PLANETARY FORMULAS, 23 Janis Way, Scotts Valley, CA 95066; tel: 800-606-6226.

Shield Chi by Jade: Tablets. Chinese herbal formula that helps protect the body's *qi* (vital life energy) against pathogens by controlling the opening and closing of pores, readjusting body temperature, and helping to warm and strengthen certain organs, muscles, and skin.

EAST EARTH HERB INC., P.O. Box 2802 Eugene, OR 97402; tel: 800-827-HERB (4372) or 541-687-0155.

Squalene: Capsules or softgels. Squalene, an extract from the liver of the Aizame shark, increases new tissue growth, which covers wounds; it also stimulates the defensive forces of the body, enhances resistance to immune system disorders, supports the activity of the liver, and acts as an adaptogen similar to ginseng and antioxidants.

OPTIMAL NUTRIENTS, 1163 Chess Drive #F, Foster City, CA 94404; tel: 800-966-8874 or 650-525-0112.

Vita Carte Bovine Cartilage: Capsules. 100% pure bovine cartilage, derived from range-grown, certified hormone-free cattle; research has proven that bovine tracheal cartilage is effective in treating arthritis by selectively stimulating the body's immune system.

PHOENIX BIOLOGICS, 2794 Loker Avenue West #104, Carlsbad, CA 92008; tel: 800-947-8482 or 760-631-7729.

Wellness Formula: Tablets. Contains a large dose of vitamin C, antioxidants, herbs, and other vitamins and ingredients to provide nutritional protection during the winter months and throughout the year.

SOURCE NATURALS, THRESHOLD ENTERPRISES, 23 Janis Way, Scotts Valley, CA 95066; tel: 800-777-5677 or 831-438-1144.

ANTIOXIDANTS

ACES Gold: Tablets. Contains coenzyme Q10, vitamins A, C, and E, and glutathione peroxidase support (selenium, glutathione, and N-acetylcysteine), superoxide dismutase support (zinc, copper, and manganese), alpha-lipoic acid, citrus bioflavonoids, quercetin, and odorless garlic (*Allium sativum*).

J.R. CARLSON LABS INC., 15 College Drive, Arlington Heights, IL 60004-1985; tel: 800-323-4141 or 708-255-1600.

Advanced Antioxidant Formula: Vegicaps. Provides vitamin, mineral, and plant-based antioxidants, plus SOD (superoxide dismutase) inducers in a food and herbal formula.

SOLGAR VITAMIN & HERB CO, INC., 500 Willow Tree Road, Leonia, NJ 07605; 800-645-2246.

Advanced Nutritional System: Tablets. Contains vitamins and minerals (including antioxidant nutrients and food-grown B vitamins), plus plant-source enzymes, herbal extracts, and a blend of superfoods.

RAINBOW LIGHT, P.O. Box 600, Santa Cruz, CA 95061; tel: 800-635-1233 or 408-429-9089.

Antioxidant Formula: Capsules. Contains antioxidants and nutrients that enhance the uptake of vitamin C and cellular function; ingredients include vitamins A, C, and E, beta and alpha carotenes, coenzyme forms of vitamins B1, B2, and B6, N-acetyl-L-cysteine, ferulic acid, malic acid, lipoic acid, calcium, copper, manganese, magnesium, selenium, zinc, pycnogenols and green tea catechins.

HEALTH PRODUCTS DISTRIBUTORS INC., 23847 Peaceful Ridge Road, Smithsburg, MD 21783; tel: 800-228-4265 or 301-416-0500.

Antioxidant Formula: Capsules. Reduces free-radical formation; contains vitamin E and beta carotene (from broccoli powder, carrot powder, and blue-green algae) in a base of antioxidant-supportive food concentrates and herbs (including extracts of grape seed, green tea, and pine bark).

ZAND HERBAL FORMULAS, 1722 14th Street #230, Boulder, CO 80302; tel: 800-800-0405 or 303-786-8558.

Basic Antiox: Capsules or tablets. Antioxidant nutrient program to help support the heart and immune system.

AMNI, 2247 National Avenue, Hayward, CA 94540-5012; tel: 800-437-8888 or 510-783-6969.

Beta-Carotene Antioxidant System: Tablets. Fights free-radical damage; contains antioxidant plant nutrients, vitamins, minerals, foods, and potent herbal extracts.

RAINBOW LIGHT, P.O. Box 600, Santa Cruz, CA 95061; tel: 800-635-1233 or 408-429-9089.

Beta Glucan NSC 24: Capsules. Activates macrophage cells, white blood cells that digest foreign proteins, cellular debris, and other wastes in the blood.

SOLARAY, NUTRACEUTICAL CORP., P.O. Box 681869, Park City, UT 84068; tel: 800-669-8877.

BioBoost: Capsules. Contains echinacea, goldenseal, and antioxidant vitamins and minerals to support your body's natural defenses.

BIODYNAMAX, 6525 Gunpark Drive #150-507, Boulder, CO 80301; tel: 800-926-7525 or 303-530-4665.

Buffered Vitamin C Powder or Beet Source "Buffered Vitamin C": Capsules or powder. Contains ascorbic acid, from a hypoallergenic, non-corn source, and buffered with the carbonates of potassium, calcium, and magnesium; some sensitive people are able to tolerate this formula if unable to tolerate other vitamin C products.

ALLERGY RESEARCH GROUP/NUTRICOLOGY, P.O. Box 55907, Hayward, CA 94544; tel: 800-545-9960 or 510-487-8526.

C Complex Plus: Tablets. Vitamin C rids the body of toxins as it travels through the bloodstream; contains vitamin C (vegetable source) and vitamin A (fish liver oil) in a base of seaweed, capsicum (cayenne), goldenseal root, yerba santa, and lemon bioflavonoids.

NATURAL ENERGY PRODUCTS, 21101 Welch Road, Snohomish, WA 98296; tel: 425-486-5956.

Cee Complete: Tablets. Contains 500 mg of vitamin C with rose hips.

NATURE'S PLUS, 548 Broadhollow Road, Melville, NY 11747-3708; tel: 800-645-9500 or 516-293-0030.

Chewable Orange Vitamin C: Tablets. Contains vitamin C (ascorbic acid) with rose hips.

AMERICAN HEALTH, 4320 Veterans Memorial Highway, Holbrook, NY 11741; tel: 800-445-7137.

Coenzyme Q10: Capsules. Powerful antioxidant and healthy heart supplement, CoQ10 also works to produce ATP (adenosine triphosphate), which is the energy molecule found in every cell in the body.

SCHIFF, WEIDER NUTRITION GROUP, 2002 South 5070 West, Salt Lake City, UT 84104; tel: 800-439-8042 or 801-975-5000.

Coenzyme Q-10 Rx (Q-Gel): Softgels. Cellular energizer that research has shown to be the only hydrosoluble coenzyme Q10 product; has up to four times more bio-availability than other delivery systems.

PHYTO-THERAPY INC., OPTIMUM HEALTH, 483 West Middle Turnpike, Manchester, CT 06040; tel: 800-228-1507.

Elan Vital: Tablets. Multiple antioxidant that also supports structural integrity, energy generation, neurotransmitter production, and liver health; contains the antioxidants NAC (N-acetyl-cysteine), vitamins C and E, beta carotene, selenium, niacin, biotin, chromium, coenzyme Q10, ginkgo, DMAE (an amino-acid complex originating from soybeans), silymarin, bilberry, N-acetyl-glucosamine, quercetin, N-acetyl L-tyrosine, and lipoic and succinic acids.

SOURCE NATURALS, THRESHOLD ENTERPRISES, 23 Janis Way, Scotts Valley, CA 95066; tel: 800-777-5677 or 831-438-1144.

E-mergen-C: Powder. Replenishes electrolytes and muscle minerals and fights off free-radical damage; contains vitamin C mineral ascorbates, vitamins B1, B2, B6, and B12, potassium, magnesium, manganese, calcium, zinc, and chromium.

ALACER CORP., 19631 Pauling, Foothill Ranch, CA 92610; tel: 800-854-0249 or 949-454-3900.

E-mergen-C Lite: Powder. Contains the same basic formula as E-mergen-C without the B vitamins or added sweeetners; no calories.

ALACER CORP., 19631 Pauling, Foothill Ranch, CA 92610; tel: 800-854-0249 or 949-454-3900.

Essential Balance: Tablets. Multivitamin/mineral with antioxidant vitamins C and E and beta carotene, which help protect the body from possible cell damage caused by oxidants.

NATURE MADE LLC, NATURE'S RESOURCE, P.O. Box 9606 Mission Hills, CA 91346-9606; tel: 800-314-HERB (4372) or 800-423-2405.

Ester C Plus: Capsules. Non-acidic form of vitamin C, which possesses antioxidant, antihistamine, anti-inflammatory, and immune-enhancing properties, and strengthens blood vessels.

PHILLIPS NUTRITIONALS, 27071 Cabot Road #122, Laguna Hills, CA 92653; tel: 800-514-5115 or 702-898-8141.

Esterol With Ester-C: Capsules. Contains ester C and three water-soluble antioxidant bioflavonoids (quercetin, rutin, and proanthocyanidins from grape seed), and calcuim; highly absorbable and non-acidic, so minimally irritating to the intestines.

ALLERGY RESEARCH GROUP/NUTRICOLOGY, P.O. Box 55907, Hayward, CA 94544; tel: 800-545-9960 or 510-487-8526.

EsterPlex: Tablets. Buffered, ester C/polyascorbate complex that has been chelated (combined with an amino acid to improve assimilation); neutral pH for individuals who cannot tolerate ascorbic acid.

NATURE'S PLUS, 548 Broadhollow Road, Melville, NY 11747-3708; tel: 800-645-9500 or 516-293-0030.

Grape Seed-Power 100: Capsules. Antioxidant and bioflavonoid; contains grape seed extract in a base of grape skin extract.

NATURE'S HERBS, 600 East Quality Drive, American Fork, UT 84003; tel: 800-437-2257 or 801-763-0700.

Green Tea Extract: Tablets. Contains one of green tea's active components, epigallocatechin gallate (EGCg), a powerful antioxidant that test results suggest is 200 times more powerful than vitamin E.

SOURCE NATURALS, THRESHOLD ENTERPRISES, 23 Janis Way, Scotts Valley, CA 95066; tel: 800-777-5677 or 831-438-1144.

KYOLIC Formula 105: Tablets. Contains 200 mg of Aged Garlic Extract (a Wakunaga product), vitamins A, C, and E, selenium, and green tea, which are known for their antioxidant properties; dairy-free.

WAKUNAGA OF AMERICA, 23501 Madero, Mission Viejo, CA 92691; tel: 800-421-2998 or 949-855-2776.

Life Maintenance Formula: Packets. Contains antioxidant ingredients to optimize immune, cardiovascular, and neurological system nutrition, while combating the effects of stress, tension, and pollution.

NATURE'S PRODUCTS, 1301 Sawgrass Corporate Parkway, Sunrise, FL 33233; tel: 800-752-7873.

Mycel Vitamin E: Liquid. Vitamin E is a fat-soluble antioxidant and is involved in the functioning of all major organ systems in the body.

ETHICAL NUTRIENTS, 971 Calle Negocio, San Clemente, CA 92673; tel: 800-668-8743 or 949-366-0818.

Natural Source Vitamin C: Tablets. Contains vitamin C from the dehydrated juice of the acerola (cherry) berry and from wild Spanish orange.

SONNE'S ORGANIC FOODS, INC., P.O. Box 2160, Cottonwood, CA 96022; tel: 800-544-8147 or 530-347-5868.

Natural Vitamin E +: Capsules. Contains dry (non-oil) vitamin E plus selenium and chromium.

INFINITY HEALTH, 1519 Contra Costa Boulevard, Pleasant Hill, CA 94523; tel: 800-733-9293 or 925-676-8982.

Original AntiOx: Capsules. Contains antioxidant nutrients with the minerals necessary to activate antioxidant enzymes plus B vitamins that act as cofactors to help support and "recharge" the antioxidant defenses.

ALLERGY RESEARCH GROUP/NUTRICOLOGY, P.O. Box 55907, Hayward, CA 94544; tel: 800-545-9960 or 510-487-8526.

Oxystat: Capsules. Contains the major antioxidants, NAC (N-acetyl-cysteine), standardized green tea (50% catechins), silymarin, choline, methionine, glutathione, chlorophyll, coenzyme Q10, calcium D-glucarate, and other nutritional cofactors.

NF FORMULAS INC., 9755 Southwest Commerce Circle, C-5, Wilsonville, OR 97070; tel: 800-547-4891 or 503-682-9755.

Phyto-Power: Capsules. Blend of antioxidant vitamins C and E, beta carotene, folic acid, phytonutrients, and herbs.

NATURE'S HERBS, 600 East Quality Drive, American Fork, UT 84003; tel: 800-437-2257 or 801-763-0700.

PhytoxyActin: Capsules. Phytonutrient complex with standardized herbs and antioxidants to nutritionally support the body's natural free-radical defense system; contains standardized vegetable extracts such as broccoli, spinach, and tomato with maximum-strength antioxidants.

NATURE'S PLUS, 548 Broadhollow Road, Melville, NY 11747-3708; tel: 800-645-9500 or 516-293-0030.

Premier Anti-Oxidant: Capsules. Formula 1 helps the body recycle anitoxidant nutrients; contains glutathione and ALA (alpha-lipoic acid). Formula 2 contains the antioxidants vitamin A, alpha carotene (which helps protect the liver), beta carotene (a precursor to vitamin A), ester C, vitamin C, standardized green tea (50% catechins), quercetin, bromelain (needed to assimilate quercetin), zinc, copper, GLA (gamma-linoleic acid), and organic selenium.

BIO-NUTRITIONAL FORMULAS, 106 East Jericho Turnpike, Mineola, NY 11501; tel: 800-950-8484.

Pycnogenol & Citrus Bioflavonoids: Capsules. Contains pycnogenol from pine bark, a powerful antioxidant that crosses the blood-brain barrier helping to protect the body and the central nervous system from the damaging effects of free radicals.

AMERICAN HEALTH, 4320 Veterans Memorial Highway, Holbrook, NY 11741; tel: 800-445-7137.

Resveratrol: Tablets. Protective compound produced by grapevines and other plants in response to infection or environmental stress; provides antioxidant protection and can help prevent platelet aggregation.

SOURCE NATURALS, THRESHOLD ENTERPRISES, 23 Janis Way, Scotts Valley, CA 95066; tel: 800-777-5677 or 831-438-1144.

Super Defense Antioxidant Formula: Capsules. Antioxidant formula containing high levels of beta carotene, vitamins C and E, and selenium.

BRONSON LABORATORIES, INC., 600 East Quality Drive, American Fork, UT 84003; tel: 800-235-3200 or 801-756-5670.

Triple Action Antioxidant +: Capsules. Combination of proanthocyanidins, citrus bioflavonoids, and vitamin C to provide protection from free radicals, nourish the body, enhance joint flexibility, and promote healthy blood vessels and pliable, youthful skin.

NUPRO, 735-L Park Street, Castle Rock, CO 80104; tel: 303-660-0562 or 800-704-8910.

Ultra Antioxidants: Tablets. Contains 21 antioxidants including selenium, zinc, grape seed extract, green tea, garlic, and other nutrients.

BIODYNAMAX, 6525 Gunpark Drive #150-507, Boulder, CO 80301; tel: 800-926-7525 or 303-530-4665.

Ultra Antioxidan Plus: Softgels. Contains pycnogenol, coenzyme Q10, SOD (superoxide dismutase), glutathione, zinc, beta carotene, vitamins C and E, and selenium to neutralize free-radical production. Clinical data has shown the damaging effects of free radicals and single oxygen on cells and body systems.

PHILLIPS NUTRITIONALS, 27071 Cabot Road #122, Laguna Hills, CA 92653; tel: 800-514-5115 or 702-898-8141.

Vitamin C With Rose Hips: Tablets. Vitamin C is an antioxidant that helps boost the immune system and neutralize free radicals; rose hips are a natural source of vitamin C.

NATURE MADE LLC, NATURE'S RESOURCE, P.O. Box 9606 Mission Hills, CA 91346-9606; tel: 800-314-HERB (4372) or 800-423-2405.

ECHINACEA AND GOLDENSEAL

Products listed in the other immune support categories also contain echinacea and/or goldenseal, but those listed here feature one or both of these herbs as the predominant ingredient.

Echinacea Astragalus: Capsules or liquid. Enhances the body's resistance to infection.

FRONTIER COOPERATIVE HERBS, 3021 78th Street, Norway, IA 52318; tel: 800-669-3275 or 319-227-7996.

Echinacea/Astragalus/Reishi: Capsules. Contains echinacea, astragalus root, and reishi mushroom.

NATURE'S WAY PRODUCTS, INC., 10 Mountain Springs Parkway, Springville, UT 84663; tel: 801-489-1500.

Echinacea Chewable With Vitamin C: Tablets. Contains *Echinacea purpurea* and *Echinacea angustifolia* root blended with antioxidant vitamins A, B6, and C, zinc, and beta carotene, in a base of sorbitol, fructose, vegetable stearin, magnesium stearate, silicon dioxide, and stevia extract.

CHAINATA CORP., 5965 205 A Street, Langley, British Columbia, Canada V3A8C4; tel: 800-406-7668 or 604-533-8883.

Echinacea Ginger Wonder Syrup. Helpful during the cold and flu season; contains echinacea, ginger, and honey.

NEW CHAPTER, 22 High Street, Brattleboro, VT 05301; tel: 800-543-7279 or 802-257-9345.

Echinacea Glycerites: Liquid. Naturally sweet alternative to the traditional bitter-tasting echinacea liquid supplements.

PLANETARY FORMULAS, 23 Janis Way, Scotts Valley, CA 95066; tel: 800-606-6226.

Echinacea-Goldenseal Combo: Capsules. Echinacea and goldenseal may stimulate resistance by helping maintain the immune system.

NATURE'S SOURCE, 15451 San Fernando Mission Boulevard, Mission Hills, CA 91345; tel: 800-423-2405 or 818-837-3633.

Echinacea • Goldenseal Compound: Liquid. For colds and flu and a strengthening, preventive tonic for those susceptible to colds and flu; contains echinacea root, goldenseal rhizome and roots, osha root, spilanthes flowering herb and root, yerba santa leaf, horseradish root, elder flower, yarrow flower, watercress herb, and wild indigo root.

HERB PHARM, 20260 Williams Highway, Williams, OR 97544; tel: 800-348-4372 or 541-846-6262.

Echinacea & Goldenseal Herbal Blend: Capsules. Blend of concentrated organically grown echinacea (*E. angustifolia*, *E. pallida*, and *E. pur-*

purea) that can boost immunity, goldenseal to help combat infections, and the supporting herbs red clover (*Trifolium pratense*), garlic, stinging nettle, and ginger; helps support the immune system during the cold and flu season.

CHAINATA CORP., 5965 205 A Street, Langley, British Columbia, Canada V3A8C4; tel: 800-406-7668 or 604-533-8883.

Echinacea Plus: Caplets. Contains two sources of echinacea, plus vitamin C for immune support.

AMERIFIT, 166 Highland Park Drive, Bloomfield, CT 06002; tel: 800-990-FIRM (3476) or 860-242-3476.

Echinacea Plus Vitamin C: Softgels.

J.R. CARLSON LABS INC., 15 College Drive, Arlington Heights, IL 60004-1985; tel: 800-323-4141 or 708-255-1600.

Echinacea PM: Liquid. Sedating, nighttime herbal syrup that stimulates the immune system to reduce the active symptoms of a cold or flu while promoting sleep; features antiviral and antibacterial herbs to reduce irritating symptoms and nervine herbs to relax the nervous system and facilitate recovery.

ZAND HERBAL FORMULAS, 1722 14th Street #230, Boulder, CO 80302; tel: 800-800-0405 or 303-786-8558.

Echinacea With Golden Seal Root: Capsules. Ingredients include *Echinacea purpurea*, the roots of *Echinacea angustifolia*, goldenseal, burdock, and gentian, cayenne (*Capsicum anuum*), and wood betony; helps support immune function and maintain good health, especially during the cold-weather season.

NATURE'S WAY PRODUCTS INC., 10 Mountain Springs Parkway, Springville, UT 84663; tel: 801-489-1500.

Echinacea With Vitamin C: Capsules. Herbal formula containing echinacea and vitamin C for healthy immune function.

NATURE'S HERBS, 600 East Quality Drive, American Fork, UT 84003; tel: 800-437-2257 or 801-763-0700.

SP-21 Echinacea-Goldenseal Blend: Capsules. Contains echinacea, goldenseal root, myrrh gum, garlic, licorice root, vervain, butternut bark, kelp, and a homeopathically prepared mineral formula.

SOLARAY, NUTRACEUTICAL CORP., P.O. Box 681869, Park City, UT 84068; tel: 800-669-8877.

GARLIC

Garlic-Power: Tablets. Concentrated garlic extract from a Chinese formula of red and white garlic equivalent to 1,200 mg of fresh garlic; contains higher allicin potential (minimum 3 mg of total allicin potential calculated as allicin content and relative allinase enzyme activity per tablet) than any other garlic supplement; odor-controlled.

NATURE'S HERBS, 600 East Quality Drive, American Fork, UT 84003; tel: 800-437-2257 or 801-763-0700.

Katsu Herbal Garlic Complex: Tablets. Concentrated extract of garlic, coix, and rice bran, with shark cartilage and vitamin C; garlic is well-known for its ability to inhibit bacteria, fungi, yeast (including *Candida*) and parasites (protozoa and worms), promote immune functions, lower cholesterol, reduce platelet aggregation, and aid digestion.

KENSHIN TRADING CORP., P.O. Box 7511, Torrance, CA 90504; tel: 800-766-1313 or 310-212-3199.

KYOLIC Formula 100: Capsules or tablets. Contains 300 mg of Aged Garlic Extract (a Wakunaga product), plus whey for normalizing colon flora.

WAKUNAGA OF AMERICA, 23501 Madero, Mission Viejo, CA 92691; tel: 800-421-2998 or 949-855-2776.

#1 Garlic Plus Ester-C and FOS: Capsules. Contains garlic, important for the immune and cardiovascular systems; ester C, a type of vitamin C that enters the bloodstream quickly; and FOS (fructo-oligosaccharides) to support the friendly intestinal bacteria.

NUTRITION NOW, 501 Southeast Columbia Shore Boulevard #350, Vancouver, WA 98661; tel: 800-929-0418 or 360-737-6800.

"GREEN" FOOD PRODUCTS

Broken Cell Chlorella: Tablets. Broken-cell chlorella is a green, microscopic freshwater plant that has a concentrated supply of vitamins, minerals, and proteins; chlorella contains a high-quality form of chlorophyll that supports the bloodstream, bowels, kidneys, and liver; helps support cellular growth, metabolic balance, and the immune system by stimulating the activity of T cells and promoting the body's production of interferon (proteins released by white blood cells to combat a virus).

SOLAR GREENS, NUTRACEUTICAL CORP., P.O. Box 681869, Park City, UT 84068; tel: 800-669-8877.

Chlorella: Tablets. Source of concentrated chlorophyll combined with rich levels of blood-building iron, folic acid, and vitamin B12, which can protect against environmental toxins.

NEW CHAPTER, 22 High Street, Brattleboro, VT 05301; tel: 800-543-7279 or 802-257-9345.

Chlorophyll Caps: Capsules. Contains water-soluble chlorophyll derived from 600 mg of organically grown alfalfa.

NATURE'S PLUS, 548 Broadhollow Road, Melville, NY 11747-3708; tel: 800-645-9500 or 516-293-0030.

Green-Power: Capsules. Contains beta carotene and folic acid in a blend of broccoli extract, the powders of cabbage, spinach, parsley, barley grass, and wheat grass, alfalfa, Japanese chlorella, and spirulina.

NATURE'S HERBS, 600 East Quality Drive, American Fork, UT 84003; tel: 800-437-2257 or 801-763-0700.

Hawaiian Spirulina: Tablets. Contains 100% Hawaiian spirulina, a blue-green algae that is a concentrated vegetarian nutrition source.

RAINBOW LIGHT, P.O. Box 600, Santa Cruz, CA 95061; tel: 800-635-1233 or 408-429-9089.

Pure Chlorella Wakasa Extract: Liquid. People using chlorella have found that it enhances their immune system, makes them more resistant to colds and flu, and decreases recovery time from illness; chlorella also cleanses, detoxifies, and balances the body.

SHOKO'S NATURAL PRODUCTS, 3402 Edgmont Avenue #373, Brookhaven, PA 19015; tel: 800-654-4394 or 610-876-9850.

Shiitake/Reishi Complex With Chlorella: Capsules. Contains chlorella combined with shiitake and reishi organic mushroom extracts.

COUNTRY LIFE, 101 Corporate Drive, Hauppauge, NY 11788; tel: 800-645-5768 or 516-231-1031.

Spirulina: Tablets. Contains blue-green algae rich in minerals, vitamins, complete biological proteins, amino acids, and essential fatty acids that support the immune system; contains over 2,000 enzymes and a full range of vitamins including 12 carotenoids.

SOLAR GREENS, P.O. Box 681869, Park City, UT 84068; tel: 800-669-8877.

Sun Chlorella: Tablets. Chlorella is one of the highest sources of DNA,

RNA, and chlorophyll and contains more than 20 different vitamins and minerals, including beta carotene (pro-vitamin A) and vitamin B12; also contains 19 amino acids, including all of the essential amino and fatty acids, and is rich in lysine.

SHOKO'S NATURAL PRODUCTS, 3402 Edgmont Avenue #373, Brookhaven, PA 19015; tel: 800-654-4394 or 610-876-9850.

Vital Green: Tablets. Contains spirulina and chlorella with alfalfa, barley, and wheat grass juice concentrates.

FUTUREBIOTICS, 145 Ricefield Lane, Hauppauge, NY 11788; tel: 800-FOR-LIFE (367-5433) or 516-273-6300.

MINERALS

Bentonite Minerals: Liquid. Contains 50% of the U.S. RDA (Recommended Daily Allowance) of zinc, copper, selenium, and chromium; bentonite minerals are more absorbable in the body, less apt to cause allergies, and allow the body to assimilate minerals, vitamins, and foods more readily.

WHITE ROCK MINERAL, P.O. Box 967, Springville, UT 84663-0967; tel: 888-328-2529 or 801-489-7138.

Dr. Powers Colloidal Mineral Source: Liquid. Contains the minerals calcium, selenium, magnesium, and zinc, plus trace amounts of more than 70 micro-colloidal minerals.

AMERICAN HEALTH, 4320 Veterans Memorial Highway, Holbrook, NY 11741; tel: 800-445-7137.

OptiZinc: Tablets. Contains zinc menomethionine (zinc combined with the essential amino acid methionine); zinc is critical for the health of the thymus gland (necessary for the body's natural defense), skin health, wound healing, and carbohydrate metabolism.

SOURCE NATURALS, THRESHOLD ENTERPRISES, 23 Janis Way, Scotts Valley, CA 95066; tel: 800-777-5677 or 831-438-1144.

Super Minerals: Liquid. Contains the minerals and trace minerals in a blend of non-ionic colloidal minerals, providing 98% bioavailability; contains chromium, calcium, copper, iodine, iron, lithium, magnesium, manganese, potassium, selenium, silica, silver, sulfur, zinc, and others.

R GARDEN, 3881 Enzyme Lane, Kettle Falls, WA 99141; tel: 800-700-7767 or 425-271-0539.

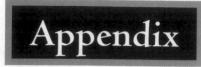

Appendix

Great Smokies Diagnostic Laboratory Tests

Consumer-direct laboratory analyses (health screens that can be ordered without a doctor's approval) are available through the BodyBalance Division of the Great Smokies Diagnostic Laboratory. This functional medicine laboratory is responsible for several advances in the medical field. Their concern with dysbiosis (imbalance in intestinal flora) led them to national recognition as pioneers in research and development of testing for digestive disorders and chronic illness.

The laboratory offers assessments of skeletal health, gastrointestinal, endocrine (hormonal), and nutritional functions. You can request an analysis kit including instructions on how to collect the sample (stool, urine, saliva, or hair) along with a pre-paid mailer. After tests are completed, an easy-to-read report is mailed directly to you, indicating whether you are within the expected normal ranges for your age and gender.

Types of Diagnostic Health Screens

Great Smokies Diagnostic Laboratory's consumer-direct tests include:

■ **HormoneChecks:** precision salivary hormone analysis for men and women. Saliva levels of hormones correlate well with tissue levels. These tests provide the precise status of your hormone levels, which can then serve as a guideline for treatment, if it is needed. *FemaleCheck* is useful for premenopausal, perimenopausal, or postmenopausal women who suspect a hormonal imbalance. It is also used by women who want to know more about their estrogen, progesterone, and testosterone levels or to monitor hormone replacement therapy. *MaleCheck* measures the hormones (testosterone and DHEA) that are necessary for a man's optimal health. *PerformanceCheck* helps the athletically inclined determine if they are getting optimal function out of their hormones by assessing testosterone, DHEA, and cortisol levels. *StressCheck* measures DHEA

To order these tests, contact: Great Smokies Diagnostic Laboratory, BodyBalance Division, 63 Zillicoa Street, Asheville, NC 28801-1074; tel: 800-522-4762; website: www.bodybalance.com.

and cortisol levels, which are essential hormones that help the body cope with stress. The last test in this category is *SleepCheck*, which measure meletonin levels. Melatonin imbalances are often linked to sleep disorders.

- **ToxicCheck** and **MineralCheck:** hair analysis to check for toxic exposure and nutrient deficiencies. Hair analysis is regarded as the best method for determining element levels in the body, as it accurately measures the long-term accumulation of toxic elements and minerals in the system. ToxicCheck analyzes hair levels of toxic elements (aluminum, arsenic, bismuth, cadmium, lead, mercury, nickel, silver, and tin). MineralCheck screens for possible deficiencies in certain essential minerals (boron, calcium, chromium, cobalt, copper, iodine, magnesium, manganese, selenium, strontium, sulfur, and zinc).

- **CandidaCheck:** a non-invasive stool culture that can determine your levels of intestinal yeast, specifically checking for any harmful overgrowth that may occur. Yeast overgrowth can lead to a variety of harmful conditions, especially digestive and gastrointestinal illnesses.

- **OsteoCheck:** osteoporosis risk assessment. This health screen analyzes a biochemical marker of bone loss in your urine. This biochemical marker, deoxypyridinoline (D-Pyd), determines the current rate of bone loss and predicts the future risk of fractures or spinal deformity. OsteoCheck is able to detect bone loss long before it shows up on conventional X rays and other scanning methods. It provides an early warning of bone loss, before it has progressed to the point of damaging the bone. The test can also be used to monitor the effectiveness of bone-loss treatment.

Endnotes

Part I
An Introduction to Supplements

1 Ralph Golan, M.D. *Optimal Wellness* (New York: Ballantine Books, 1995), 120.

2 James F. Balch, M.D., and Phyllis A. Balch, C.N.C. *Prescription for Nutritional Healing* (Garden City Park, NY: Avery Publishing Group, 1997), 34-36.

3 Stephen T. Sinatra, M.D. *Optimum Health: A Natural Lifesaving Prescription for Your Body and Mind* (New York: Bantam Books: 1996), 89.

4 Anthony Cichoke, D.C. *The Complete Book of Enzyme Therapy* (Garden City Park, NY: Avery Publishing Group, 1999), 3.

5 Stephen T. Sinatra, M.D. *Optimum Health* (New York: Bantam Books, 1996), 89.

6 Michael T. Murray, N.D. *Encyclopedia of Nutritional Supplements* (Rocklin, CA: Prima Publishing, 1996), 151-152.

7 Stephen T. Sinatra, M.D. *Optimum Health* (New York: Bantam Books, 1996), 89.

8 Melvyn R. Werbach, M.D. *Nutritional Influences on Illness* (Tarzana, CA: Third Line Press, 1988), 253.

9 Stephen T. Sinatra, M.D. *Optimum Health* (New York: Bantam Books, 1996), 89.

10 F. Cai et al. "Preliminary Report of Efficacy of Diabetic Polyneuropathy Treated with Large Dose Inositol." *Hua Hsi I Ko Ta Hsueh Hsueh Pao* 21:2 (June 1990), 201-203.

11 Stephen T. Sinatra, M.D. *Optimum Health* (New York: Bantam Books, 1996), 89.

12 Ibid.

13 R.L. Baehner and L.A. Boxer. "Role of Membrane Vitamin E and Cytoplasmic Glutathione in the Regulation of Phagocytic Functions of Neutrophils and Monocytes." *American Journal of Pediatric Hematology/Oncology* 1:1 (1979), 71-76.

14 T.N. Kaul et al. "Antiviral Effect of Flavonoids on Human Viruses." *Journal of Medical Virology* 15 (1985), 71-79. E. Middleton, Jr., and G. Drzewiecki. "Flavonoid Inhibition of Human Basophil Histamine Release Stimulated by Various Agents." *Biochemical Pharmacology* 33:21 (1984), 3333.

15 Christopher Hobbs. *Foundations of Health: Healing With Herbs and Foods* (Capitola, CA: Botanica Press, 1992), 229.

16 K. Folkers and A. Wolaniuk. "Research on Coenzyme Q10 in Clinical Medicine and in Immunomodulation." *Drugs Under Experimental and Clinical Research* 11:8 (1985), 539-545.

17 R. Walters. "DMSO Therapy." In *Options: The Alternative Cancer Therapy Book* (Garden City Park, NY: Avery Publishing Group, 1993), 249.

18 R. Bauer and H. Wagner. "Echinacea Species as Potential Immunostimulatory Drugs." *Econ Med Plant Res* 5 (1991), 253-321. P.H. List and L. Hoerhammer. *Hagers Handbuch der Pharmazeutischen Praxis*, Volumes 2-5 (Berlin: Springer-Verlag).

19 U.N. Das. "Antibiotic-like Action of Essential Fatty Acids." *Canadian Medical Association Journal* 132 (1985), 1350.

20 S.R. Glore et al. "Soluble Fiber and Serum Lipids: A Literature Review." *Journal of the American Dietetic Association* 94 (1994), 425-436.

21 D.B. Mowrey, Ph.D. *The Scientific Validation of Herbal Medicine* (New Canaan, CT: Keats Publishing, 1986), 158.

22 E. Lehmann et al. "Efficacy of a Special Kava Extract (*Piper methysticum*) in Patients With States of Anxiety, Tension, and Excitedness of Non-mental Origin." *Phytomedicine* 3 (1996), 113-119.

23 J.G. Brook et al. "Dietary Soya Lecithin Decreases Plasma Triglyceride Levels and Inhibits Collagen- and ADP-induced Platelet Aggregation." *Biochemical Medicine and Metabolic Biology* 35 (1986), 31-39. J. Wojcicki et al. "Clinical Evaluation of Lecithin as a Lipid-Lowering Agent." *Phytotherapy Research* 9 (1995), 597-599.

24 J.C. Carraro et al. "Comparison of Phytotherapy (Permixon®) with Finasteride in the Treatment of Benign Prostatic Hyperplasia: A Randomized International Study of 1098 Patients." *Prostate* 29 (1996), 231-240. Donald Brown, N.D. "Comparing Saw Palmetto Extract and Finasteride for BPH." *Quarterly Review of Natural Medicine* (Spring 1997), 13-14.

25 Ronald G. Reichert, N.D. "St. John's Wort Extract as a Tricyclic Medication Substitute for Mild to Moderate Depression." *Quarterly Review of Natural Medicine* (Winter 1995), 275-278. Michael Murray, N.D. "The Clinical Use of *Hypericum perforatum*." *American Journal of Natural Medicine* 2:3 (April 1995), 8-12, 17.

26 P.M. Altman. "Australian Tea Tree Oil." *Australian Journal of Pharmacy* 69 (1988), 276-278.

Part II
An A to Z of Health Conditions: Nutrients and Herbal Remedies

1 Linda Rector Page, N.D., Ph.D. *Healthy Healing* (Sonora, CA: Healthy Healing Publications, 1997), 78-79.

2 Michael T. Murray, N.D. *Encyclopedia of Nutritional Supplements* (Rocklin, CA: Prima Publishing, 1996), 449. James C. Breneman, M.D. *Basics of Food Allergy* (Springfield, IL: Charles C. Thomas, 1984), 63-71.

3 E. Middleton Jr. and G. Drzewiecki. "Flavonoid Inhibition of Human Basophil Histamine Release Stimulated by Various Agents." *Biochemical Pharmacology* 33:21 (1984), 3333. C.A. Clemetson. "Histamine and Ascorbic Acid in Human Blood." *Journal of Nutrition* 110:44 (1980), 662-668. K. Folkers et al. "Biochemical Evidence for a Deficiency of Vitamin B6 in Subjects Reacting to Monosodium-L-Glutamate by the Chinese Restaurant Syndrome." *Biochemical and Biophysical Research Communications* 100 (1981), 972-977. S.W. Simon. "Vitamin B12 Therapy in Allergy and Chronic Dermatoses." *Journal of Allergy* 2 (1951), 183-185. P. Mittman. "Randomized, Double-Blind Study of Freeze-dried *Urtica dioica* in the Treatment of Allergic Rhinitis." *Planta Medica* 56 (1990), 44-47. N.A. Hayes and J.C. Foreman. "The Activity of Compounds Extracted from Feverfew on Histamine Release from Rat Mast Cells." *Journal of Pharmacy and Pharmacology* 39 (1987), 466-467. A.C. Markey et al. "Platelet Activating Factor-Induced Clinical and Histopathologic Responses in Atopic Skin and Their Modification by the Platelet Activating Factor Antagonist BN52063." *Journal of the American Academy of Dermatology* 23:2 (1990), 263-268.

4 D.G. Tinkelman and S.E. Avner. "Ephedrine Therapy in Asthmatic Children." *Journal of the American Medical Association* 237 (1977), 553-537.

5 R.E. Hodges et al. "Hematopoietic Studies in Vitamin A Deficiency." *American Journal of Clinical Nutrition* 31 (1978), 876-885.

6 E.R. Monsen. "Ascorbic Acid: An Enhancing Factor in Iron Absorption." In Constance Kies, ed. *Nutritional Bioavailability of Iron* (Washington, DC: American Chemical Society, 1982), 85-95.

7 A.G. Bechensteen et al. "Erythropoietin, Protein, and Iron Supplementation and the Prevention of Anaemia of Prematurity." *Archives of Disease in Childhood* 69:Special No. 1 (July 1993), 19-23. J.W. Lawless et al. "Iron Supplementation Improves Growth in Anemic Kenyan Primary School Children." *Journal of Nutrition* 124:5 (May 1994), 645-654. D.S. Silverberg et al. "Intravenous Iron Supplementation for the Treatment of the Anemia of Moderate to Severe Chronic Renal Failure Patients Not Receiving Dialysis." *American Journal of Kidney Disease* 27:2 (February 1996), 234-238.

8 D.B. Mowrey, Ph.D. *The Scientific Validation of Herbal Medicine* (New Canaan, CT: Keats Publishing, 1986), 207.

9 Melvyn R. Werbach, M.D. *Nutritional Influences on Illness* (Tarzana, CA: Third Line Press, 1988), 37-38.

10 S.K. Bhattacharya and S.K. Mitra. "Anxiolytic Activity of *Panax ginseng* Roots: An Experimental Study." *Journal of Ethnopharmacology* 34 (1991), 87-92. C. Hallstrom et al. "Effect of Ginseng on the Performance of Nurses on Night Duty." *Comparative Medicine East and West* 6 (1982), 277-282. S.J. Fulder. "Ginseng and the Hypothalamic-Pituitary Control of Stress." *American Journal of Chinese Medicine* 9 (1981), 112-118.

11 Personal report by Jeffry L. Anderson, M.D., of Corte Madera, California, based on his clinical use of Stabilium with patients. T. Dorman et al. "The Effectiveness of *Garum armoricum* (Stabilium) in Reducing Anxiety in College Students." *Journal of Advancement in Medicine* 8:3 (Fall 1995), 193-200.

12 D.B. Mowrey, Ph.D. *Herbal Tonic Therapies* (New Canaan, CT: Keats Publishing, 1993), 200-201.

13 D.B. Mowrey, Ph.D. *The Scientific Validation of Herbal Medicine* (New Canaan, CT: Keats Publishing, 1986), 12.

14 E. Lehmann et al. "Efficacy of a Special Kava Extract (*Piper methysticum*) in Patients with States of Anxiety, Tension, and Excitedness of Non-Mental Origin." *Phytomedicine* 3 (1996), 113-119.

15 Linda Rector Page, N.D., Ph.D. *Healthy Healing* (Sonora, CA: Healthy Healing Publications, 1990), 86.

16 A. di Fabio. *Treatment and Prevention of Osteoarthritis, Parts I and II* (Franklin, TN: The Rheumatoid Disease Foundation, 1989).

17 J.E. Pizzorno and M.T. Murray. *Encyclopedia of Natural Medicine* (Rocklin, CA: Prima Publishing, 1991).

18 A. di Fabio. *Gouty Arthritis* (Franklin, TN: The Rheumatoid Disease Foundation, 1989). J.E. Pizzorno and M.T. Murray. *Encyclopedia of Natural Medicine* (Rocklin, CA: Prima Publishing, 1991).

19 J.M. Kremer. "Clinical Studies of Omega-3 Fatty Acid Supplementation in Patients Who Have Rheumatoid Arthritis." *Rheumatic Diseases Clinics of North America* 17:2 (May 1991), 391-402. P. Geusens et al. "Long-term Effect of Omega-3 Fatty Acid Supplementation in Active Rheumatoid Arthritis. A 12-Month, Double-Blind, Controlled Study." *Arthritis and Rheumatism* 37:6 (June 1994), 824-829. D.F. Horrobin. "The Importance of Gamma-Linolenic Acid and Prostaglandin E1 in Human Nutrition and Medicine." *Journal of Holistic Medicine* 3 (1981), 118-139. T.M. Hansen et al. "Treatment of Rheumatoid Arthritis with Prostaglandin E1 Precursors Cis-Linoleic Acid and Gamma-Linolenic Acid." *Scandinavian Journal of Rheumatology* 12 (1983), 85.

20 Maurice Shils, M.D., Sc.D., and Vernon Young, Ph.D. *Modern Nutrition in Health and Disease* (Philadelphia, PA: Lea and Febiger, 1988), 286-287.

21 A.Y. Leung. *Encyclopedia of Common Natural Ingredients* (New York: Wiley Publishing, 1980).

22 *British Herbal Pharmacopoeia* (West Yorks, England: British Herbal Medicine Association, 1983). R.F. Chandler et al. "Herbal Remedies of the Maritime Indians: Sterols and Triterpenes of *Achillea Millefolium L.* (Yarrow)." *Journal of Pharmaceutical Sciences* 71:6 (1982), 690-693.

23 C. Cochran, D.C. *At Last Collastin* (San Marcos, CA: Reprints, 1997).

24 Joel Wallach, B.S, D.V.M, N.D., and Ma Lan, M.D., M.S. *Rare Earths: The Forbidden Cures* (Bonita, CA: Double Happiness Publishing, 1994), 351.

25 Garbe Edeltraut, M.D., et al. "Inhaled and Nasal Glucocorticoids and the Risks of Ocular Hypertension or Open-Angle Glaucoma." *Journal of the American Medical Association* 277 (1997), 722-727. World Health Organization (WHO). *Bronchodilators and Other Medications for the Treatment of Wheeze-Associated Illnesses in Young Children: Programme for the Control of Acute Respiratory Infections* (Geneva, Switzerland: World Health Organization, 1993), 11; available on the WHO website: www.who.ch/chd/pub/ari/broncho.htm.

26 Melvyn R. Werbach, M.D. *Nutritional Influences on Illness* (Tarzana, CA: Third Line Press, 1988), 92-94.

27 D.G. Tinkelman and S.E. Avner. "Ephedrine Therapy in Asthmatic Children." *Journal of the American Medical Association* 237 (1977), 553-537.

28 M.C.S. Kennedy and J.P.P. Stock. "The Bronchodilator Action of Khellin." *Thorax* 7 (1952), 43-65.

29 S. Mansuri et al. "Some Pharmacological Characteristics of Ganglionic Activity of Lobeline." *Arzneimittel-Forschung* 23 (1973), 1271-1275.

30 S. Gupta et al. "*Tylophora indica* in Bronchial Asthma: A Double-Blind Study." *Indian Journal of Medical Research* 69 (1979), 981-989.

31 N.M. Newman and R.S.M. Ling. "Acetabular Bone Destruction Related to Nonsteroidal Anti-inflammatory Drugs." *The Lancet* ii (1985), 11-13. L. Solomon. "Drug Induced Arthropathy and Necrosis of the Femoral Head." *Journal of Bone and Joint Surgery* 55B (1973), 246-251.

32 G. Crolle and E. D'este. "Glucosamine Sulfate for the Management of Arthrosis: A Controlled Clinical Investgation." *Current Medical Research Opinoin* 7 (1980), 104-109. A. Reichelt et al. "Efficacy and Safety of Intramuscular Glucosamine Sulfate in Osteoarthritis of the Knee. A Randomized, Placebo-Controlled, Double-Blind Study." *Arzneimittel-Forschung* 44 (1994), 75-80.

33 Melvyn R. Werbach, M.D. *Nutritional Influences on Illness* (Tarzana, CA: Third Line Press, 1988), 253-261.

34 Ibid., 260.

35 R. Neubauer. "A Plant Protease for the Potentiation of and Possible Replacement of Antibiotics." *Experimental Medicine and Surgery* 19 (1961), 143-160.

36 A.H. Amin et al. "Berberine Sulfate: Antimicrobial Activity, Bioassay, and Mode of Action." *Canadian Journal Microbiology* 15:9 (1969), 1067-1076.

37 I. Ofek et al. "Anti-*Escherichia coli* Adhesin Activity of Cranberry and Blueberry Juices." *New England Journal of Medicine* 324 (1991), 1599.

38 R. Bauer and H. Wagner. "Echinacea Species as Potential Immunostimulatory Drugs." *Econ Med Plant Res* 5 (1991), 253-321.

39 D.B. Mowrey, Ph.D. *The Scientific Validation of Herbal Medicine* (New Canaan, CT: Keats Publishing, 1986), 158.

40 Allan Sachs, D.C., C.C.N. *The Authoritative Guide to Grapefruit Seed Extract* (Mendocino, CA: LifeRhythm, 1997), 17-19.

41 Morton Walker, D.P.M. "Antimicrobial Attributes of Olive Leaf Extract." *Townsend Letter for Doctors and Patients* (July 1996), 80-85.

42 P.M. Altman. "Australian Tea Tree Oil." *Australian Journal of Pharmacy* 69 (1988), 276-278.

43 *Merck Manual of Diagnosis and Therapy*, Home Edition (Whitehouse Station, NJ: Merck, 1997), 168.

44 Linda Rector Page, N.D., Ph.D. *Healthy Healing* (Sonora, CA: Healthy Healing Publications, 1997), 250.

45 *Merck Manual of Diagnosis and Therapy*, 15th Edition. (Rahway, NJ: Merck Sharp & Dohme

Research Laboratories, 1987), 635.

46 Morton Walker, D.P.M. "Antimicrobial Attributes of Olive Leaf Extract." *Townsend Letter for Doctors and Patients* (July 1996), 80-85.

47 James, C. Brenneman, MD. *Basics of Food Allergy* (Springfield, IL: Charles C. Thomas, 1984), 65, 69.

48 Nancy Appleton, Ph.D. *Lick the Sugar Habit* (Garden City Park, NY: Avery Publishing, 1988).

49 Earl Ubell. "Are Our Children Overmedicated?" *Parade Magazine* (October 12, 1997), 4-6.

50 Ann-Christine Nyquist, M.D., M.S.P.H., et al. "Antibiotic Prescribing for Children With Colds, Upper Respiratory Tract Infections, and Bronchitis." *Journal of the American Medical Association* 279 (1998), 875-877. Editorial. "Why Do Physicians Prescribe Antibiotics for Children With Upper Respiratory Tract Infections?" *Journal of the American Medical Association* 279 (1998), 881-882.

51 B. Feingold. *Why Your Child Is Hyperactive* (Westminster, MD: Random, 1975). Herbert Needleman, M.D., and Philip Landrigan, M.D. *Raising Children Toxic Free* (New York: Farrar, Straus and Giroux, 1994), 70-71.

52 R. Klich and B. Gladbach. "Childhood Behavior Disorders and Their Treatment." *Medizinische Welt* 26:25 (1975), 1251-1254.

53 James F. Balch, M.D., and Phyllis A. Balch, C.N.C. *Prescription for Nutritional Healing* (Garden City Park, NY: Avery Publishing, 1997), 358.

54 Burton Goldberg and the Editors of *Alternative Medicine Digest. Alternative Medicine Guide to Heart Disease* (Tiburon, CA: Future Medicine Publishing, 1998), 45-46.

55 J.A. Simon. "Vitamin C and Cardiovascular Disease: A Review." *Journal of the American College of Nutrition* 11 (1992), 107-125. J.R. DiPalma and W.S. Thayer. "Use of Niacin as a Drug." *Annual Review of Nutrition* 11 (1991), 169-187.

56 A.L. Welsh and M. Ede. "Inositol Hexanicotinate for Improved Nicotinic Acid Therapy. *Int Record Med* 174 (1961), 9-15. A.M.A. El-Enein et al. "The Role of Nicotinic Acid and Inositol Hexaniacinate as Anticholesterolemic and Antilipemic Agents." *Nutr Rep Intl* 28 (1983), 899-911.

57 Maurice Shils, M.D., Sc.D., and Vernon Young, Ph.D. *Modern Nutrition in Health and Disease* (Philadelphia: Lea and Febiger, 1988), 74.

58 S.R. Glore et al. "Soluble Fiber and Serum Lipids: A Literature Review." *Journal of the American Dietetic Association* 94 (1994), 425-436.

59 S. Nityanand et al. "Clinical Trials with Gugulipid: A New Hypolipidemic Agent." *Journal of the Association of Physicians of India* 37:5 (1989), 323-328. S.K. Verma and A. Bordia. "Effect of

Commiphora mukul (Gum Guggul) in Patients of Hyperlipidemia with Special Reference to HDL-Cholesterol." *Indian Journal Medical Research* 87 (1988), 356-360.

61 Linda Rector Page, N.D., Ph.D. *Healthy Healing* (Sonora, CA: Healthy Healing Publications, 1997), 115. Burton Goldberg and the Editors of *Alternative Medicine Digest. Alternative Medicine Guide to Chronic Fatigue, Fibromyalgia, and Environmental Illness* (Tiburon, CA: Future Medicine Publishing, 1998).

61 Scott J. Gregory. *A Holistic Protocol for the Immune System* (Joshua Tree, CA: Tree of Life Publications, 1995), 92.

62 Morton Walker, D.P.M. "Antimicrobial Attributes of Olive Leaf Extract." *Townsend Letter for Doctors and Patients* (July 1996), 80-85.

63 Ibid.

64 James F. Balch, M.D., and Phyllis A. Balch, C.N.C. *Prescription for Nutritional Healing* (Garden City Park, NY: Avery Publishing, 1997), 223.

65 Joel Wallach, B.S, D.V.M, N.D., and Ma Lan, M.D., M.S. *Rare Earths: The Forbidden Cures* (Bonita, CA: Double Happiness Publishing, 1994), 418.

66 C.J. Gibson and A. Gelenberg. "Tyrosine for the Treatment of Depression." *Advances in Biological Psychiatry* 10 (1983), 148-159.

67 Personal report by Jeffry L. Anderson, M.D., of Corte Madera, California, based on his clinical use of Stabilium with patients. T. Dorman et al. "The Effectiveness of *Garum armoricum* (Stabilium) in Reducing Anxiety in College Students." *Journal of Advancement in Medicine* 8:3 (Fall 1995), 193-200.

68 D. Satter. "Diabetes Called Sure Fate for Obese People." *Los Angeles Times* (February 13, 1972), Section C.

69 J.W. Anderson and K. Ward. "High-carbohydrate, High-Fiber Diets for Insulin-Treated Men with Diabetes Mellitus." *American Journal of Clinical Nutrition* 32 (1979), 2312-2321.

70 H. Freund et al. "Chromium Deficiency During Total Parenteral Nutrition." *Journal of the American Medical Association* 241:5 (1979), 496-498. O.B. Martinez et al. "Dietary Chromium and Effect of Chromium Supplementation on Glucose Tolerance of Elderly Canadian Women." *Nutrition Research* 5 (1985), 609-620. E. Offenbacher and F. Stunyer. "Beneficial Effect of Chromium-Rich Yeast on Glucose Tolerance and Blood Lipids in Elderly Patients." *Diabetes* 29 (1980), 919-925.

71 L.M. Klevay et al. "Diminished Glucose Tolerance in Two Men Due to a Diet Low in Copper." *American Journal of Clinical Nutrition* 37 (1983), 717.

"Manganese and Glucose Tolerance." *Nutrition Review* 26:7 (1968), 207-209. S.J. Solomon and J.C. King. "Effect of Low Zinc Intake on Carbohydrate and Fat Metabolism in Men." *Federation Proceedings* 42 (1983), 391.

72 Melvyn R. Werbach, M.D. *Nutritional Influences on Illness* (Tarzana, CA: Third Line Press, 1988), 171-172.

73 P. Sandhya and U.N. Das. "Vitamin C Therapy for Maturity Onset Diabetes Mellitus: Relevance to Prostaglandin Involvement." *IRCS Journal of Medical Science* 9:7 (1981), 618.

74 G. Paolisso et al. "Pharmacologic Doses of Vitamin E Improve Insulin Action in Healthy Subjects and Non-Insulin-Dependent Diabetic Patients." *American Journal of Clinical Nutrition* 57:5 (May 1993), 655-656. B. Caballero. "Vitamin E Improves the Action of Insulin." *Nutrition Review* 51:11 (November 1993), 339-340.

75 Y. Shigeta et al. "Effect of Coenzyme-Q7 Treatment on Blood Sugar and Ketone Bodies of Diabetics." *Journal of Vitaminology* 12 (1966), 293. CoQ7 is interchangeable with coQ10 in the body.

76 "Abstracts: The Netherlands Society for the Study of Diabetes, March 17 and 23, 1984, Utrecht." *Netherlands Journal of Medecine* 29:2 (1986), 65-70. M.M. KKandgraf-Leurs et al. "Pilot Study on Omega-3 Fatty Acids in Type I Diabetes Mellitus." *Diabetes* 39:3 (March 1990), 369-375. G.A. Jamal et al. "Gamma-Linolenic Acid in Diabetic Neuropathy." *The Lancet* 1 (1986), 1098.

77 A. Scharrer and M. Ober. "Anthocyanosides in the Treatment of Retinopathies." (In German.) *Klinische Monatsblatter Augenheilkunde* 178 (1981), 386-389. G. Lagrue et al. "Pathology of the Microcirculation in Diabetes and Alterations of the Biosynthesis of Intracellular Matrix Molecules." *Frontiers of Matrix Biology* 7 (1979), 324-325.

78 Y. Srivastava et al. "Antidiabetic and Adaptogenic Properties of *Momordica charantia* Extract: An Experimental and Clinical Evaluation." *Phytotherapy Research* 7 (1993), 285-289. R.D. Sharma et al. "Effect of Fenugreek Seeds on Blood Glucose and Serum Lipids in Type I Diabetes. *European Journal of Clinical Nutrition* 44:4 (1990), 301-306.

79 K. Baskaran et al. "Antidiabetic Effect of a Leaf Extract from *Gymnema sylvestre* in Non-Insulin-Dependent Diabetes Mellitus Patients." *Journal of Ethnopharmacology* 30 (1990), 295-305. E.R.B. Shanmugasundaram et al. "Use of *Gymnema sylvestre* Leaf in Insulin-Dependent Diabetes Mellitus." *Journal of Ethnopharmacology* 30 (1990), 281-294.

80 *Merck Manual of Diagnosis and Therapy*, Home Edition (Whitehouse Station, NJ: Merck and Co.,

1997), 1012.

81 D.B. Mowrey, Ph.D. *The Scientific Validation of Herbal Medicine* (New Canaan, CT: Keats Publishing, 1986), 216-217.

82 Earl L. Mindell. *The MSM Miracle: Enhance Your Health With Organic Sulfur* (New Canaan, CT: Keats Publishing, 1997).

83 D. Bryce-Smith and R.I.D. Simpson. "Anorexia, Depression and Zinc Deficiency." *The Lancet* 2 (1984), 1162. R. Bakan. "The Role of Zinc in Anorexia Nervosa: Etiology and Treatment." *Medical Hypotheses* 5 (1979), 731-736.

84 H. Glatzel. "Treatment of Dyspeptic Disorders with Spice Extracts." *Hippokrates* 40:23 (1969), 916-919. R. Deininger. "Amarum-Bitter Herbs. Common Bitter Principle Remedies and Their Action." *Krankenpflege* 29:3 (1975), 99-100.

85 P.F. Jacques and L.T. Chylack, Jr. "Epidemiologic Evidence of a Role for the Antioxidant Vitamins and Carotenoids in Cataract Prevention." *American Journal of Clinical Nutrition* 53:1 Suppl (January 1991), 352S-355S. J.M. Robertson et al. "A Possible Role for Vitamins C and E in Cataract Prevention." *American Journal of Clinical Nutrition* 53:1 Suppl (January 1991), 346S-351S.

86 A. Ceriello et al. "Hypomagnesemia in Relation to Diabetic Retinopathy." *Diabetes Care* 5 (1982), 558-559.

87 H.J. Merte and W. Merkle. "Long-Term Treatment with *Ginkgo biloba* Extract of Circulatory Disturbances of the Retina and Optic Nerve." (In German.) *Klinische Monatsblatter fur Augenheilkunde* 177:5 (1980), 577-583.

88 Earl L. Mindell. *The MSM Miracle: Enhance Your Health With Organic Sulfur* (New Canaan, CT: Keats Publishing, 1997).

89 D.A. Newsome et al. "Oral Zinc in Macular Degeneration." *Archives of Ophthalmology* 106:2 (February 1988), 192-198.

90 Nancy Appleton, Ph.D. *Lick the Sugar Habit* (Garden City Park, NY: Avery Publishing, 1988), 31.

91 E. Cheraskin et al. "Daily Vitamin C Consumption and Fatigability." *Journal of the American Geriatric Society* 24:3 (1976), 136-137.

92 D.B. Mowrey. "Capsicum, Ginseng, and Gotu Kola in Combination." *The Herbalist* (1975), 22-28. D.B. Mowrey. "The Effects of Capsicum, Gotu Kola, and Ginseng on Activity: Further Evidence." *The Herbalist* 1:1 (1976), 51-54.

93 Chuck Cochran, D.C. *Cetyl Myristoleate* (New York: Healing Wisdom Publications, 1997).

94 G. Abraham. "Management of Fibromyalgia: Rationale for the Use of Magnesium and Malic Acid. *Journal of Nutritional Medicine* 3 (1992), 49-59.

95 G.F. Kroker. "Chronic Candidiasis and Allergy." In J.

Brostoff and S.J. Challacome, eds. *Food Allergy and Intolerance* (Philadelphia: W.B. Saunders, 1987), 850-872. W.G. Crook. *The Yeast Connection* 2nd ed. (Jackson, TN: Professional Books, 1984).

96 James F. Balch, M.D., and Phyllis A. Balch, C.N.C. *Prescription for Nutritional Healing* (Garden City Park, NY: Avery Publishing, 1997), 52.

97 E.L. Keeney. "Sodium Caprylate: A New and Effective Treatment of Moniliasis of the Skin and Mucous Membrane." *Bulletin of Johns Hopkins Hospital* 78 (1946), 333-339.

98 Amber Ackerson, N.D., and Corey Resnick, N.D. "The Effects of L-Glutamine, N-Acetyl-D-Glucosamine, Gamma-Linolenic Acid and Gamma-Oryzanol on Intestinal Permeability." *Townsend Letter for Doctors* (January 1993), 20, 22.

99 "Some Experience With Deglycyrrhizinated Licorice in the Treatment of Gastric and Duodenal Ulcers With Special Reference to its Spasmolytic Effect." *Gut* 9 (1968), 48-51.

100 Paul Pitchford. *Healing With Whole Foods* (Berkeley, CA: North Atlantic Books, 1993), 188.

101 James F. Balch, M.D., and Phyllis A. Balch, C.N.C. *Prescription for Nutritional Healing* (Garden City Park, NY: Avery Publishing, 1997), 52.

102 R.C. Wren, F.L.S. Potter's *New Cyclopaedia of Botanical Drugs and Preparations* (Saffron Walden/C.W. Daniel, 1994), 283.

103 J.J. Murphy et al. "Randomised Double-Blind Placebo-Controlled Trial of Feverfew in Migraine Prevention." *The Lancet* 2:8604 (July 23, 1988), 189-192. E.S. Johnson et al. "Efficacy of Feverfew as Prophylactic Treatment of Migraine." *British Medical Journal* 291:6495 (August 31, 1985), 569-573.

104 James R. Privitera, M.D. *Clots: Life's Biggest Killer* (Unpublished manuscript, 1992).

105 Burton Goldberg and The Editors of *Alternative Medicine. Alternative Medicine Guide To Heart Disease* (Tiburon, CA: Future Medicine Publishing, 1998), 33.

106 Melvyn R. Werbach, M.D. *Nutritional Influences on Illness* (Tarzana, CA: Third Line Press, 1988), 238-239.

107 Gary Null, Ph.D. The *Clinician's Handbook of Natural Healing* (New York: Kensington Publishing, 1997), 46-53.

108 Ibid., 286-306.

109 R.F. Weiss. *Herbal Medicine* (Gothenburg, Sweden: A.B. Arcanum, 1988).

110 Gary Null, Ph.D. *The Clinician's Handbook of Natural Healing* (New York: Kensington Publishing, 1997), 398-401.

111 R. Pompei et al. "Glycyrrhizic Acid Inhibits Virus Growth and Inactivates Virus Particles." *Nature* 281:5733 (October 25, 1979), 689-690.

112 T.N. Kaul et al. "Antiviral Effect of Flavonoids on Human Viruses." *Journal of Medical Virology* 15 (1985), 71-79.

113 D.E. Walsh et al. "Subjective Response to Lysine in the Therapy of Herpes Simplex." *Journal of Antimicrobial Chemotherapy* 12:5 (November 1983), 489-496.

114 I. Brody. "Topical Treatment of Recurrent Herpes Simplex and Post-Herpetic Erythema Multiforme with Low Concentrations of Zinc Sulphate Solution." *British Journal of Dermatology* 104:2 (February 1981), 191-194. W. Kneist et al. "Clinical Double-Blind Trial of Topical Zinc Sulfate for Herpes Labialis Recidivans." (In German.) *Arzneimittel-Forschung* 45:5 (May 1995), 624-626.

115 NIH Consensus Conference Panel on Impotence. "Impotence." *Journal of the American Medical Association* 270 (1993), 83-90.

116 Melvyn R. Werbach, M.D., and Michael T. Murray, N.D. *Botanical Influences on Illness* (Tarzana, CA: Third Line Press, 1988), 199.

117 R. Sikora et al. "*Ginkgo biloba* Extract in the Therapy of Erectile Dysfunction." *Journal of Urology* 141 (1989), 188A.

118 J.G. Susset et al. "Effect of Yohimbine Hydrochloride on Erectile Impotence: A Double-Blind Study." *Journal of Urology* 141:6 (1989), 1360-1363. K. Reid et al. "Double-Blind Trial of Yohimbine in Treatment of Psychogenic Impotence." *The Lancet* ii (1987), 421-423.

119 H.K. Choi et al. "Clinical Efficacy of Korean Red Ginseng for Erectile Dysfunction." *International Journal of Impotence Research* 7:3 (September 1995), 181-186.

120 J. Waynberg. "Aphrodisiacs: Contribution to the Clinical Validation of the Traditional Use of *Ptychopetalum guyanna.*" Presented at the First International Congress on Ethnopharmacology, Strasbourg, France (June 5-9, 1990).

121 Maurice Shils, M.D., Sc.D., and Vernon Young, Ph.D. *Modern Nutrition in Health and Disease* (Philadelphia: Lea and Febiger, 1988), 148.

122 E. Howell. *Enzyme Nutrition: The Food Enzyme Concept* (Garden City Park, NY: Avery Publishing, 1985), 10-13.

123 A. Bu-Abbas et al. "Marked Antimutagenic Potential of Aqueous Green Tea Extracts: Mechanism of Action." *Mutagenesis* 9 (1994), 325-331. C.S. Yang and Z.Y. Wang. "Tea and Cancer." *Journal of the National Cancer Institute* 85:13 (1993), 1038-1049.

124 P. Pitchford. *Healing With Whole Foods* (Berkeley,

CA: North Atlantic Books, 1993), 187-189.

125 Michael T. Murray, N.D. *Encyclopedia of Nutritional Supplements* (Rocklin, CA: Prima Publishing, 1996), 332-334.

126 James F. Balch, M.D., and Phyllis A. Balch, C.N.C. *Prescription for Nutritional Healing* (Garden City Park, NY: Avery Publishing, 1997), 358.

127 Gabriel Cousens, M.D. *Conscious Eating* (Santa Rosa, CA: Vision Books International, 1992).

128 James, C. Brenneman, MD. *Basics of Food Allergy* (Springfield, IL: Charles C. Thomas, 1984), 65.

129 Michael T. Murray, N.D. and Joseph E. Pizzorno, N.D. *Encyclopedia of Natural Medicine* (Rocklin, CA: Prima Publishing, 1991), 59.

130 Paul Pitchford. *Healing With Whole Foods* (Berkeley, CA: North Atlantic Books, 1993), 401. Michael T. Murray, N.D. *The Healing Power of Herbs* (Rocklin, CA: Prima Publishing, 1992), 88. Michael Tierra, C.A., N.D., O.M.D. *Planetary Herbology* (Santa Fe, NM: Lotus Press, 1988), 175.

131 Maesimund B. Panos, M.D. and DeeAnn Hench. *A Guide to Homeopathic Remedies for Home Care* (Los Angeles, CA: Standard Homeopathic Co., 1993).

132 Christine Ammer. *The New A to Z of Women's Health: A Concise Encyclopedia* (New York: Hunter House, 1989), 270.

133 Notably John R. Lee, M.D., of Sebastopol, California. See his book, *What Your Doctor May Not Tell You About Menopause* (New York: Warner Books, 1996).

134 R.S. Kaldas and C.L. Hughes. "Reproductive and General Metabolic Effects of Phytoestrogens in Mammals." *Reproductive Toxicology* 3 (1989), 81-89. M. Messina and S. Barnes. "The Roles of Soy Products in Reducing Risk of Cancer." *Journal of the National Cancer Institute* 83 (1991), 541-546. Peter Jaret. "The Miracle Bean." *Health Magazine* (October 1995), 30, 32.

135 Rebecca Flynn, M.S. and Mark Roest. *Your Guide to Standardized Herbal Products* (Prescott, AZ: One World Press, 1995), 1.

136 P.H. List and L. Hoerhammer. *Handbuch der Pharmazeutischen Praxis*, Volumes 2-5 (Berlin: Springer-Verlag).

137 R.G. Hunter et al. "The Action of Papain and Bromelain on the Uterus." *American Journal of Obstetrics and Gynecology* 73 (1957), 867-880. D. Colombo and R. Vescovini. "Controlled Trial of Anthocyanosides from *Vaccinium myrtillus* in Primary Dysmenorrhea." *G Ital Obstet Ginecol* 7 (1985), 1033-1038. P.H. List and L. Hoerhammer. *Handbuch der Pharmazeutischen Praxis*, Volumes 2-5 (Berlin: Springer-Verlag).

138 F.P. Porcher. "Report on the Indigenous Medical Plants of South Carolina." *Transactions of the American Medical Association II* (1849). C.F. Millspaugh. *American Medicinal Plants* (New York: Dover Publications, 1974).

139 Cynthia Wilson. *Chemical Exposure and Human Health* (Jefferson, NC: McFarland and Company, 1993), 123.

140 L.G. Hochman et al. "Brittle Nails: Response to Daily Biotin Supplementation." *Cutis* 51 (1993), 303-307.

141 Linda Rector Page, N.D., Ph.D. *Healthy Healing* (Sonora, CA: Healthy Healing Publications, 1997), 371. James F. Balch, M.D., and Phyllis A. Balch, C.N.C. *Prescription for Nutritional Healing* (Garden City Park, NY: Avery Publishing, 1997), 400. Michael T. Murray, N.D. *Encyclopedia of Nutritional Supplements* (Rocklin, CA, Prima Publishing, 1996), 411.

142 John R. Lee, M.D. *Natural Progesterone: The Multiple Roles of a Remarkable Hormone* (Sebastopol, CA: BLL Publishing, 1993), 42, 57.

143 Ibid, 56.

144 Nancy Appleton, Ph.D. *Healthy Bones: What You Should Know About Osteoporosis* (Garden City Park, NY: Avery Publishing, 1991).

145 S.L. Meacham. "Effect of Boron Supplementation on Blood and Urinary Calcium, Magnesium, and Phosphorus, Urinary Boron in Athletic and Sedentary Women." *American Journal of Clinical Nutrition* 61 (1995), 341-345.

146 Maurice Shils, M.D., Sc.D., and Vernon Young, Ph.D. *Modern Nutrition in Health and Disease* (Philadelphia, PA: Lea and Febiger, 1988), 148.

147 S. Gupte. "Use of Berberine in the Treatment of Giardiasis." *American Journal of Diseases of Childhood* 129 (1975), 866. J. Haginiwa and M. Harada. "Pharmacological Studies on Crude Drugs V: Comparison of the Pharmacological Actions of Berberine-Type Alkaloid-Containing Plants and Their Components." *Yakugaku Zasshi* 81 (1961), 1387, and *Yakugaku Zasshi* 82 (1962), 726-731.

148 W.R. Harris. "Practice of Medicine and Surgery by the Canadian Tribes in Champlain's Time." *27th Ann Archeol Rep Min Educ* (Ontario, 1915). A.Y. Leung. *Chinese Herbal Remedies* (New York: Universe Books, 1984).

149 D.B. Mowrey, Ph.D. *The Scientific Validation of Herbal Medicine* (New Canaan, CT: Keats Publishing, 1986), 230.

150 J. Dobbing, ed. *Prevention of Spina Bifida and Other Neural Tube Defects* (London: Academic Press, 1983). M. Tolarova. "Periconceptional Supplementation With Vitamins and Folic Acid to Prevent Recurrence of Cleft Lip." *The Lancet* 2 (1982), 217.

151 R.V. Sutton. "Vitamin E in Habitual Abortion."

British Medical Journal (October 4, 1958), 858. W.M. Jacobs. "Citrus Bioflavonoid Compounds in Rh-Immunized Gravidas: Results of a 10-Year Study." *Obstetrics and Gynecology* 25 (1965), 648.

152 Editorial. "Vitamin A and Teratogenesis." *The Lancet* 1:8424 (February 1985), 319-320.

153 James F. Balch, M.D., and Phyllis A. Balch, C.N.C. *Prescription for Nutritional Healing* (Garden City Park, NY: Avery Publishing, 1997), 269.

154 S. Heller et al. "Vitamin B6 Status in Pregnancy." *American Journal of Clinical Nutrition* 26:12 (1973), 1339-1348.

155 Elson Haas, M.D. *Staying Healthy With Nutrition* (Berkeley, CA: Celestial Arts, 1992), 706.

156 Melvyn R. Werbach, M.D. *Nutritional Influences on Illness* (Tarzana, CA: Third Line Press, 1988), 357-358.

157 Arthur C. Guyton. *Textbook of Medical Physiology* (Philadelphia: W.B. Saunders, 1986), 995.

158 D.B. Mowrey, Ph.D. *The Scientific Validation of Herbal Medicine* (New Canaan, CT: Keats Publishing, 1986), 110, 334.

159 Joe Thornton. "Chlorine, Human Health and the Environment: The Breast Cancer Warning, A Greenpeace Report." (Washington, DC: Greenpeace, 1993) 9-15.

160 M.K. Berman et al. "Vitamin B6 in Premenstrual Syndrome." *Journal of the American Dietary Association* 90 (1990), 859-861. J. Kliejnen et al. "Vitamin B6 in the Treatment of Premenstrual Syndrome—A Review." *British Journal of Obstetrics and Gynaecology* 97 (1990), 847-852.

161 J. Durlach, ed. *First International Symposium on Magnesium Deficiency in Human Pathology* (Paris: Springer Verlag, 1973), 261-263. D.L. Rosenstein. "Magnesium Measures Across the Menstrual Cycle in Premenstrual Syndrome." *Biological Psychiatry* 35 (1994), 557-561. F. Facchinetti et al. "Oral Magnesium Successfully Relieves Premenstrual Mood Changes." *Obstetrics and Gynecology* 78 (1991), 177-181.

162 Ralph Golan, M.D. *Optimal Wellness* (New York: Ballantine Books, 1995), 407.

163 Gary Null, Ph.D. *The Complete Encyclopedia of Natural Healing* (New York: Kensington Publishing, 1998), 313.

164 D. Awang. "Milk Thistle." *Canadian Pharmaceutical Journal* 422 (1993), 403-404. H. Hikino et al. "Antihepatotoxic Actions of Flavonolignans from *Silybum marianum* Fruits." *Planta Medica* 50 (1984), 28-250.

165 Linda Rector Page, N.D., Ph.D. *Healthy Healing* (Sonora, CA: Healthy Healing Publications, 1997), 390.

166 M. Fahim et al. "Zinc Treatment for the Reduction of Hyperplasia of the Prostate." *Federation Proceedings* 35 (1976), 361.

167 Allan L. Miller, N.D. "Benign Prostatic Hyperplasia, Nutritional and Botanical Therapeutic Options." *Alternative Medicine Review* 1:1 (1996), 18-25.

168 "*Serenoa repens*: A Phytotherapeutic Agent for Benign Prostatic Hypertrophy." *Drugs & Therapy Perspectives* 10:3 (1997), 1-4.

169 C. Carani et al. "Urological and Sexual Evaluation of Treatment of Benign Prostatic Disease Using *Pygeum africanum* at High Doses." *Archivio Italiano Urologia, Nefrologia, Andrologia* 63:3 (1991), 341-345. A. Barlet et al. "Efficacy of *Pygeum africanum* Extract in the Medical Therapy of Urination Disorders Due to Benign Prostatic Hyperplasia: Evaluation of Objective and Subjective Parameters." *Wiener Klinische Wochenschrift* 102:22 (November 23, 1990), 667-673.

170 Allan L. Miller, N.D. "Benign Prostatic Hyperplasia, Nutritional and Botanical Therapeutic Options." *Alternative Medicine Review* 1:1 (1996), 18-25.

171 B.E. Carbin et al. "Treatment of Benign Prostatic Hyperplasia With Phytosterols." *British Journal of Urology* 66 (1990), 639-641.

172 D.B. Mowrey, Ph.D. *The Scientific Validation of Herbal Medicine* (New Canaan, CT: Keats Publishing, 1986), 234-235.

173 Michael T. Murray, N.D. *Encyclopedia of Nutritional Supplements* (Rocklin, CA: Prima Publishing, 1996), 481.

174 James F. Balch, M.D., and Phyllis A. Balch, C.N.C. *Prescription for Nutritional Healing* (Garden City Park, NY: Avery Publishing, 1997), 452.

175 James F. Balch, M.D., and Phyllis A. Balch, C.N.C. *Prescription for Nutritional Healing* (Garden City Park, NY: Avery Publishing, 1997), 24.

176 Ibid., 28.

177 D.F. Birt. "Update on the Effects of Vitamins A, C, and E and Selenium on Carcinogenesis." *Proceedings of the Society for Experimental Biology and Medicine* 183:3 (December 1986), 311-320.

178 James F. Balch, M.D., and Phyllis A. Balch, C.N.C. *Prescription for Nutritional Healing* (Garden City Park, NY: Avery Publishing, 1997), 29.

179 A.V. Strosser and L.S. Nelson. "Synthetic Vitamin A in the Treatment of Eczema in Children." *Annals of Allergy* 10 (1952), 703-704. S. Wright and J.L. Burton. "Oral Evening-Primrose-Seed Oil Improves Atopic Eczema." *The Lancet* (November 20, 1982), 1120-1122.

180 A.C. Markey et al. "Platelet Activating Factor-Induced Clinical and Histopathologic Responses

in Atopic Skin and Their Modification by the Platelet Activating Factor Antagonist BN52603." *Journal of the American Academy of Dermatology* 23:2 (1990), 263-268.

181 V.A. Ziboh et al. "Effects of Dietary Supplementation of Fish Oil on Neutrophil and Epidermal Fatty Acids: Modulation of Clinical Course of Psoriatic Subjects." *Archives of Dermatology* (November 1986), 1277-1282.

182 Melvyn R. Werbach, M.D., and Michael T. Murray, N.D. *Botanical Influences on Illness* (Tarzana, CA: Third Line Press, 1988), 290.

183 Melvyn R. Werbach, M.D. *Nutritional Influences on Illness* (Tarzana, CA: Third Line Press, 1988), 488, 490.

184 James F. Balch, M.D., and Phyllis A. Balch, C.N.C. *Prescription for Nutritional Healing* (Garden City Park, NY: Avery Publishing, 1997), 351.

185 C. Straube. "The Meaning of Valerian Root in Therapy." *Therapie der Gegenwart* 107 (1968), 555-562.

186 D. Steinman. *Diet for a Poisoned Planet* (New York: Ballantine Books, 1990), 203. T.H. Maugh, II. "Experts Downplay Cancer Risk of Chlorinated Water." *Los Angeles Times* (July 2, 1992).

187 V.F. Fairbanks and E. Beutler. "Iron." In M.E. Shils and V.R. Young, eds. *Modern Nutrition in Health and Disease* (Philadelphia: Lea and Febiger, 1988), 193-226.

188 C.K. Reddy et al. "Studies on the Metabolism of Glycosaminoglycans Under the Influence of New Herbal Anti-Inflammatory Agents." *Biochemical Pharmacology* 20 (1989), 3527-3534.

189 Simon Mills. *The Dictionary of Modern Herbalism* (Rochester, NY: Healing Arts Press, 1988), 67.

190 Michael T. Murray, N.D. *The Healing Power of Herbs* (Rocklin, CA: Prima Publishing, 1992), 273, 317.

191 D.B. Mowrey, Ph.D. *The Scientific Validation of Herbal Medicine* (New Canaan, CT: Keats Publishing, 1986), 26-27.

192 Personal report by Jeffry L. Anderson, M.D., of Corte Madera, California, based on his clinical use of Stabilium with patients. T. Dorman et al. "The Effectiveness of *Garum armoricum* (Stabilium) in Reducing Anxiety in College Students." *Journal of Advancement in Medicine* 8:3 (Fall 1995), 193-200.

193 Peggy Huddleston. *Prepare for Surgery, Heal Faster* (Cambridge, MA: Angel River Press,1996), 3.

194 B.E. Cohen et al. "Reversal of Post-Operative Immunosuppression in Man by Vitamin A." *Surgery, Gynecology and Obstetrics* 149:5 (November 1979), 658-662. W.M. Ringsdorf, Jr., and E. Cheraskin. "Vitamin C and Human Wound Healing." *Oral Surgery, Oral Medicine, and Oral Pathology* 53:3 (March 1982), 231-236. A. Barbul et al. "Wound Healing and Thymotropic Effects of Arginine: A Pituitary Mechanism of Action." *American Journal of Clinical Nutrition* 37 (1983), 786-794.

195 Linda Rector Page, N.D., Ph.D. *Healthy Healing* (Sonora, CA: Healthy Healing Publications, 1997), 339.

196 Alan R. Gaby, M.D. and Jonathan V. Wright, M.D. *Nutritional Therapy in Medical Practice* (Baltimore, MD: The Wright/Gaby Nutrition Institute, 1994), 6.

197 James F. Balch, M.D., and Phyllis A. Balch, C.N.C. *Prescription for Nutritional Healing* (Garden City Park, NY: Avery Publishing, 1997), 156.

198 L. Gibson et al. "Effectiveness of Cranberry Juice in Preventing Urinary Tract Infections in Long-Term Care Facility Patients." *Journal of Naturopathic Medicine* 2:1 (1991), 45-47. P.N. Prodromos et al. "Cranberry Juice in the Treatment of Urinary Tract Infections." *Southwest Medicine* 47 (1968), 17. I. Ofek et al. "Anti-*Escherichia coli* Adhesin Activity of Cranberry and Blueberry Juices." *New England Journal of Medicine* 324:22 (1991), 1599.

199 R. Bauer and H. Wagner. "Echinacea Species as Potential Immunostimulatory Drugs." *Econ Med Plant Res* 5 (1991), 253-321.

200 D.B. Mowrey, Ph.D. *The Scientific Validation of Herbal Medicine* (New Canaan, CT: Keats Publishing, 1986), 122, 158.

201 J. Bernstein et al. "Depression of Lymphocyte Transformation Following Oral Glucose Ingestion." *American Journal of Clinical Nutrition* 30 (1977), 613. W.R. Beisel. "Single Nutrients and Immunity." *American Journal of Clinical Nutrition* 35:Suppl (1982), 417-468.

202 H. Hemila. "Vitamin C and the Common Cold." *British Journal of Nutrition* 67:1 (January 1992), 3-16. J.C. Godfrey et al. "Zinc for Treating the Common Cold: Review of All Clinical Trials Since 1984." *Alternative Therapies in Health and Medicine* 2:6 (November 1996), 63-72.

203 I. Beladi et al. "*In vitro* and *in vivo* Antiviral Effects of Flavonoids." In L. Farkas et al., eds. *Flavonoids and Bioflavonoids* (New York: Elsevier, 1982), 443-450.

204 Morton Walker, D.P.M. "Antimicrobial Attributes of Olive Leaf Extract." *Townsend Letter for Doctors and Patients* (July 1996), 80-85.

205 NIH Technology Assessment Conference Panel. "Methods for Voluntary Weight Loss and Control." *Annals of Internal Medicine* 116:11 (June 1992), 942-949.

206 Michael T. Murray, N.D. *The Healing Power of Herbs* (Rocklin, CA: Prima Publishing, 1992), 111.

207 M.F. McCarthy. "Hypothesis: Sensitization of Insulin-Dependent Hypothalamic Glucoreceptors May Account for the Fat-Reducing Effects of Chromium Picolinate." *Journal of Optimal Nutrition* 21 (1993), 36-53.

208 Michael T. Murray, N.D. *Encyclopedia of Nutritional Supplements* (Rocklin, CA: Prima Publishing, 1996), 306.

209 H.W. Johnston. "Composition of Edible Seaweeds." *Proceedings of the Seventh International Seaweed Symposium* (New York: Wiley and Sons, 1972), 429-435.

210 G.A. Spiller. *Dietary Fiber in Health and Nutrition* (Boca Raton, FL: CRC Press, 1994).

211 Michael T. Murray, N.D. *Encyclopedia of Nutritional Supplements* (Rocklin, CA: Prima Publishing, 1996), 319.

212 Melvyn R. Werbach, M.D. *Nutritional Influences on Illness* (Tarzana, CA: Third Line Press, 1988), 320-321.

213 Maurice Shils, M.D., Sc.D., and Vernon Young, Ph.D. *Modern Nutrition in Health and Disease* (Philadelphia: Lea and Febiger, 1988), 82.

214 Melvyn R. Werbach, M.D., and Michael T. Murray, N.D. *Botanical Influences on Illness* (Tarzana, CA: Third Line Press, 1988), 250.

215 W.D. Drucker et al. "Biologic Activity of Dehydroepiandrosterone Sulfate in Man." *Journal of Clinical Endocrinology* 35 (1972), 48-54.

Part III

Supplements as Preventive Medicine

1 Dharma Singh Khalsa, M.D. *Brain Longevity* (New York: Warner Books, 1997), 262.

2 Ibid., 51.

3 H. Baker et al. "Vitamin Profiles in Elderly Persons Living at Home or in Nursing Homes, Versus Profiles in Healthy Subjects." *Journal of the American Geriatric Society* 27 (1979) 444.

4 James F. Balch, M.D., and Phyllis A. Balch, C.N.C. *Prescription for Nutritional Healing* (Garden City Park, NY: Avery Publishing, 1997), 15.

5 Ibid., 16-17, 51.

6 Dharma Singh Khalsa, M.D. *Brain Longevity* (New York: Warner Books, 1997), 267.

7 Ibid., 251.

8 Alex Schauss. *Minerals and Human Health: The Rationale for Optimal and Balanced Trace Element Levels* (Hurricane, UT: Life Sciences Press, 1995), 1-3.

9 Melvyn R. Werbach, M.D. and Michael T. Murray, N.D. *Botanical Influences on Illness* (Tarzana, CA: Third Line Press, 1998), 119.

10 R.C. Wren, F.L.S. *Potter's New Cyclopaedia of Botanical Drugs and Preparations* (Saffron Walden/C.W. Daniel Company Limited, 1994), 128-129.

11 The Burton Goldberg Group. *Alternative Medicine: The Definitive Guide* (Tiburon, CA: Future Medicine Publishing, 1995), 521-522.

12 Russell L. Blaylock, M.D. *Excitotoxins: The Taste That Kills* (Sante Fe, NM: Health Press, 1997), 90, 104, 122, 127, 133, 143.

13 Dharma Singh Khalsa, M.D. *Brain Longevity* (New York: Warner Books, 1997), 263.

14 Jack Masquelier. "Recent Advances in the Therapeutic Activity of Procyanidins, Natural Products as Medicinal Agents." In J.L. Beal and E. Reinhard, eds. *Supplement of Plant Medica, Journal of Medicinal Plant Research,* and *Journal of Natural Products* (July 1980), 244-255.

15 Personal communication from W. Lee Cowden, M.D., Richardson, Texas.

16 Richard Anderson, N.D., N.M.D. "The Key to Excellent Health: Cleansing the Colon" *Alternative Medicine* 28 (February/March 1999), 18-22.

17 Ralph Golan, M.D. *Optimal Wellness* (New York: Ballantine Books, 1993), 174.

18 Daniel B. Mowrey, Ph.D. *Herbal Tonic Therapies* (New Canaan, CT: Keats Publishing, 1993), 229.

19 Ralph Golan, M.D. *Optimal Wellness* (New York: Ballantine Books, 1995), 178-180.

20 Gary Null, Ph.D. *The Clinician's Handbook of Natural Healing* (New York: Kensington Publishing, 1997).

21 Melvyn R. Werbach, M.D. *Nutritional Influences on Illness* (Tarzana, CA: Third Line Press, 1988), 247-248.

Index

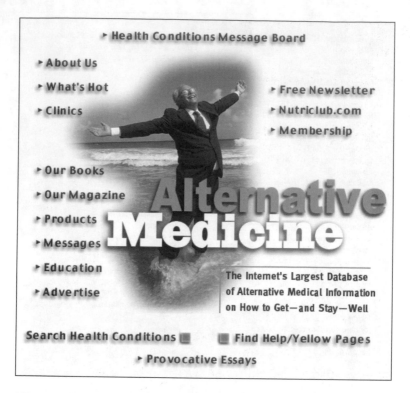

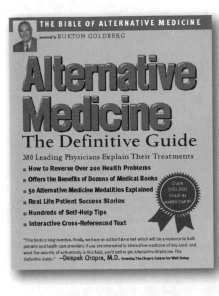

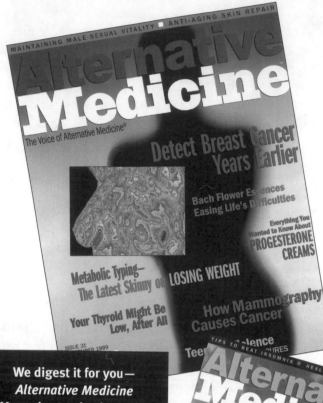

TO ORDER,
CALL 800-333-HEAL

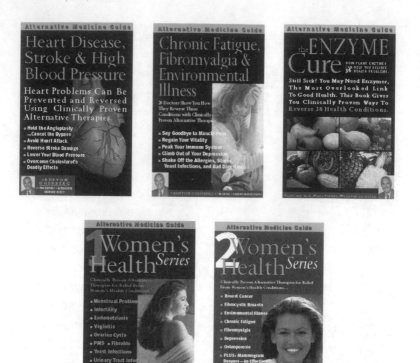

These titles are part of our *Alternative Medicine Guide* paperback series—healing-edge advice that may mean the difference between sickness and robust health. We distill the advice of hundreds of leading alternative physicians from all disciplines and put it into a consumer-helpful for-mat—medical knowledge without the jargon. Essential reading before—or instead of—your next doctor's visit. Because you need to know your medical alternatives.

TO ORDER, CALL 800-333-HEAL